SURGERY
CASEBOOK

The National Medical Series for Independent Study

NMS

SURGERY CASEBOOK

Bruce E. Jarrell, M.D.
Professor, Department of Surgery
University of Maryland
College of Medicine
Baltimore, Maryland

◆ LIPPINCOTT WILLIAMS & WILKINS
A **Wolters Kluwer** Company

Philadelphia • Baltimore • New York • London
Buenos Aires • Hong Kong • Sydney • Tokyo

Editor: Neil Marquardt
Managing Editor: Emilie Linkins
Marketing Manager: Scott Lavine
Production Editor: Christina Remsberg
Compositor: Peirce Graphic Services
Printer: Data Reproductions

Printed in the United States of America

Library of Congress Cataloging-in-Publication Data

Surgery casebook / editor, Bruce E. Jarrell.
     p. ; cm.—(The national medical series for independent study)
    Includes index.
    ISBN 13: 978-0-7817-3219-2
    ISBN 10: 0-7817-3219-0
    1. Surgery, Operative—Case studies. I. Jarrell, Bruce E. II. Series
    [DNLM: 1. Surgical Procedures, Operative—Case Report. 2. Surgery—Case
Report. WO 18.2 S96013 2002]
    RD32 .S825 2002
    617'.91—dc21   2002070247

*The publishers have made every effort to trace the copyright holders for
borrowed material. If they have inadvertently overlooked any, they will
be pleased to make the necessary arrangements at the first opportunity.*

To purchase additional copies of this book, call our customer
service department at **(800) 638-3030** or fax orders to **(301) 824-
7390.** International customers should call **(301) 714-2324.**

Visit Lippincott Williams & Wilkins on the Internet:
http://www.LWW.com. Lippincott Williams & Wilkins customer service representatives are available from 8:30 am to 6:00
pm, EST.

20 19 18 17 16 15 14 13

DEDICATION

This book is dedicated to several important people that have strongly influenced my ability to pursue a medical student-oriented career.

To Brigadier General Fritz Plugge, MC, USAF (Ret), who has been amazingly kind in his support of this department

To Lazar Greenfield, M.D., who has been a wonderful role model for many of us in surgery

To Donald Wilson, M.D., James Dalen, M.D., Joe Gonella, M.D., and Frank Calia, M.D., my deans, who have each given me the opportunity to be with medical students my entire life

And to my family, Leslie, Noble, Kevin, Gwynneth, Jerry, Dad and Mom, who have always helped me out

Bruce E. Jarrell, M.D.

PREFACE

Over the past 22 years I have worked with medical students in their clinical years. During this time, my students have stimulated me to think about how I can do a better job of teaching. This book is one way of trying to attain that goal. The cases in this book represent how I, as an experienced surgeon, think and make decisions about a clinical problem. I have attempted to write it in a way that allows me to talk to you as you read it, so that the book will be the next best thing to teaching in person.

The cases are organized into body systems, and they represent common presentations. The history and physical examination clues help you reach a diagnosis. Illustrations are used liberally to help you detect visual clues. Case variations are also presented to help you consider treatment of patients with various complications and co-existing conditions.

This book is of use to 3rd and 4th year medical students in their surgery rotation as well as interns and residents planning to enter the field of surgery. Using this book alone or in combination with *NMS Surgery* will help you apply your knowledge to decision-making in clinical situations, and master all of the steps in managing a patient.

CONTRIBUTORS

Marshall E. Benjamin, MD
Associate Professor of Surgery
University of Maryland School of Medicine
Baltimore, Maryland

Wendy Berg, MD
Chief of Breast Imaging
Department of Diagnostic Radiology
University of Maryland School of Medicine
Baltimore, Maryland

Daniel J. Bochicchio, MD, FCCP
Assistant Professor
Anesthesiology and Critical Care Medicine
University of Maryland School of Medicine
Baltimore, Maryland

Molly M. Buzdon, MD
Resident in Surgery
Laparoscopic Fellowship
University of Maryland School of Medicine
Baltimore, Maryland

W. Bradford Carter, MD
Associate Professor
Department of Surgery
University of Maryland School of Medicine
Baltimore, Maryland

John L. Flowers, MD, FACS
Associate Professor of Surgery
Division Head, General Surgery
Director, Maryland Center for Videoscopic
 Surgery
University of Maryland School of Medicine
Baltimore, Maryland

Joseph S. McLaughlin, MD
Professor
Division of Cardiac Surgery
University of Maryland School of Medicine
Baltimore, Maryland

Thomas M. Scalea, MD
Physician-in-Chief,
R. Adams Cowley Shock Trauma Center
Professor of Surgery
Director, Program in Trauma
University of Maryland School of Medicine
Baltimore, Maryland

Katherine H. Tkaczuk, MD
Association Professor of Medicine and
 Oncology
University of Maryland School of Medicine
Acting Director, University of Maryland
 Breast Evaluation and Treatment Program
University of Maryland Cancer Center
Baltimore, Maryland

CONTENTS

Special Thanks to Radiologists who assisted in numerous chapters:
   Barry Daly, M.D.
   Robert Pugatch, M.D.
   Charles White, M.D.

PART ONE GENERAL ISSUES

| C H A P T E R 1 |

Preoperative Care

Bruce E. Jarrell M.D., Molly Buzdon M.D., Daniel Bochicchio M.D.

CASE 1.1. ▶ Routine Surgery in a Healthy Patient

A 42-year-old fairly active man who works as a mechanic has a right inguinal hernia and is planning to undergo elective repair. He has had no other operations. However, his medical history reveals mild hypertension that is currently untreated. His family history is also important; his father died as the result of an acute myocardial infarction (MI) at 68 years of age. In addition, his social history is significant for 20 pack-years of smoking.

Review of systems is negative. His blood pressure (BP) is 140/88 mm Hg. With the exception of an easily reducible right inguinal hernia, examination is otherwise negative.

▶ *How would you assess the patient's operative risk?*

▶ The **American College of Cardiology/American Heart Association (ACC/AHA) has proposed several clinical predictors of increased perioperative cardiovascular risk** (Tables 1–1 and 1–2). This patient has none of the risk factors for coronary artery disease, as defined by Table 1–1 but does have hypertension, a positive family history, and a significant smoking history.

▶ *What preoperative tests are necessary?*

▶ Standard preoperative tests include a complete blood count (CBC), electrolyte panel, electrocardiogram (ECG), and chest radiograph (CXR). An ECG is generally indicated in men older than age 40 years and women older than age 50–55 years, unless there is a known history or symptoms suggestive of cardiac disease; in this case, the test should be performed regardless of age. A CXR is especially appropriate in this patient, who has a 20-pack-year smoking history (Table 1–3).

You decide to proceed with the hernia repair.

▶ *How would you categorize the patient's anesthesia risk?*

▶ All anesthetic techniques are associated with some risk. The American Society of Anesthesiologists (ASA) has attempted to classify anesthetic morbidity and mortality based on physical status **(ASA classes 1–5)** [Table 1–4]. This patient presents an ASA 2 risk.

▶ *How would you decide whether to use local, spinal, or general anesthesia?*

▶ **The decision concerning the most appropriate type of anesthesia is multifaceted and should be made in consultation with an anesthesiologist.**

TABLE 1-1

Clinical Predictors of Increased Perioperative Cardiac Risk*

Major Risk
Unstable or severe angina, with MI in past 7–30 days
Decompensated CHF
Significant arrhythmias
    High-grade atrioventricular block
    Symptomatic ventricular arrhythmias
    Uncontrolled supraventricular arrhythmias
Severe valvular disease

Intermediate Risk
Mild angina
Previous MI or Q waves on ECG
Compensated CHF
Diabetes mellitus

Minor Risk
Advanced age
Abnormal ECG (left ventricular hypertrophy, LBBB, ST-T wave abnormalities)
Nonsinus rhythm (e.g., atrial fibrillation)
Poor exercise tolerance
History of stroke
Uncontrolled hypertension

From American College of Cardiology/American Heart Association Task Force Report. Guidelines for perioperative evaluation of noncardiac surgery. *J Am Coll Cardiol* 1996;27:910–948.
  *Including MI, CHF, and death.
  CHF = congestive heart failure, ECG = electrocardiogram, LBBB = left bundle branch block, MI = myocardial infarction.

Most anesthesiologists believe that it is not the technique itself but how well it is used that determines its risk.

Local anesthesia is associated with fewer physiologic consequences than with regional or general anesthetics if a good anesthetic block is achieved. However, with poor local anesthesia, patients experience increased pain, which is stressful and requires large doses of intravenous (IV) sedatives to offset. This significantly increases the risk.

Good spinal anesthesia may lead to fewer pulmonary complications than general anesthesia.

However, it may be more dangerous in patients with coronary artery disease, marginal cardiac reserve with low ejection fraction, valvular heart disease, or diabetic peripheral vascular disease with neuropathy. This danger is secondary to either a loss of peripheral vasoconstrictor ability or ability to increase cardiac output when necessary. Thus, hypotension may occur as a result of the vasodilation caused by spinal anesthesia. To restore BP and relieve hemodynamic instability, IV drugs will have to be used, thus increasing

TABLE 1-2

Risk of Cardiac Events* for Noncardiac Surgical Procedures

High Risk (>5%)
Emergent major operations in elderly
Aortic reconstruction
Major peripheral vascular procedures
Procedures with major fluid shifts or blood loss

Intermediate Risk (1%–5%)
Carotid endarterectomy
Major head and neck resections
Laparotomy
Thoracotomy
Major orthopedic procedures
Open prostatectomy

Low Risk (<1%)
Endoscopy
Breast procedures
Cataract extraction

From American College of Cardiology/American Heart Association Task Force Report. Guidelines for perioperative evaluation of noncardiac surgery. *J Am Coll Cardiol* 1996;27:910–948.
   *Including nonfatal myocardial infarction.

the risk. In addition, if a spinal anesthetic fails to provide good anesthesia, patients will require additional IV sedation or even general anesthesia, further increasing the risk.

 General anesthesia allows excellent analgesia and amnesia while maintaining **good physiologic control.**

In addition, it provides a secure airway.

 Major drawbacks of general anesthesia are an **increased incidence of pulmonary complications** and the **mild cardiodepression** that all anesthetics can cause.

In this particular patient, minimal risk and excellent outcome should be expected regardless of the type of anesthesia used, assuming it is properly administered.

CASE 1.2. ▶ Common Risk Factors Associated with Routine Surgery

You evaluate a patient similar to the man in Case 1.1, who is also in need of an inguinal hernia repair.

▶ *How would your preoperative assessment and proposed management change in each of the following situations?*

TABLE 1-3

Criteria for Preoperative Testing

Complete Blood Count
History of anemia or polycythemia
Procedure with predictable blood loss
Surgery for malignancy

Electrolytes, Glucose, and Creatinine
Older patients (>50 years of age)
Conditions associated with fluid and electrolyte disorders
    Chronic diarrhea
    Chronic renal failure
    Diuretic therapy
    Diabetes
    Steroid therapy
    Chronic liver therapy

Liver Function Tests
Hepatobiliary diseases
Malignancy

PT/ PTT/ Platelet Count*
Positive history of bleeding
Anticoagulant therapy
Liver disease

Urinalysis
Conditions or procedures involving urinary tract

Electrocardiogram (ECG)
Age (men >40 years, women >55 years)
Known cardiac disorders
Serious operative procedures
Systemic conditions with a high incidence of cardiac diseases (e.g., diabetes, hypertension)
Therapy with cardiac medications
Therapy with cardiotoxic drugs (e.g., doxorubicin)

Chest Radiograph (CXR)
Active pulmonary disease or history of such disease
Serious operative procedures

*Coagulation tests are not indicated if a careful history reveals no evidence of coagulopathic disorders. Studies are usually not indicated in chronic renal failure, because the abnormality is platelet dysfunction, which is detected with the bleeding time, not the PT, PTT, or platelet count.
  PT = prothrombin time, PTT = thromboplastin time.

Case Variation 1.2.1. The patient takes one aspirin per day.

▶ Aspirin and nonsteroidal anti-inflammatory drugs (NSAIDs) can cause platelet dysfunction due to inhibition of cyclo-oxygenase, preventing prostaglandin synthesis.

 Aspirin has an irreversible effect on platelet aggregation for at least 7–10 days. NSAIDs have a reversible effect;

TABLE 1-4

American Society of Anesthesiologists' Classification of Perioperative Mortality

Class	Definition
1	A normal healthy patient.
2	A patient with mild systemic disease and no functional limitations.
3	A patient with moderate to severe systemic disease that results in some functional limitation.
4	A patient with severe systemic disease that is a constant threat to life and functionally incapacitating.
5	A moribund patient who is not expected to survive 24 hours with or without surgery.
6	A brain-dead patient whose organs are being harvested.
E	If the procedure is an emergency, the physical status is followed by "E" (for example, "2E").

Class	Mortality Rate
1	0.06%–0.08%
2	0.27%–0.4%
3	1.8%–4.3%
4	7.8%–23%
5	9.4%–51%

From Morgan GE Jr, Mikhail MS. *Clinical anesthesiology. 3rd ed. Lang Medical Books-McGraw Hill: NY, 2002, pg 8–9.*

in 2 days after cessation of medication, platelets have recovered normal function. Thus, for an elective procedure, aspirin should be discontinued for 7 to 10 days prior to the procedure and NSAIDs discontinued for 2 days.

Case Variation 1.2.2. The patient's father and brother both died from acute MIs at 45 years of age.

▶ The man's positive family history should prompt concentrated study of his cardiac history. He should be asked if he has ever experienced anginal symptoms or shortness of breath. An ECG should be performed. An exercise stress test may also be advisable in patients with a strong family history.

Case Variation 1.2.3. The patient's most recent serum cholesterol is 320 mg/dL.

▶ Hypercholesterolemia increases the risk of coronary artery disease, but this factor alone should not postpone surgery.

Case Variation 1.2.4. The patient's preoperative ECG provides evidence of a previous inferior MI, but he has no knowledge of this MI and is chest pain–free on careful examination.

▶ A previous MI increases the risk of postoperative MI. Appropriate workup includes a **cardiology consultation** and perhaps an exercise stress test to identify stress-induced ischemia. If signs of ischemia are apparent, cardiac catheterization may be necessary to determine if coronary revascularization is required prior to surgery.

Case Variation 1.2.5. The patient has diabetes.

▶ This particular patient, who will be "nothing by mouth" (NPO) after midnight, should be given IV fluids with dextrose.

QUICK CUTS Patients who are taking oral hypoglycemic agents should not receive their medication the morning of surgery.

Individuals with insulin-dependent diabetes mellitus (IDDM) should have their glucose levels checked the morning of surgery to ensure that they are not hyper- or hypoglycemic. As a general rule, a slightly elevated glucose level is preferred to a reduced level. If the glucose level is greater than 250 mg/dL, most clinicians would give **two-thirds** of the morning dose of neutral protamine hagadorn (NPH) and regular insulin. If the glucose level is less than 250 mg/dL, you could administer **one-half** of the morning dose.

Case Variation 1.2.6. The patient's hematocrit is 34%, and his other laboratory tests are normal.

▶ **The patient is anemic, and the reason for the anemia must be determined.** The surgery should be postponed. The most common cause of anemia is colorectal cancer, but other causes should be investigated if the workup for gastrointestinal (GI) blood loss is negative.

Case Variation 1.2.7. The patient's hematocrit is 55%.

▶ This result suggests that the patient has either hypovolemia or polycythemia due to some other condition.

QUICK CUTS Regardless of the cause, **the polycythemia should be evaluated and the risk assessed prior to surgery.**

If dehydration is present, surgery should be delayed until the patient is well hydrated. Physical signs of dehydration include poor skin turgor and dry mouth.

Important but less common causes of polycythemia such as polycythemia vera, chronic obstructive pulmonary disease (COPD), and erythropoietin-secreting tumors (e.g., renal cell carcinoma, hepatocellular carcinoma) should be diagnosed and treated prior to elective surgery. If patients with polycythemia vera need surgery, the operative risk for thrombotic complications is increased unless the hematocrit is normalized; a combination of hydration and phlebotomy can be used.

Case Variation 1.2.8. The patient is obese (100 lb overweight) and reports becoming winded easily when climbing stairs.

QUICK CUTS Obese patients have a **higher incidence of hypertension and cardiovascular disease. Severe cases result in hypoventilation, hypercapnia, and pulmonary hypertension. These individuals are also at increased risk for adult-onset diabetes mellitus and deep venous thrombosis (DVT).**

A complete medical evaluation is necessary, including an evaluation of pulmonary status prior to surgery and optimization of functional capacity with bronchodilators and antibiotics as appropriate. At a minimum, this will involve arterial blood gases (ABGs), as well as pulmonary function studies if ABGs are abnormal. Because the hernia repair is elective, postponing the surgery may be an option if the patient is willing to participate in a weight-loss program. Otherwise, **epidural anesthesia and aggressive postoperative pulmonary care** may be used to avoid atelectasis.

 Sequential compression stockings and/or prophylactic subcutaneous heparin are also important in the **prevention of DVT.**

CASE 1.3. ▶ Common Problems in a Patient Waiting to Enter the Operating Room

You plan to repair an inguinal hernia in a male patient. He arrives at the hospital, and you re-assess him just before he is moved into the operating room.

▶ *How would your proposed management change in each of the following situations?*

Case Variation 1.3.1. The patient is known to be diabetic, and this morning his blood glucose is 320 mg/dL.

▶ Perioperative blood glucose levels should be 100–250 mg/dL, and

 surgery should be delayed until the glucose level is brought under control.

The man may need subcutaneous insulin or an insulin drip to lower his glucose level, and he may also require IV drip of a dextrose solution to prevent his blood glucose level from becoming too low. Infection may also be a problem;

 patients with poorly controlled diabetes mellitus have a higher incidence of postoperative wound infections.

Case Variation 1.3.2. The patient has cellulitis from an infected hair follicle in his axilla.

 Surgery performed in the presence of an active infection is associated with a significant increase in wound infection.

Elective surgery should be postponed until the acute infection is resolved, regardless of its location. Unrecognized toe and foot infections are not uncommon in diabetics, who should be examined carefully.

Case Variation 1.3.3. The patient experiences burning on urination.

▶ A urinalysis and a urine culture should be performed. If the urinalysis is positive for infection, the surgery should be postponed until the urinary tract infection (UTI) has been successfully treated with antibiotics. A repeat urinalysis and culture indicates resolution of the infection. Urologic consultation may be needed to determine the cause of the UTI.

Case Variation 1.3.4. His BP, which was 140/88 mm Hg in your office, has risen to 180/110 mm Hg.

QUICK CUTS — **Diastolic blood pressure greater than or equal to 110 mm Hg is a risk factor for development of cardiovascular complications such as malignant hypertension, acute MI, and congestive heart failure.**

Patients with hypertension have a 25% incidence of perioperative hypotension or hypertension. Significant data suggest that β-blockers may help reduce the risk of cardiac complications following surgery. This patient should be maintained on antihypertensive medications on the day of surgery. (β-blockers, in particular, have a high rate of rebound hypertension if withheld.) Studies have found that postponing surgery for mild hypertension (diastolic BP <110 mm Hg) does not reduce perioperative risk.

CASE 1.4. ▶ Surgery in a Patient with Pulmonary Symptoms

A 58-year-old man has suffered several bouts of biliary colic in the past 10 days. An ultrasound study 4 days ago showed multiple small gallstones. The man's surgeon says he needs a cholecystectomy.

▶ *How would you interpret the following findings, and how would they affect your proposed management?*

Case Variation 1.4.1. The patient has daily production each day and has had this for many years. He smokes 2 packs per day.

▶ Questions should be asked about the number of cigarettes smoked daily, the duration of smoking, and any recent change in sputum quality.

QUICK CUTS — **The relative risk of postoperative complications in smokers is 2–6 times that of nonsmokers,**

because cigarette smoking is toxic to respiratory epithelium and cilia, resulting in impaired mucous transport, and therefore decreased resistance to infection.

Bronchial ciliary function returns to normal after 2 days of smoking cessation, and sputum volume decreases to normal after 2 weeks of smoking cessation. However, studies indicate

QUICK CUTS — **no improvement in postoperative respiratory morbidity until after 6–8 weeks of abstinence.**

Because the planned cholecystectomy is elective surgery, this patient should be advised that abstaining from cigarettes 6–8 weeks prior to surgery will decrease the risk of post-operative complications.

Case Variation 1.4.2. The patient normally has daily sputum production, but his sputum has been green for 3 weeks.

▶ If this symptom represents **bronchitis limited to the upper airways** as assessed on chest auscultation in the absence of fever, **oral antibiotics** can be given, and the **surgery can be rescheduled after treatment is complete.** Acute or systemic symptoms from pneumonia or other serious diseases warrant further evaluation.

Case Variation 1.4.3. The patient's sputum has been blood-streaked for 3 weeks.

▶ Blood-tinged sputum in patients with a significant smoking history may suggest **active infection or lung carcinoma.** A full workup, including a CXR and most likely a computed tomography (CT) scan of the chest, should be performed prior to surgery to determine the cause of the problem. Bronchoscopy is also necessary to check for endobronchial lesions and obtain samples for cytology.

CASE 1.5. ▶ Urgent Surgery in a Patient with Severe, Acute Pulmonary Function Problems

You are asked to see a man in the emergency department who is quite ill, with **right upper quadrant (RUQ) pain** and a **temperature of 103°F.** He states that he is a heavy smoker and that he becomes short of breath on mild exertion. He has **scant sputum production**—a thin, white secretion. Examination indicates a barrel chest with decreased breath sounds bilaterally and scattered wheezes, as well as acute tenderness over the RUQ at Murphy's point. CXR findings are typical of **advanced COPD,** and an abdominal ultrasound study shows gallstones and a thickened, inflamed gallbladder. You diagnose his abdominal problem as **acute cholecystitis.**

▷ *How would you manage the patient's pulmonary problem?*

▶ To determine the degree of pulmonary disease, **ABGs,** preferably on room air, are necessary. A PaO_2 of less than 60 mm Hg correlates with pulmonary hypertension, and a $PaCO_2$ of more than 45 mm Hg is associated with increased perioperative morbidity.

   Knowledge of patients' preoperative pulmonary status helps determine intra- and postoperative management. If this patient's septic picture worsens, he will need to go to the operating room regardless of his pulmonary function. If his septic picture improves, spirometry,

 QUICK CUTS preoperative bronchodilator therapy, and other efforts to improve pulmonary status prior to surgery may be appropriate (Table 1–5).

   It is most likely that the sepsis is secondary to biliary infection from gallstones, **and the patient may respond to hydration and IV fluids. The surgery can be postponed until the patient is in better condition. However, the course of the disease is unknown at this time, and prompt evaluation is essential.**

The man says that he is normally very short of breath at rest but that his current breathing problems are much worse than usual. **He cannot speak an entire sentence without gasping for air.** On room air, **his PO_2 is 49 mm Hg, and his PCO_2 is 65 mm Hg.**

▶ *How would your management plans change if the patient has severe COPD in addition to acute cholecystitis?*

▶ This patient is at high risk for **acute pulmonary failure with surgery.** Further workup should include a CXR to rule out underlying pneumonia. In addition, the man must be asked whether he requires oxygen at home, and to determine whether his current respiratory status is at baseline, if he has had any previous pulmonary studies. If the surgery is absolutely necessary, the patient should be taught incentive spirometry before the surgery, and perioperative bronchodilators may be used. It is also important to minimize the duration of anesthesia. To prevent atelectasis, the patient should be mobilized postoperatively as soon as possible.

The **choice of operation** may also substantially influence the postoperative course. **Open cholecystectomy** is one option, which may be prudent in this case. **Cholecystostomy** is another option. Under local anesthesia, a small incision is made in the abdomen, the gallbladder is identified, and a large drain is placed in it for drainage. Drainage to the exterior usually resolves the acute sepsis, avoiding the need for cholecystectomy at this time.

QUICK CUTS   **Laparoscopy** may lead to increased CO_2 absorption into the blood, which then requires excretion through the lungs and increased pulmonary work. This further compromises a patient's pulmonary status and would be contraindicated in this patient.

TABLE 1-5

Pulmonary Function Values Suggesting Increased Perioperative Risk of Pulmonary Complications*

Test	Value	Significance
Forced expiratory volume in 1 sec (FEV$_1$)	<70% of predicted	Moderate risk (major surgery)
	<35% of predicted	High risk (major surgery)
	0.6 L	Pulmonary wedge resection only can be tolerated
	1 L	Major pulmonary resection up to a pulmonary lobectomy can be tolerated
	2 L	Major pulmonary resection up to a pneumonectomy can be tolerated
Forced vital capacity (FVC)	<50%–75% of predicted	Moderate risk
Pulmonary arterial pressure (PAP)	<25 mm Hg	Moderate to high risk
Arterial blood PaCO_2	>45 mm Hg	Moderate risk

Adapted from Pett SB, Wernly JA. Respiratory function in surgical patients: perioperative evaluation and management. *Surg Annual* 1988;20:36.

*Pulmonary risk includes postoperative atelectasis, pneumonia, pneumothorax, inability to wean patient from ventilator, right heart failure, and death.

CASE 1.6. ▶ **Cardiac and Neurologic Risk Associated with Surgery for Peripheral Vascular Disease**

A 74-year-old man presents with a recent onset of rest pain in his right foot. He has had non–insulin dependent diabetes mellitus (NIDDM) for the past 8 years, smokes two packs of cigarettes per day, and has a history of mild hypertension that is well controlled with an angiotensin-converting enzyme (ACE) inhibitor. On physical examination, obvious ischemia of the right foot is evident, with absent popliteal and pedal pulses, dependent rubor, loss of lower leg hair, and shiny skin. The ankle–brachial index is 0.4, indicating severe ischemia of the leg. You recommend a revascularization procedure to salvage the leg. An angiogram indicates that a bypass from the femoral artery to the distal tibial vessels is necessary for adequate revascularization. To proceed safely, you should evaluate the man's medical risk.

▷ *How would the following findings alter your plans for evaluation and management?*

Case Variation 1.6.1. The man tells you that he has no cardiac problems.

▶ The patient's cardiac risk should still be evaluated.

> **QUICK CUTS** **Atherosclerosis is a disease that is not confined to the lower extremities in patients with peripheral vascular disease.** Coronary artery disease or carotid artery disease is often present as well.

To determine the degree of disease in other systems, a thorough workup is necessary before any bypass surgery is performed. To achieve a successful outcome, the benefits of peripheral revascularization must exceed the risks underlying the surgery. **Five factors** are used to predict risk for cardiac complications after vascular surgery. They are:

1. **Q waves** on ECG
2. History of **ventricular ectopy** that requires treatment
3. History of **angina**
4. **Diabetes mellitus** that requires more than dietary therapy
5. **Age 70** or older

Because this man has diabetes and is older than 70 years, he is classified as an intermediate risk for a cardiac event. Therefore, he should have a rapid cardiac workup prior to surgery. This should include **a comparison of the previous ECG with the current ECG.** Because the man has rest pain, he would not tolerate an exercise stress test, but he should undergo a **persantine thallium stress test or dobutamine echocardiogram** to assess his current cardiac status.

> **QUICK CUTS** If **reversible ischemia** is present, he may need a **cardiac catheterization** to determine whether a coronary revascularization procedure is necessary prior to bypass.

Case Variation 1.6.2. The man tells you that he had an acute MI 3 years ago.

The most common cause of early postoperative death following lower extremity revascularization is MI.

Studies have found that the rate of **reinfarction** with **prior history of MI is as high as 15%** in patients undergoing vascular surgery and rises to **37%** in patients who have had a **recent MI.** The risk of cardiac death or recurrent MI decreases as the duration from surgery increases (i.e., the time interval between MI and surgery).

The patient should undergo a stress test. If reversible ischemia is present, he should undergo cardiac catheterization. If only an irreversible defect is present, no cardiac catheterization is necessary if no other abnormalities are present. The reversible defect is most likely due to his old MI.

Case Variation 1.6.3. The man tells you that he had an acute MI 3 months ago.

▶ In 1996, the ACC/AHA proposed a set of guidelines to estimate coronary risk related to noncardiac surgery (Table 1–6). This patient has 10 points by these guidelines. This would place him in the lower but less predictable risk (<3%) for a cardiac complication. To better define that risk, he should be evaluated for the "low cardiac risk" variables (footnote 2 in Table 1–6). Since he is having a vascular procedure performed, he should have a cardiology evaluation and stress test performed. Occurrence of MI more than 30 days before noncardiac surgery is an intermediate risk factor.

He tells you that he had an acute MI 3 weeks ago.

▶ The ACC/AHA criteria stipulate that MI within 30 days of noncardiac surgery is a major risk factor for perioperative cardiac complications. If possible, the **surgery should be delayed.**

Case Variation 1.6.4. The man tells you that he had a non–Q-wave MI 9 months ago.

▶ Non–Q-wave MIs generally signify a **nontransmural infarct,** which leaves peri-infarct myocardium at risk for further infarction during and after surgery. This patient should have a persantine thallium stress test to determine whether reversible ischemia is present. If so, coronary bypass is necessary before surgery.

Case Variation 1.6.5. The patient's ECG shows left bundle branch block (LBBB).

 LBBB is never a normal variant and is highly suggestive of underlying ischemic heart disease.

The presence of this conduction disturbance should prompt a **careful evaluation for underlying cardiopulmonary disease.** If invasive intraoperative monitoring is necessary in patients with LBBB, placement of a pulmonary artery catheter rarely increases the risk of concurrent right bundle branch block (RBBB), so transthoracic pacing capabilities should be readily available. **RBBB** is a normal variant in up to 10% of the general population, but it is more frequently seen in patients with **significant pulmonary disease.**

Case Variation 1.6.6. The patient had a coronary artery bypass graft (CABG) 2 years ago.

TABLE 1-6

Modified Cardiac Risk Index*

Value	No. of Points
Coronary artery disease	
MI <6 months earlier	10
MI >6 months earlier	5
Angina	
With 1–2 blocks or 1 flight of stairs	10
Inability to perform physical activity without angina	20
Alveolar pulmonary edema	
Within past week	10
Ever	5
Suspected critical aortic stenosis	20
Arrhythmias	
Rhythm other than sinus	5
Arterial premature beats	5
More than 5 PVCs	5
Poor medical condition	
(PO_2 <60 mm Hg, PCO_2 >5 mm Hg, serum potassium <3 mEq/L, BUN >50 mg/dL, creatinine >2.6 mg/dL)	5
Age >70 years	5
Emergency surgery	10

*The points are used to determine whether further cardiac evaluation is necessary prior to surgery.

1. Patients with scores of ≥20 points are at high risk (10%–15%) for a cardiac complication. They should be evaluated by a cardiologist, have a stress test, and have appropriate management to improve their cardiac risk prior to elective surgery.

2. Patients with <20 points are at a lower but less predictable risk (<3%) for a cardiac complication. To further define their risk, they should then be evaluated for another set of risk factors, the "low cardiac risk" variables. These include: age >70 years, history of angina, diabetes, Q waves on ECG, history of MI, ST-segment abnormalities on resting ECG, hypertension with significant left ventricular hypertrophy, and history of CHF.

3. Patients who have no more than one cardiac risk variable may proceed with surgery; they are at low risk for a cardiac event.

4. Patients who have more than one cardiac risk variable who are undergoing a nonvascular procedure may proceed with surgery without further workup. If they are undergoing a vascular procedure, they are at a higher risk (3%–15%) for a cardiac event. They should be evaluated by a cardiologist, have a stress test, and have appropriate management to improve their cardiac risk prior to elective surgery.

From American College of Cardiology/American Heart Association. Guidelines for assessing and managing the perioperative risk from coronary artery disease associated with major noncardiac surgery. *Ann Intern Med* 1997;127:309–312.

BUN = blood urea nitrogen, PVC = premature ventricular contraction.

▶ There is evidence that **prior coronary artery revascularization may reduce the risk of cardiac complications in patients who are undergoing other surgery.** This situation is most likely in patients who had the cardiac surgery 6 months to 5 years before the noncardiac surgery and who have no symptoms of ischemia with physical activity. In part, this may result from the increased use of internal mammary arterial grafts in the past decade.

Case Variation 1.6.7. The patient had a CABG 10 years ago.

▶ The benefit of CABG is less clear in patients who have had a coronary revascularization procedure more than 5 years prior. **With saphenous vein bypass, the graft occlusion rates** are 12%–20% at 1 year after CABG, 20%–30% at 5 years, and 40%–50% at 10 years. A stress test should be performed to determine whether this patient has reversible ischemia.

Case Variation 1.6.8. The patient had a percutaneous transluminal coronary angioplasty (PTCA) 2 years ago.

▶ The incidence of **coronary restenosis** after PTCA is 25%–35% at 6 months, so a cardiac evaluation with a stress test would be necessary.

Case Variation 1.6.9. The man had a PTCA 2 days ago.

▶ **Noncardiac surgery should probably be delayed for several weeks following coronary angioplasty,** if feasible, because the risk of coronary thrombosis is increased during the first month postsurgery. The recent PTCA may induce a procoagulant state that might be detrimental to a fresh arterial intervention.

Case Variation 1.6.10. The patient has angina on moderate exertion and uses nitroglycerin.

▶ Because this patient displays evidence of coronary artery disease, **coronary angiography would be appropriate** to determine the extent of disease and whether PTCA or coronary artery revascularization are indicated.

Case Variation 1.6.11. The patient's ECG shows six premature ventricular contractions (PVCs) per minute.

▶ Early studies by Goldman and coworkers in the 1970s showed that preoperative ECGs with more than five PVCs per minute were associated with increased cardiac mortality. Later studies reported that these findings do not necessarily indicate a high likelihood of intraoperative or postoperative ventricular tachycardia. More likely, the cardiac risk of arrhythmia is related to underlying **ventricular dysfunction.** A stress test and an echocardiogram to evaluate left ventricular function and check for underlying cardiac disease would be appropriate. Prophylactic antiarrhythmic therapy has not proved beneficial.

Case Variation 1.6.12. The patient's ECG indicates atrial fibrillation.

▶ If patients have no previous diagnosis of atrial fibrillation, an underlying cause such as **coronary artery disease, congestive heart failure, or valvular heart disease** must be sought. Heart rate must be well controlled, and therapy may involve cardioversion to normal sinus rhythm or β-blockers to control heart rate. Both cardioversion and chronic atrial fibrillation may require anticoagulation to minimize the risk of embolization. Therapeutic decisions must be made in conjunction with a cardiologist and the surgery planned around them. Oral anticoagulants may also need to be used postoperatively.

Case Variation 1.6.13. The patient has a loud right carotid bruit.

▶ A carotid duplex study should be performed to evaluate for carotid artery disease. Studies have found that one-third of patients with carotid bruits have severe internal carotid stenosis. **For patients with a high-grade stenosis (80%–99%), carotid endarterectomy might be considered** prior to lower extremity revascularization.

 QUICK CUTS The primary cause of morbidity and mortality remains myocardial ischemia and infarction.

The risk of neurologic events associated with noncardiac vascular surgery is low (i.e., about 0.4%–0.9%).

Case Variation 1.6.14. The patient had a stroke 2 years ago.

▶ A carotid duplex study should be performed in patients who have had a previous stroke with good neurologic recovery to assess the carotid arteries.

 Carotid endarterectomy is likely to be beneficial for stroke patients with good recovery of function and 70%–99% stenosis of the ipsilateral carotid artery.

In stroke patients with significant residual neurologic deficit, no further evaluation is necessary.

Case Variation 1.6.15. The man's ankle brachial index (ABI) is 0.2, and he has a large, infected right toe.

▶ An infected extremity puts patients at higher risk for gangrene and subsequent amputation, because the peripheral circulation does not allow the limb to heal. This particular patient should still have a workup for coronary artery disease, but his need for **peripheral revascularization is more urgent** than in an individual with rest pain and an ABI of 0.4. Thus, it may be necessary to proceed with revascularization despite an incomplete workup of his cardiac disease. If so, the man should be treated as if he were at risk for myocardial ischemia and his anesthesia managed accordingly.

CASE 1.7. ▶ Surgery in a Patient with Liver Failure

A 47-year-old man with a large umbilical hernia, which has been progressively increasing in size, would like to have it repaired. His history is significant for chronic liver failure secondary to alcohol abuse; he states that currently he is not using alcohol. He is taking a diuretic for control of the ascites. On physical examination, moderate ascites and a 5-cm umbilical hernia are evident. In your assessment, you believe he has alcoholic cirrhosis.

▷ *What factors affect the patient's operative risk, and how are they evaluated?*

▶ The major factors that influence the operative risk relate to the state of compensation and the severity of cirrhosis. Well-compensated patients can tolerate most surgical procedures, but poorly compensated patients cannot tolerate even mild sedatives. The severity of cirrhosis can be estimated by physical examination and laboratory studies (Table 1–7).

A careful examination and laboratory assessment is necessary to assess the risk fully. In this case, the patient has advanced liver failure and is somewhat decompensated, as evidenced by the ascites. In addition, the ascites is probably part of the cause of the hernia; the constant pressure exerted by the ascitic fluid is certainly making the hernia worse.

Careful examination indicates no evident hepatic encephalopathy and no infections but some mild muscle wasting. Laboratory studies reveal serum albumin, 3.2 g/dL; bilirubin, 2.5 mg/dL; prothrombin time (PT), 15 seconds; and platelet count, 110,000/mm².

▷ *How is Child's classification used to determine the patient's operative risk?*

▶ **Child's classification was originally designed to stratify risk in patients undergoing portosystemic shunting procedures,** but the risk appears similar in patients undergoing

TABLE 1-7

Clinical and Laboratory Evidence of Severe Liver Failure

Clinical Indicators
Jaundice
Ascites
Muscle wasting
Asterixis
Advanced encephalopathy
Caput medusa (dilated periumbilical vessels)
Splenomegaly
History of gastric or esophageal varices

Laboratory Indicators*
Decreased serum albumin
Increased serum bilirubin
Elevated PT
Thrombocytopenia

*Also indicators of marginal hepatic reserve.

nonhepatic procedures. The system, which combines three laboratory studies with two clinical findings, remains the most accurate measure of hepatic reserve (Table 1–8). This patient satisfies the majority of the criteria for **Group B** and therefore presents an intermediate operative risk.

▶ *Would you proceed with the surgery?*

▶ As previously stated, patients with chronic liver failure can tolerate most surgical procedures well if they are in a relatively **compensated state preoperatively.** They should **abstain from alcohol** for 6–12 weeks before surgery. If the hernia is repaired but the ascites remains uncontrolled, there is a significant chance of hernia recurrence and bacterial peritonitis. Thus, patients should be **medically optimized** before repair. **Ascites should be controlled** with potassium-sparing diuretics, as well as sodium and water restriction.

In this case, the patient's **serum electrolytes** should be restudied **preoperatively,** be-

TABLE 1-8

Child's Classification of Liver Failure

	Group A	Group B	Group C
Bilirubin (mg/dL)	<2.0	2.0–3.0	>3
Albumin (g/dL)	>3.5	3.0–3.5	<3
Ascites	None	Easily controlled	Poorly controlled
Encephalopathy	None	Minimal	Advanced
Nutrition	Excellent	Good	Poor
Mortality	0%–5%	10%–15%	>25%

From Jarrell BE. *NMS surgery.* 4th ed. Philadelphia: Lippincott Williams & Wilkins, 2000:274.

cause diuretic therapy can cause abnormalities. If possible, the patient's **nutrition status should be improved. In addition, improvement in the man's Child's status** will improve his chance for a successful outcome. Lastly, he has a very **abnormal Protime,** which should be normalized with vitamin K, if possible, prior to surgery.

▶ *What factors might prompt a delay in the patient's surgery?*

▶ Classification in **Child's group C** and presence of **acute alcoholic hepatitis** make patients generally poor operative candidates. Time and alcohol abstinence allow alcoholic hepatitis to resolve. If surgery can be delayed, efforts to improve a patient's Child's status can also be instituted.

You decide to delay the man's surgery and begin efforts to improve his ascites and normalize his Protime.

▶ *How would your proposed management change in each of the following situations?*

Case Variation 1.7.1. The patient has a small ulcerated area on the hernia.

▶ The skin over an umbilical hernia can ulcerate due to pressure necrosis, thus increasing the **risk of rupture,** which has a mortality rate of 11%–43%. This hernia should be repaired in an expedient manner, after proper inpatient management of ascites.

Case Variation 1.7.2. The patient returns to the emergency department in a confused, disoriented, and mildly lethargic state.

▶ Evaluation for **mental status change** is necessary. Possible causes include **electrolyte abnormalities, GI bleeding, sepsis, and an intracranial event (e.g., subdural hematoma or hepatic encephalopathy)** related to liver failure. Development of **spontaneous bacterial peritonitis** or **peritonitis related to cellulitis** or infection on the umbilical hernia skin is also possible. The ascites should be tapped, and the patient should be treated with antibiotics if the fluid contains more than 250 white blood cells (WBCs)/mm^3.

Case Variation 1.7.3. The patient returns to the emergency department with serous fluid leaking from a small ulcer on the hernia.

▶ **Ascitic fluid leaking** from the umbilical hernia leads to an increased risk of bacterial peritonitis. The mortality rate is high, primarily due to infection. The serous fluid should be sent for cell count and culture, and IV antibiotics should be initiated before culture results return. The hernia should be **repaired urgently.**

Case Variation 1.7.4. You smell alcohol on the patient in the office.

▶ The **surgery should be delayed** until the patient has abstained from alcohol and undergone withdrawal. **Alcohol withdrawal** during the postoperative period is associated with high morbidity and mortality.

Case Variation 1.7.5. The patient tells you that he has severe hemorrhoids he wants removed. Examination confirms several moderate-sized internal hemorrhoids.

▶ Hemorrhoid removal requires **great caution** in patients with cirrhosis and possible **portal hypertension.** Uncontrollable hemorrhage during surgical repair may occur as a result of portal hypertension.

CASE 1.8. ▶ Surgery in a Patient with Chronic Kidney Problems

A 52-year-old man with aseptic necrosis of his right leg requires hip replacement. His history is significant for chronic renal failure for 10 years secondary to glomerulonephritis. Initial management involved a kidney transplant from a living relative and immunosuppression with cyclosporine and **prednisone.** Recently, he has experienced progressive chronic rejection and has a creatinine of 3.5 mg/dL. On physical examination, multiple stigmata of steroid management, including striae, moon facies, and easy bruisability, are evident. He has mild ankle edema. The patient experiences pain on passive motion of the right hip.

▷ *Would you recommend proceeding with the hip replacement at this time?*

▶ The decision regarding the timing of hip replacement surgery is best made in conjunction with an orthopedist who is experienced in treating patients with renal problems. In patients with progressive deteriorating renal function, repair of the hip should be delayed until the transplant function has stabilized or the necessary dialysis has begun. Once a patient's renal status is stable, the hip can be reassessed and a plan determined. **Repairing the hip during transplant deterioration may complicate or aggravate the rejection process and hasten the need for dialysis.**

▷ *How would you prepare the patient for surgery?*

▶ The major objective is to **resolve any correctable problems** before taking a patient with chronic renal failure to the operating room.

QUICK CUTS	**Well-dialyzed patients** have the most normalized platelet function, hydration state, BP control, and electrolyte status.

Thus, dialysis immediately before surgery is desirable. **Transplant patients** should be adequately hydrated and have well-controlled BP. Infection control is desirable in both types of patients. Many of these patients also have been on steroids in the recent past. If so, **perioperative steroids** should be given. Typical replacement therapy is methylprednisone 125 mg IV every 8 hours for 3 doses.

Preoperative laboratory tests from 2 days ago reveal a serum potassium of 5.1 mEq/L, and the patient is in the holding area ready for the operating room.

▷ *Is a 2-day-old potassium value an adequate preoperative measurement?*

▶ This measurement is **too old** to rely on for surgery because the potassium can rise to dangerous levels in short periods of time in chronic renal failure. A repeat potassium level needs to be obtained immediately—before the patient proceeds to the operating room.

You decide to proceed with surgery and encounter intraoperative bleeding due to a "capillary ooze."

▷ *How would you manage the bleeding?*

QUICK CUTS	**Platelet dysfunction due to uremia can contribute to intraoperative bleeding. Transfusion of platelets will not help.**

Several substances can be used to improve platelet function. Desmopressin (ddAVP) may be used acutely. It has a rapid effect of short duration and may induce tachyphylaxis (loss of hemostatic effect with multiple doses); its action is related to release of von Willebrand's factor from endothelial cells, and it increases the spreading and aggregation of platelets. Fresh frozen plasma also temporarily corrects the platelet defect. Conjugated estrogens, which have a slow onset of action, may be effective for up to 2 weeks. Finally, postoperative hemodialysis may reduce the uremia and improve platelet function.

The patient becomes hypotensive, with a BP of 80/60 mm Hg, in the operating room. There is no evidence of surgical bleeding.

▶ *In addition to the usual methods to correct hypotension, are there any special measures you might take in this patient?*

▶ The hypotension must be explained; this condition has many causes. **Glucocorticoid deficiency** is one important cause of such low blood pressure in many renal failure patients who have previously taken steroids. The hypotension should be treated with hydrocortisone 25 mg intraoperatively, followed by 100 mg in the next 24 hours.

You successfully replace the man's hip. In the recovery room, his postoperative potassium level returns to 7.1 mEq/L, and he is producing 10 mL/hr of urine.

▶ *How would you manage the patient?*

▶ The patient has oliguria and **hyperkalemia.** He should be adequately hydrated, and his high potassium concentration should be treated. **Peaked T waves** on the ECG suggest that the hyperkalemia is physiologically important and warrants **immediate treatment.** IV **calcium gluconate** should be given to stabilize cardiac membranes. **IV insulin and glucose** should be given to reduce potassium levels, but **hemodialysis** will probably also be necessary.

CASE 1.9. ▶ Surgery in a Patient with Cardiac Valvular Disease

▶ You are asked to see a female patient who needs an elective cholecystectomy. She has known valvular heart disease.

▶ *How would you manage the following preoperative conditions?*

Case Variation 1.9.1. The patient has chronic mitral valve stenosis that is currently well compensated.

▶ Stenosis of the mitral valve leads to increased left atrial pressure, which may result in passive **pulmonary hypertension and right heart failure,** leading to symptoms of fatigue, dyspnea on exertion, or hemoptysis. The distended atrium is susceptible to **atrial fibrillation or other arrhythmias.** Many surgeons would obtain a cardiology opinion and an echocardiogram to evaluate cardiac function if there is any doubt about the patient's cardiac status. The perioperative mortality for all patients with hemodynamically significant mitral stenosis is as high as 5%.

Because this patient has well-compensated mitral valve stenosis, surgery could proceed. Intravascular volume should be maintained, and hypoxemia, hypercapnia, and acidosis, which all increase pulmonary vascular resistance, should be avoided. Tachycardia should also be avoided, because it decreases diastolic filling time. Like all patients with valvular heart disease, this woman should also receive **prophylactic antibiotics** for the prevention of subacute bacterial endocarditis.

Case Variation 1.9.2. The patient had chronic mitral valve stenosis and an episode of congestive heart failure (CHF) 1 month ago.

▶ Mitral valve stenosis with underlying CHF increases mortality to as high as 20%. More **extensive cardiac workup** and perioperative monitoring may be necessary, and ECG and echocardiography are indicated to determine the extent of disease. If urgent surgery is needed, **intraoperative monitoring** may include an arterial line and transesophageal echocardiography. The pulmonary artery catheter is of limited usefulness, because the pressure gradient across the mitral valve distorts the relationship between the pulmonary capillary wedge pressure and the left ventricular end-diastolic pressure.

Case Variation 1.9.3. The patient has known aortic stenosis and a grade IV systolic murmur.

▶ The obstruction to left ventricular outflow leads to left ventricular hypertrophy and increased left ventricular end-diastolic pressure, which may cause angina, dyspnea, syncope, or **sudden death.** The outflow obstruction causes an inability to increase cardiac output. In patients who need **elective surgery, cardiac assessment** and possibly valve replacement would take priority. In patients who need urgent surgery, **perioperative hemodynamic monitoring** with a pulmonary artery catheter, an arterial line, and transesophageal echocardiography should be considered.

CASE 1.10. ▶ Endocarditis Prophylaxis in a Surgical Patient with Valvular Heart Disease

A 58-year-old woman with mitral valve disease secondary to rheumatic fever is scheduled to undergo a hemicolectomy for diverticular disease.

▷ *When would you consider bacterial endocarditis prophylaxis?*

▶ Antimicrobial prophylaxis for bacterial endocarditis is recommended for patients who are undergoing GI procedures that are likely to cause significant trauma (Table 1–9). Many different microorganisms are responsible for bacterial endocarditis, including streptococcus, staphylococcus, and enterococcus. Because GI surgery may cause the release of anaerobic organisms in the bloodstream, prophylaxis consisting of ampicillin and gentamicin is directed against enterococci (Table 1–10).

CASE 1.11. ▶ Surgery in a Patient with Cardiomyopathy

You are asked to see a woman with colon cancer who needs a left colectomy. She has a known cardiomyopathy, with mild shortness of breath and fine rales in both lung bases.

▷ *How would you manage the patient perioperatively?*

 Patients with cardiomyopathy are at risk for complications such as **arrhythmias, CHF, cardiac outflow obstruction, and sudden death.**

TABLE 1-9

Conditions Associated with Bacterial Endocarditis

CARDIAC CONDITIONS*

High Risk (prophylaxis recommended)
Prosthetic heart valves
Previous endocarditis
Complex congenital heart defects
Prosthetic vascular grafts

Moderate Risk (prophylaxis recommended)
Rheumatic valvular disease
Mitral valve prolapse with regurgitation
Hypertrophic cardiomyopathy

Negligible Risk (prophylaxis not recommended)
Previous coronary artery bypass graft surgery
Repair of atrial and ventricular septal defects
Mitral valve prolapse without regurgitation
Physiologic heart murmurs
Cardiac pacemakers

NONCARDIAC PROCEDURES (prophylaxis recommended with moderate and high cardiac risk)

Dental Work
Extractions
Periodontal procedures
Cleaning where bleeding is expected

Respiratory Tract
Tonsillectomy
Rigid bronchoscopy
Procedures involving tracheobronchial tree and lung

Gastrointestinal Tract
Esophageal variceal banding
Dilation of strictures
Endoscopic retrograde cholangiopancreatography
Biliary tract surgery
Surgery involving intestinal tract

Genitourinary Tract
Prostatic surgery
Cystoscopy
Dilation of strictures
Major open procedures

*From Dagani AS, Taubert K, Wilson W, et al. Prevention of bacterial endocarditis recommendations by the American Heart Association. *JAMA* 1997;277:1794–1801.

Because this patient needs elective surgery, she should be carefully evaluated by a cardiologist. Patients who require urgent surgery should have their fluid status carefully controlled and possible arrhythmias monitored. Pulmonary artery catheterization and/or transesophageal echocardiography may be necessary to manage volume status properly.

TABLE 1-10

Prophylactic Regimens for Bacterial Endocarditis

Dental, Oral, Respiratory Tract, and Esophageal Procedures
Amoxicillin 1 hour before procedure
> *OR*

Clindamycin or cephalosporin or clarithromycin 1 hour before procedure for penicillin-allergic patients (cephalosporin may cross-react in penicillin-allergic patients)

Gastrointestinal and Genitourinary Procedures
High-risk patients
- Ampicillin and gentamicin 30 minutes before and ampicillin 6 hours after procedure
> *OR*
- Vancomycin and gentamicin infusion completed 30 minutes before procedure with no follow-up dose in penicillin-allergic patients

Moderate-risk patients
- Amoxicillin or ampicillin 1 hour before procedure with no follow-up dose
> *OR*
- Vancomycin 1–2 hours before procedure with no follow-up dose in penicillin-allergic patients

*From Dagani AS, Taubert K, Wilson W, et al. Prevention of bacterial endocarditis recommendations by the American Heart Association. *JAMA* 1997;277:1794–1801.

CASE 1.12. ▶ Preparation of the Colon for Colectomy

A 55-year-old man with diabetes has adenocarcinoma of the sigmoid colon. The day before an elective colectomy, he is undergoing a **bowel "prep."**

▶ *What is the purpose of a bowel "prep"?*

▶ The purpose of preoperative bowel preparation is to decrease fecal mass and bacterial content in the colon. High bacterial counts are related to complications in colon surgery (e.g., wound infections, anastomotic dehiscence). Bowel "preps" usually begin on the day prior to surgery, along with a clear liquid diet.

 Most important is the mechanical removal of stool, which is usually accomplished with cathartics and enemas.

Oral nonabsorbable antibiotics such as neomycin and erythromycin are also used to decrease the bacterial load in the bowel.

Several cathartics are commonly used, including Golytely, Fleets Phospho-Soda, or an oral laxative such magnesium citrate.

▶ *What are the fluid and electrolyte consequences of bowel "preps," and what should be done to avoid these complications?*

Golytely (polyethylene glycol electrolyte solution)

▶ This formula contains potassium chloride, sodium bicarbonate, sodium chloride, and sodium sulfate. This concentration of electrolytes causes **no net absorption or secretion of ions** and thus no change in the electrolyte or water balance. Patients ingest 4 L by mouth the day before surgery. The large volume of fluid remains in the bowel and effects a "volume washout" of the colon, which is equivalent in effectiveness to enemas. Studies have shown that Golytely is safe, well tolerated, and cost-effective. However, older patients should be watched during this treatment because they can become dehydrated.

Fleets Phospho-Soda

▶ Fleets Phospho-Soda is **contraindicated in diabetics** (it contains sugar) and in patients on salt-restricted diets, so it should not be used in this patient. This **hypertonic** sodium phosphate solution (hyperosmotic saline) works by **drawing large amounts of fluid into the intestinal lumen.** Compared to plasma, fecal fluid contains less sodium and chloride and more potassium and bicarbonate. With significant **losses of bicarbonate, patients can become predisposed to metabolic acidosis.** Such deprivation also exacerbates potassium loss, because a cation shift occurs as potassium leaves the cell in exchange for sodium and hydrogen ions in the body's attempt to form more bicarbonate. These electrolyte imbalances can lead to signs of confusion, irregular heart rate, muscle cramping, weakness, and fatigue. It is imperative to watch for signs of dehydration, and administration of IV fluids may be required.

Magnesium Citrate

▶ **Magnesium is poorly absorbed** from the intestinal lumen; therefore, this preparation works as an **osmotic agent that draws fluid into the bowel lumen.** As previously stated, it is important with any form of osmotic diarrhea to monitor patients for signs of dehydration and electrolyte imbalance. **Patients with renal failure** who are unable to clear large amounts of magnesium from the bloodstream may suffer other complications. Signs of toxicity include flushing, hypotension, respiratory depression, bradycardia, central nervous system (CNS) depression, muscle paralysis, loss of deep tendon reflexes, and worsening renal failure. If levels of magnesium reach more than 5 mEq/L, patients should receive calcium gluconate to alleviate the **hypermagnesemic** symptoms.

CHAPTER 2

Postoperative Care

Bruce E. Jarrell M.D., Molly Buzdon M.D.

CASE 2.1. ▶ Postoperative Fluid and Electrolyte Management

A 55-year-old diabetic man who has an adenocarcinoma of the sigmoid colon undergoes a colectomy. The operation goes smoothly, and he returns to the recovery room in good condition with a nasogastric (NG) tube in place.

▶ *How would you determine whether the intraoperative fluid replacement was adequate?*

▶ Determination of intraoperative replacement requirements involves knowledge of the extent of both measurable, or sensible, and unmeasurable, or insensible, fluid losses. Measurable losses include estimated blood loss (EBL), amount of fluid given intraoperatively, and urine output. Assuming the patient received no blood in the operating room, replacement of every 1 mL of EBL with 3 mL of isotonic fluid is necessary; approximately two-thirds of the intravenous (IV) fluid administered to the patient rapidly leaves the intravascular space (Table 2–1).

> **QUICK CUTS** Postoperative fluid replacement requires replacement of fluid lost during a procedure; provision of maintenance requirements; and consideration of ongoing losses through drains, nasogastric tubes, and fistulas.

Insensible losses, which occur through evaporation and other processes, are not easily quantifiable. Large amounts of such losses take place in patients who undergo long procedures, particularly when the peritoneal cavity is open. Insensible losses must be estimated using clinical judgment, based on vital signs, urine output, and other physiologic measurements obtained through central venous catheters.

▶ *How would you estimate the patient's routine postoperative fluid and electrolyte requirements?*

▶ Maintenance fluid requirements can be easily calculated using a formula based on body weight (Table 2–2). The combination of $D_5 0.5$ NS plus KCl 20 mEq/L satisfies the sodium, potassium, and chloride requirements of the average patient. After a large intraoperative blood loss, lactated Ringer's solution or 0.9 NS may be chosen for the first 24 hours. (Because the fluid lost is isotonic, it is replaced by isotonic fluid.) Regardless, the patient's volume and electrolyte status should always be estimated frequently, particularly in the first 24–48 hours after surgery. This involves careful bedside observation, together with analysis of vital signs and laboratory values.

▶ *How would you determine the volume of fluids and electrolytes needed to replace those lost from the patient's NG tube?*

TABLE 2-1

Sample Calculation of Intraoperative Fluid Requirements

Measured losses

EBL:	500 mL
IV fluids given in OR:	1000 mL
Urine output:	200 mL

(EBL × 3 mL isotonic fluid/1 mL blood loss) + 200 − 1000 = 700
700 mL of isotonic fluid (lactated Ringer's or normal saline) should be replaced.

EBL = estimated blood loss; IV = intravenous; OR = operating room.

▶ Gastrointestinal (GI) fistulas and tubes placed in certain sites typically drain fluids of a predictable concentration. The amount lost should be replaced milliliter for milliliter (Table 2–3). IV fluids of a known concentration are commonly used for fluid replacement (Table 2–4).

▷ *How do the patient's fluid requirements change during the postoperative course?*

▶ As the man regains GI function and recovers from the surgery, he will begin to mobilize fluid from third-space accumulation. This excess fluid, which must be excreted by the kidneys, represents an additional volume in the intravascular space. Thus, IV fluid requirements decrease during the recovery period. Failure to reduce IV intake may result in fluid overload, edema, and even pulmonary edema.

CASE 2.2. ▶ Postoperative Acute Renal Failure

A 75-year-old man with a history of benign prostatic hypertrophy undergoes a minor ambulatory surgical procedure on his foot. He presents to the emergency department 12 hours later with acute urinary retention. A urinary catheter is placed, and 1200 mL of clear urine is removed. He is admitted to the hospital.

▷ *How would your evaluation and management change in each of the following situations?*

TABLE 2-2

Estimate of Maintenance Fluid Requirements

Body Weight (kg)	Fluid Requirements (mL/kg/24 hr)
First 10	100
Next 10	50
Beyond 20	20 per kilogram

EXAMPLE: 70-kg patient
(100 mL/kg × 10 kg) + (50 mL/kg × 10 kg) + (20 mL/kg × 50 kg)
1000 mL + 500 mL + 1000 mL = **2500 mL/24 hr** (approximately 100 mL/hr)

TABLE 2-3

Electrolyte Content of Gastrointestinal Fluids

Gastrointestinal Fluid	Na$^+$ (mEq/L)	K$^+$ (mEq/L)	Cl$^-$ (mEq/L)	HCO$_3^-$ (mEq/L)
Gastric aspirate	100	10	140	0
Pancreatic juice	140	5	75	100
Bile	140	5	100	60
Small bowel drainage	110	5	105	30
Distal ileum and cecum	140	5	70	50
Colon	60	70	15	30

Case Variation 2.2.1. The patient's urine output is 50 mL/hr over the next 4 hours.

▶ This value represents **normal urine output,** which should be 0.5–1 mL/kg/hr. The patient must remain adequately hydrated; sufficient oral or IV fluids must be given to replace all fluid losses and provide maintenance fluid requirements.

Case Variation 2.2.2. The patient diureses 400 mL/hr over the next 4 hours and develops a blood pressure (BP) of 80/60 mm Hg.

▶ This development could be secondary to a number of potential causes, including **preexisting renal disease with inability to concentrate urine, diabetes insipidus, or a combination of causes. Postobstructive diuresis,** another cause, may account for the increased urine output with resultant dehydration and hypotension. Certain conditions make patients more prone to postobstructive diuresis; these include chronic obstruction, edema, congestive heart failure, hypertension, weight gain, and azotemia.

> **QUICK CUTS** The diuresis may be either physiologic—caused by retained urea, sodium, and water—or pathologic—caused by impaired concentrating ability or impaired sodium reabsorption.

The hypotension must be promptly treated with more aggressive hydration and monitoring.

TABLE 2-4

Electrolyte Composition of Various Solutions

Solution	Glucose (mg/dL)	Na$^+$ (mEq/L)	K$^+$ (mEq/L)	Ca^{2+} (mEq/L)	Cl$^-$ (mEq/L)	Lactate (mg/dL)
D$_5$W	50	—	—	—	—	—
D$_{10}$W	100	—	—	—	—	—
0.9 NS	—	154	—	—	154	—
0.45 NS	—	77	—	—	77	—
Lactated Ringer's solution	—	130	4	3	110	28

When a patient such as this diureses more than 200 mL/hr for two consecutive hours, the urine should be collected over a timed period to determine the cause of diuresis. **Urine with a low osmolality probably indicates a pathologic concentrating defect, whereas urine with a higher osmolality suggests osmotic diuresis.** In most instances, postobstructive diuresis is self-limited, and the blood urea nitrogen (BUN) and creatinine (Cr) return to normal in 1 to 2 days. In general, urologists believe that it is best to keep the patient's volume expanded during the polyuric phase.

Case Variation 2.2.3. The patient's urine output is 10 mL/hr for the next 4 hours.

▶ Most commonly, severe oliguria is caused by either a mechanical problem with the catheter or severe dehydration of the patient. First, the catheter should be irrigated, and position confirmed. If no mechanical problem is evident, **volume resuscitation** should be tried. If this fails to increase the patient's urine output, placement of a central venous pressure (CVP) line or pulmonary artery catheter may be necessary to assess the adequacy of the attempts at volume repletion.

Case Variation 2.2.4. The patient's urine output is 10 mL/hr, and his CVP is 12 cm H_2O.

▶ A **pulmonary artery catheter may be indicated** to ensure that preload and cardiac output are adequate. Other laboratory tests to determine the etiology of oliguria include the fractional excretion of sodium (FeNa), BUN:Cr ratio, urine electrolytes, and osmolality. Obstruction should be ruled out by renal ultrasound (Table 2–5).

Case Variation 2.2.5. The man's first urine sample is cloudy, and he appears confused and disoriented.

▶ This scenario suggests **urosepsis.** The urine should be sent for urinalysis as well as culture, and broad-spectrum antibiotics should be initiated.

Case Variation 2.2.6. The patient develops gross hematuria as the first 1000 mL of urine are drained from the bladder.

▶ Hematuria is not uncommon following obstruction due to overdistention of the bladder and bladder wall injury, but a man of this age should also have a urology consult to rule out more serious causes, including malignancy. Infection, kidney stones, trauma, prostatitis, and medications known to cause cystitis (e.g., cyclophosphamide) may also produce hematuria. If the urine output drops, the bladder should be irrigated to dislodge any clots. If clotting occurs and persists, the patient may need constant bladder irrigation with a three-way Foley catheter.

TABLE 2-5

Measurements Used in the Evaluation of Oliguria

Cause of Oliguria	Urine osmolality (mOsm/kg)	Urine [Na$^+$] (mEq/L)	FeNa (%)	BUN/Cr ratio
Prerenal	>500	<20	<1	>20
Postrenal	250–300	>40	>3	<10

FeNa = fractional excretion of sodium.

Case Variation 2.2.7. Four hours after insertion of the catheter, the man has a temperature of 104°F and a BP of 80/60 mm Hg. He is confused.

▶ The patient most likely has urosepsis and needs urgent monitoring and fluid resuscitation in the intensive care unit. In addition, he requires a sepsis workup, broad-spectrum antibiotics, and possibly a pulmonary artery catheter.

CASE 2.3. ▶ Postoperative Fever

A 45-year-old woman has had a colon resection. You are called to see her on her fifth postoperative day. For the past 24 hours, she has had a temperature of 101°F.

▶ *How would you evaluate this patient?*

▶ A thorough history and physical examination are necessary; they are the most important part of the workup. All sources of fever should be considered. Possible sources of fever in hospitalized or postoperative patients include pneumonia, upper respiratory infection, urinary tract infection (UTI), deep venous thrombosis (DVT), infected indwelling catheters, and drug-related fever. The patient should be asked about sputum production, cough, abdominal pain, nausea, vomiting, pain at the wound site, drainage from the wound, bowel function, difficulty urinating, or blood in the urine.

▶ *How would your evaluation and management change in each of the following situations?*

Case Variation 2.3.1. On lung examination, the patient has fine crackles bilaterally.

▶ The **patient probably has atelectasis,** which is collapse of portions of the alveolar structures in the lung.

 The most common cause of fever in the immediate postoperative period is atelectasis.

This condition can be diagnosed on physical examination and with chest radiography (CXR). Treatment involves a vigorous pulmonary toilet and incentive spirometry. Use of these modalities immediately after surgery can prevent this complication. Antibiotics are not used in the treatment of atelectasis.

Atelectasis is the most common reason for a postoperative fever, but several other possibilities should be considered. Pneumonia is diagnosed by the appearance on CXR, as well as sputum suggestive of infection. Antibiotics should be started as soon as the diagnosis of pneumonia is made. Pulmonary edema should also be considered. Although this condition does not typically cause fever, it does occur postoperatively. Pulmonary edema frequently occurs several days into the postoperative period when the patient is beginning to mobilize third-space fluids.

Case Variation 2.3.2. The man reports burning on urination, and he has noticed some blood in his urine. Urinalysis reveals 10–20 white blood cells (WBCs)/hpf and 3+ leukocyte esterase.

▶ This patient has a **UTI,** which may be related to the use of a Foley catheter or urinary retention.

QUICK CUTS Urinary tract infection is a second common cause of postoperative fever, especially around day 3.

Retention can be diagnosed by physical examination, bladder ultrasound, or insertion of a catheter. Most infections can be treated with oral trimethoprim–sulfamethoxazole or ciprofloxacin. A urine culture should be performed.

Care should be taken with patients who are elderly or diabetic or show any signs of illness such as nausea, vomiting, or abdominal or flank pain. It may be important to administer the antibiotics intravenously and make certain that patients are well hydrated.

Case Variation 2.3.3. The man reports some purulent drainage from his wound site with some tenderness. His staples are still in place.

▶ In this case, **the wound must be evaluated carefully** for signs of cellulitis or fluctuance.

QUICK CUTS If the wound exhibits fluctuance, which is suggestive of a fluid collection beneath the skin, some staples should be removed and pus should be drained.

The wound should be cultured and treated locally, which often means irrigation and packing with wet to dry dressings twice a day. If significant cellulitis is present, administration of an appropriate oral antibiotic is necessary.

Case Variation 2.3.4. On examination, you note that the man has an indwelling IV in his right forearm with induration, edema, and tenderness at the site.

▶ The catheter should be removed. In most cases, after catheter removal, the inflammation will resolve. If significant cellulitis is present, antibiotics should be considered. Most surgeons recommend that all IV insertion sites be rotated every 4 days to prevent this problem.

Case Variation 2.3.5. You also discover a drop of pus on the skin at the venipuncture exit site.

▶ This condition is termed **suppurative phlebitis** and is caused by the presence of an infected thrombus in the vein and around the indwelling catheter. Affected patients are apt to have high fevers and positive blood cultures. In addition to removing the catheter, suppurative phlebitis is treated by surgically excising the infected vein.

QUICK CUTS In addition to removal of the catheter, excision of the affected vein to the first patent, noninfected collateral branch is necessary. Intravenous antibiotics should be administered, and the wound should be left open.

CASE 2.4. ▶ Management of a Small Bowel Fistula

A 65-year-old woman has had a segment of necrotic bowel resected. On the fifth postoperative day, you notice intestinal contents draining from the wound.

▶ *How would you manage this complication?*

▶ Enteric contents could originate from a leak at the jejunostomy insertion site, breakdown of the small bowel anastomosis, or a missed enterotomy.

 QUICK CUTS   A patient who shows clinical signs of peritonitis needs operative reexploration.

Surgical reexploration may be necessary if the patient has signs of peritonitis. Otherwise, a computed tomography (CT) scan is required to rule out an intra-abdominal collection, which can usually be drained percutaneously under CT guidance.

 QUICK CUTS   Percutaneous or operative drainage can then be performed if an undrained collection is present.

If no intra-abdominal fluid collection is evident, and the fistula appears to be draining adequately, this condition can be managed nonoperatively as an enterocutaneous fistula (Figure 2–1). Treatment involves giving the patient nothing by mouth (making the patient NPO), administering total parenteral nutrition (TPN), and measuring the fistula output daily. Frequent measurement of serum electrolytes is necessary to avoid electrolyte imbalance from a high fistula output. As a result of this management, most fistulas will heal in several weeks. However, in certain circumstances, fistulas will not heal. The mnemonic "FRIEND" can be used to remember these conditions (Figure 2–2).

Once the GI fistula has become established and is not rapidly closing, a fistulogram or small bowel series may be necessary to examine for explanations of persistent drainage. If the GI fistula persists after 5 or 6 weeks and the patient is free of infection, a definitive repair should be planned.

CASE 2.5. ▶ High Fever in the Immediate Postoperative Period

A 35-year-old man has received a shotgun wound to the abdomen in which he sustained a blast injury to the abdominal wall and a colon injury. Twelve hours after a right hemicolectomy with ileostomy and mucous fistula, he develops a high fever. You receive a call from a nurse because his temperature is 105°F.

▶ *How would you manage this condition?*

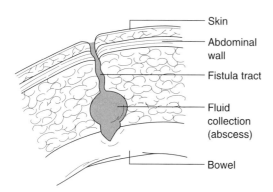

FIGURE 2-1. A gastrointestinal fistula.

F	**F**oreign body in the wound
R	**R**adiation damage to the area
I	**I**nfection or inflammatory bowel disease
E	**E**pithelialization of the fistulous tract
N	**N**eoplasm
D	**D**istal bowel obstruction

FIGURE 2-2. The *mnemonic* "FRIEND," which can be used to remember the factors associated with failure of a fistula to heal.

▶ A postoperative fever of this magnitude requires prompt attention because it is a potentially life-threatening problem. It is critical that a wound infection from a gas-forming organism be ruled out. Immediate examination of the patient and performance of a careful physical examination must take place. Removal of the abdominal wound bandages and inspection of the wound are necessary.

   Atelectasis, the most common cause of postoperative fever immediately after surgery, could account for this patient's high temperature. However, for atelectasis to cause such a fever, the patient would have to have massive collapse of an entire lobe or the entire lung. Atelectasis can be evaluated by physical examination and CXR.

The wound appears erythematous, with an advancing edge of brown skin discoloration and bleb formation. There is a thin, watery brown discharge with a foul odor and crepitus near the wound.

▶ *What diagnosis do you suspect?*

▶ A serious wound infection is likely.

 QUICK CUTS A gas-forming organism such as *Clostridium* can cause a serious wound infection and necrotizing fasciitis.

Occasionally, crepitus is a later finding, and its absence should not delay diagnosis because the disease spreads very rapidly along fascial planes.

▶ *How should you treat this infection?*

▶ The wound should be opened and cultured immediately. Clostridial myositis and cellulitis (gas gangrene) is most commonly caused by *Clostridium perfringens.*

 QUICK CUTS If gram-positive, spore-producing rods are found, the diagnosis of a clostridial wound infection is made.

Administration of high-dose penicillin G should occur, and debridement is necessary. Hyperbaric oxygen therapy may also help stop infection and inhibit the germination of heat-activated spores. Hemolysis is possible from hemagglutinin and hemolysin toxins produced by *Clostridium.* Tetanus immunization is also necessary. Multiorganism infections with streptococcus, staphylococcus, and gram-negative rods can produce similar findings.

CHAPTER 3

Wound Healing

Bruce E. Jarrell M.D.

CASE 3.1. ▶ Wound Management and Complications

A 60-year-old man undergoes lysis of adhesions for small bowel obstruction. The wound is closed primarily with staples.

▷ *How would you describe the process of wound healing in this case?*

▶ This is an example of wound healing by **primary intention.** The wound edges are closed with sutures, allowing very rapid coverage by epithelium and rapid wound healing. Certain events occur in the wound during the first several weeks of healing (Figure 3–1).

▷ *What factors are known to delay the process of wound healing?*

▶ **Good nutrition, absence of infection, and good physiological condition are necessary for normal wound healing.** Several factors are known to delay the process of wound healing (Table 3–1).

Two weeks later, at a return visit, the man asks you when he can return to his job as a loading dock worker.

▷ *What do you tell him?*

▶ You reiterate that the man should not lift significant weight until about the sixth week following surgery.

▷ *What processes are occurring in the patient's wound during the first few weeks postsurgery that support this recommendation?*

▶ Collagen production and cross-linking are still occurring during this phase. Until the collagen matures and reaches a near-final tensile strength, the wound is prone to injury and disruption. Thus, during this phase, the patient should avoid stressing the wound (Figure 3–2).

The man returns to see you in 3 months. He had no wound complications and his wound has healed. However, he is unhappy with how the wound looks and feels.

▷ *How would you manage the following physical findings at the wound?*

Case Variation 3.1.1. You feel a hard, knot-like structure beneath his skin.

▶ This is most likely a **suture knot.** If absorbable sutures were used in the operation, it may resolve with time. If nonabsorbable sutures were used, you would wait several more months for the wound to completely heal. If the man is still concerned, the knot can be removed under local anesthesia.

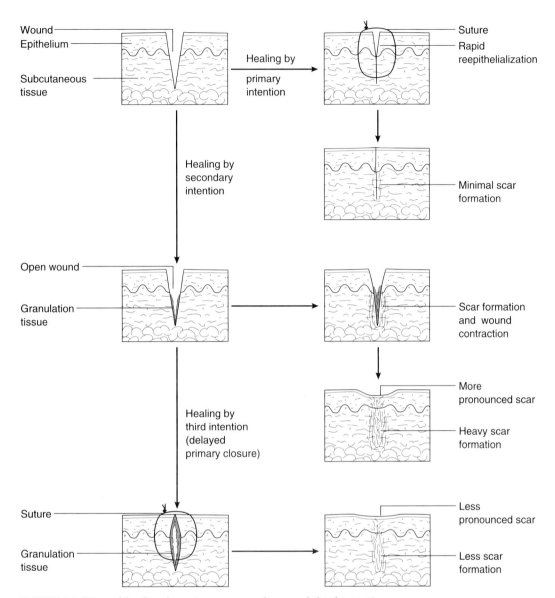

FIGURE 3-1. Wound healing by primary, secondary, and third intention.

Case Variation 3.1.2. The patient has a small, sore, red area that intermittently drains a small amount of pus and then seals over.

▶ A **stitch abscess,** which is an infection of a suture, should be suspected. Usually, this involves the knot and represents a low-grade but persistent infection. Under local anesthesia, the opening can be explored with a hemostat and the suture grasped and removed. This will usually solve the problem.

Case Variation 3.1.3. The man has a 4-cm defect in the fascia that bulges when he coughs.

PART TWO SPECIFIC DISORDERS

CHAPTER 4

Thoracic and Cardiothoracic Disorders

Bruce E. Jarrell M.D., Joseph S. MacLaughlin M.D.

CASE 4.1. ▶ Asymptomatic Abnormality Seen on Chest Radiography

A 50-year-old man with an abnormality seen on chest radiography (CXR) seeks a referral before undergoing planned repair of an inguinal hernia. He has no chest-related symptoms.

▶ *How would you describe this lesion?(Figure 4–1)*

▶ This lesion is a round, well-circumscribed lesion in the periphery of the lung. It would be called a **"coin"** lesion. For individuals who are 50 years of age, the chance that the lesion is malignant is 50%. Under 50 years, the chance decreases progressively, and above 50 years, the chance increases progressively. Different coin lesions have distinct appearances (Figure 4–2).

 Benign lesions usually have a **smooth** surface, in contrast to **malignant lesions,** which often have an **irregular** or spiculated surface.

▶ Granulomas may contain calcium, but cancers rarely do; bull's-eye configurations are almost certainly benign; and hamartomas, which are benign, typically have a "popcorn" appearance (see Figure 4–2).

▶ *What history, physical examination, or laboratory studies may help establish a definitive diagnosis?*

▶ Information about previous pulmonary illness or previous CXR abnormalities is worth seeking, and review of **previous films,** if possible, is essential. **Coin lesions** are common in the areas in which **fungal disease** is prevalent such as in the southwestern United States, where coccidioidomycosis occurs, as well as in the middle Atlantic region and the Ohio Valley, where histoplasmosis occurs. Physical examination may reveal evidence of a **primary tumor.** Testicular, breast, renal, and colon cancer may manifest as **lung metastases** (Tables 4–1, 4–2, and 4–3).

▶ *What is the next step in reaching a diagnosis?*

▶ **Computed tomography (CT)** is indicated; it clearly defines the characteristics of the lesion and can evaluate the mediastinum for the presence or absence of enlarged lymph

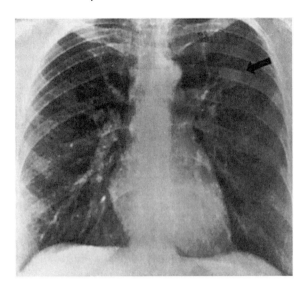

FIGURE 4-1. Chest radiograph (CXR) of the patient in Case 1. (Reprinted with permission from Greenfield LJ, Mulholland M, Oldham KT, et al *Surgery: scientific principles and practice.* 2nd ed. Philadelphia: Lippincott Williams & Wilkins, 1997: 1422.)

nodes (Figure 4–3). Using CT guidance, needle aspiration is possible for cytologic examination of the tumor.

 QUICK CUTS The chances of definitive diagnosis with **needle biopsy** are 90% or better.

▶ If the lesion is **malignant or indeterminate** on needle biopsy, **resection** is indicated. The major complication of needle biopsy is pneumothorax. If the pneumothorax is small, it may resolve on its own; however, it may require aspiration.

CASE 4.2. ▶ Symptomatic Abnormality Seen on Chest Radiography

A 60-year-old man with a history of 40 pack-years of **cigarette smoking** presents with **cough and hemoptysis.** Physical examination reveals absent breath sounds in the right lower chest. Laboratory chemistries, including coagulation studies and a liver profile, are normal. Radiographic examination reveals a 2 cm lesion of the right middle lobe (Figure 4–4A). A CT scan confirms the presence of a 2-cm mass within the right middle lobe and demonstrates a **2-cm lymph node** at the *takeoff* of the right mainstem bronchus (see Figure 4–4B).

▶ *What are the **next steps** in patient evaluation?*

QUICK CUTS **Bronchoscopy** is used to **obtain a tissue diagnosis** and to determine the **location** of the lesion in the bronchial tree. **Mediastinoscopy** is used to determine the state of the mediastinal **lymph nodes.**

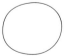

Smooth wall   Calcium spicules   Bull's eye   Spiculated surface   Popcorn

FIGURE 4-2. Radiographic appearances of various types of coin lesions.

TABLE 4-1

Assessment of Solitary Pulmonary Nodules

Evaluation	Favors Benign Status	Favors Malignant Status
History	Age <40 years	Age >40 years
	Nonsmoker	Smoker
	Previous tuberculosis exposure	No previous tuberculosis exposure
	Lives in or frequently travels to endemic, histoplasmosis, or fungal regions	Does not live or travel to endemic, histoplasmosis, or fungal regions
	No previous malignancy	Previous malignancy
Physical examination	No lymphadenopathy	Lymphadenopathy
	No organomegaly	Hepatomegaly; splenomegaly
	OB (−) stools; no hematuria	OB (+) stools; no hematuria
Skin test	PPD (+); histoplasmosis (+)	PPD (−); histoplasmosis (−) or (+)
Laboratory workup	Fungal serum titers (+)	Titers may be + or −
	Sputum acid-fast bacilli (+)	Sputum acid-fast bacilli (−)
Radiology	<3 cm on chest radiography	>3 cm on chest radiography
	Distinct margins	Hazy, spiculated, or lobulated margins
	Has not changed in size in 2 years	Has increased in size
	Doubling time <5 weeks or >465 days	Doubling time 5 weeks to 280 days
	Calcification on chest radiography, tomography, or fine-cut CT scans	Noncalcified or rarely eccentrically calcified on chest radiography, tomography, or fine-cut CT scans
	High CT density number (>164)	Low CT density number (<100)

CT = computed tomography; OB = occult bleeding; PPD = purified protein derivative.
(From Levine BA, Copeland EM III, Howard RJ, et al. *Current practice of surgery.* Vol 2. New York: Churchill Livingstone, 1993: 13. With permission.)

Usually, both bronchoscopy and mediastinoscopy are performed using the same general anesthetic. Bronchoscopy involves a flexible fiberoptic scope inserted through the endotracheal tube used for the anesthesia. Mediastinoscopy involves making a small incision above the manubrium; the scope follows the anterior wall of the trachea down to the carina and the origin of the mainstem bronchi (**Figure 4–5**).

The bronchoscopy and mediastinoscopy indicate an **adenocarcinoma of the middle lobe bronchus** 2 cm below the origin of the right middle lobe bronchus. The **enlarged lymph node is a result of benign enlargement with inflammation.**

▷ *What is the **stage** of the tumor?*

▶ Staging is an important modality; it directs treatment and allows comparison of various treatment regimens.

> **QUICK CUTS** The tumor–node–metastasis (TNM) system is used to stage lung tumors. T refers to tumor size and characteristics, N to lymph node spread, and M to the presence of metastasis.

TABLE 4-2

Masses Simulating Malignancy

Lesion	Clinical or Radiologic Features Suggesting Other Than Malignancy
Actinomycosis	Associated dental abscess or sinus Chest wall involvement
Histoplasmosis	Concentric or homogeneous calcification Endemic area
Coccidiomycosis	Thin-walled cavity often with air fluid level Endemic area
Blastomycosis	Associated chronic skin ulcers Endemic area
Cryptococcosis	Superinfection in immunocompromised patient Frequent meningeal involvement
Aspergillosis	Mycetoma with "air-crescent" sign (Fungus ball)
Hamartoma	Well-defined border with slight lobulations
Round atelectasis	Adjacent to thickened pleura "Comet-tail" vessel pattern

(From Levine BA, Copeland EM III, Howard RJ, et al. *Current practice of surgery.* Vol 2. New York: Churchill Livingstone, 1993: With permission.)

▶ By combining T, N, and M, it is possible to determine the stage of the tumor. **Stage I** indicates that the tumor is **localized** to the lung, **stage II** indicates that the tumor involves **lymph nodes** within the lung, and **stage III** indicates that the tumor has **spread beyond the lung** (Figure 4–6). In this case, T = 1, N = 0, and M = 0. Therefore, this patient's tumor is $T_1N_0M_0$, or **stage I,** and **it is potentially curable by surgical resection.**

▶ *How does cell type affect **prognosis**?*

TABLE 4–3

Common Metastatic Pulmonary Tumors

Primary	5-Year Survival (%)
Colorectal	13–38
Breast	27–50
Renal	24–54

(Adapted from Jarrell BD, Carabasi RA, Radomski JS. *NMS Surgery.* 4th ed. Philadelphia: Lippincott Williams & Wilkins, 2000.)

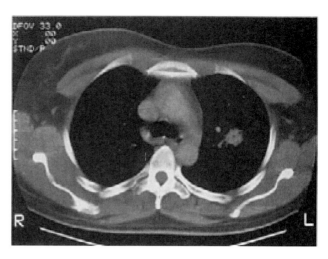

FIGURE 4-3. Computed tomography (CT) scan of a coin lesion. (Reprinted with permission from Greenfield LJ, Mulholland M, Oldham KT, et al. *Surgery: scientific principles and practice.* 2nd ed. Philadelphia: Lippincott Williams & Wilkins, 1997: 1422.)

▶ Lung cancer is generally categorized as small-cell carcinoma or non–small-cell carcinoma. **Small-cell carcinoma** is considered a **systemic disease** that begins in the lung. Because small-cell carcinoma usually has spread beyond the lung by the time it is diagnosed, the disease is rarely amenable to surgical resection. **Chemotherapy** is the primary treatment. **Non–small cell carcinoma** begins as a more **local disease that spreads to local and regional lymph nodes** before becoming systemic. Most common non–small-cell cancers are **adenocarcinoma and epidermoid (squamous-cell) carcinoma,** which occur in about equal proportions.

QUICK CUTS   **Surgical resection** is the primary mode of therapy for non–small-cell cancer, with irradiation and chemotherapy playing adjuvant roles.

Because this patient has a stage I adenocarcinoma of the lung, you proceed to thoracotomy. After exploring the mediastinum, you find no spread outside the lung and can safely perform a right middle lobectomy.

▷ *What are this patient's chances of **survival**?*

▶ For patients with **stage I** tumors, like this patient, the chance of cure via resection is **70% or better.** For patients with **stage II** tumors, the 5-year survival rate is **40%–50%.** For patients with **stage III** tumors, survival rates are **lower,** depending on how extensively the mediastinal **lymph nodes** are involved and the amount of **distant metastatic disease** present.

CASE 4.3. ▶ Symptomatic Abnormality Located in the Hilum on Chest Radiography

A 55-year-old man who smokes two packs of cigarettes per day presents with increased cough, hemoptysis, and a 10-pound weight loss. A CXR reveals a **3.5-cm mass adjacent to the right hilum** (Figures 4–7 and 4–8). **Bronchoscopy demonstrates a tumor growing out of the upper lobe bronchus,** and mediastinoscopy is negative for lymph node metastasis. No peripheral metastasis is evident. Histologic examination reveals undifferentiated squamous-cell carcinoma (**non–small-cell carcinoma**).

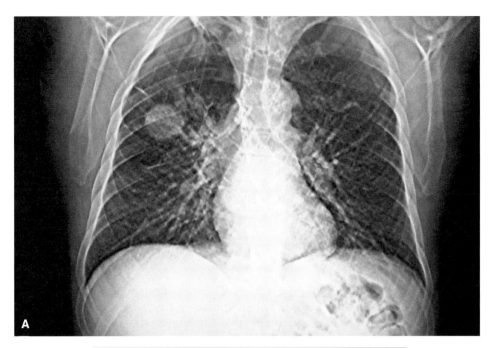

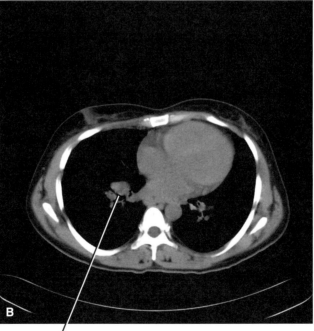

R hilar lymph node

FIGURE 4-4. (*A*) Chest radiograph of the patient in Case 2. (*B*) Computed tomography (CT) scan of the same patient confirming the presence of a right hilar lymph node.

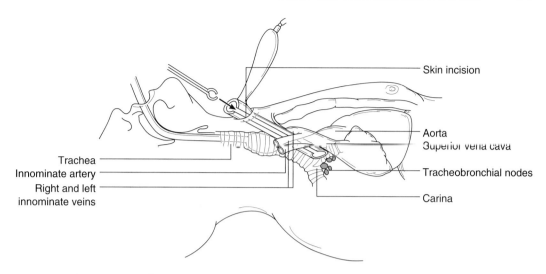

FIGURE 4-5. Description of mediastinoscopy sampling nodes anterior to the trachea down to the level of the carina. (From McKenney M, Moylan JM, Mangonon P. *Understanding surgical disease; The Miami manual of surgery.* Philadelphia: Lippincott-Raven Publishers, 1998: 250.)

▷ *What **cancer stage** does this represent?*

▶ This is a stage I tumor because it is not associated with hilar metastasis even though it is a T_2 primary lesion.

▷ *What **management procedure** would you recommend?*

▶ The patient should still undergo an exploratory thoracotomy, as in Case 2. However, the situation is different here, because the mass is **centrally located and involves the right mainstem bronchus.** It will probably require a **pneumonectomy** for complete removal.

Your assessment of the workup suggests that from a surgical point of view, this patient is a potential candidate for curative resection.

▷ *From a **medical point of view,** how would you determine if the patient will tolerate a pulmonary resection?*

▶ The **extent of the operation** is one important factor in determining the risk of the procedure. The majority (98%) of individuals in otherwise good health will tolerate a lobectomy or lesser resection. On the other hand, a pneumonectomy is associated with a far more serious physiologic risk; the risk of perioperative death ranges from 5%–10%, especially in patients greater than 70 years of age (Table 1–5).

> **QUICK CUTS** Patients with significant **cardiac** abnormalities or **obstructive airway disease** are at particularly high risk, and both cardiac and pulmonary systems require evaluation.

▶ Cardiac disease is assessed by evaluating evidence of cardiac ischemia, assessing arrythmias, and evaluating ejection fraction and wall motion. To evaluate the lungs, pulmonary function studies are useful. **Ventilation–perfusion ($\dot{V}/\dot{Q}$) scans** can determine the per-

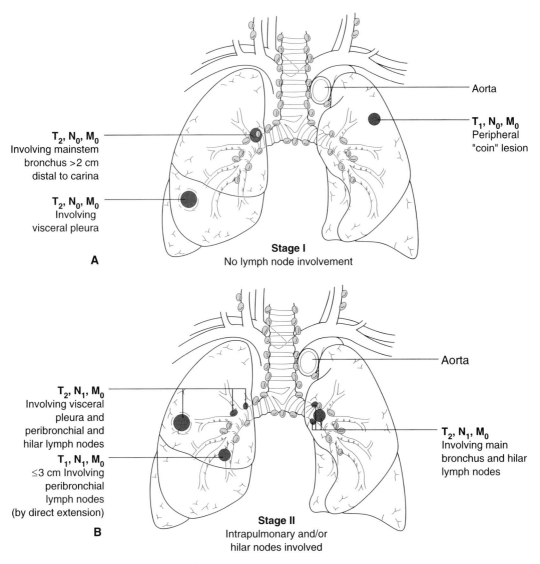

FIGURE 4-6. Staging diagram for carcinoma of the lung. (*A*) Stage IA: A T_1 lesion is 3 cm or less; Stage IB: A T_1 lesion is greater than 3 cm. (*B*) Stage IIA: A T_1 lesion with a peribronchial lymph node; Stage IIB: Hilar node involvement or limited extrapulmonary extension. (*C*) Stage IIIA: Mediastinal or subcarinal node involvement. (*D*) Stage IIIB: Extensive extrapulmonary tumor invasion of local structures. (Stage N_1: Nodal disease; N_2: Nodal disease—not pictured.) [From McKenney M, Moylan JM, Mangonon P. *Understanding surgical disease; The Miami manual of surgery.* Philadelphia: Lippincott-Raven Publishers, 1998: 261–262. Adapted from Mountain CF, Libshitz HI, Hermes KE. *Lung cancer: a handbook for staging, imaging, and lymph node classification* (*revised international system for staging and regional lymph node classification*). Houston, TX: CF Mountain and HI Libshitz, 1999: 28–38.]

centage of functioning lung tissue that remains following resection, and **spirometry** provides useful information about the mechanics of ventilation.

After determining that the risks are acceptable, you decide to perform a thoracotomy. As a result of this procedure, you learn that the tumor involves the upper lobe with **extension into**

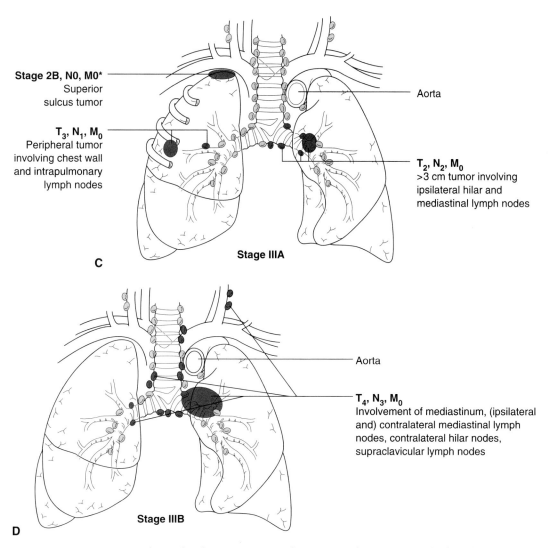

Stage 2B, N0, M0*
Superior
sulcus tumor

Aorta

T_3, N_1, M_0
Peripheral tumor
involving chest wall
and intrapulmonary
lymph nodes

T_2, N_2, M_0
>3 cm tumor involving
ipsilateral hilar and
mediastinal lymph nodes

Stage IIIA

C

Aorta

T_4, N_3, M_0
Involvement of mediastinum, (ipsilateral
and) contralateral mediastinal lymph
nodes, contralateral hilar nodes,
supraclavicular lymph nodes

Stage IIIB

D

FIGURE 4-6. (CONTINUED) *Since this figure was created superior sulcus tumor and other chest wall invasive tumors without nodal spread have been reclassified as Stage II B.

the mainstem bronchus. Sampling of the lymph nodes of the hilum and mediastinum is negative for cancer.

*What are the **surgical options?***

Essentially, there are two options: a pneumonectomy or a lobectomy with a "sleeve" resection. A **pneumonectomy** involves (1) dividing the right mainstem bronchus just distal to the carina and sewing or stapling it closed and (2) dividing the pulmonary artery and the two main pulmonary veins. A **sleeve lobectomy** involves (1) dividing the mainstem bronchus above and below the origin of the right upper lobe bronchus and (2) reattaching the bronchus by suture technique. The vessels to the right upper lobe are divided, but the blood supply to the middle and lower lobes is left intact. **Although pneumonectomy is easier to perform, it has a higher initial mortality rate. Sleeve lobectomy is safer,** but it may not be feasible because of local invasion of the main pulmonary artery.

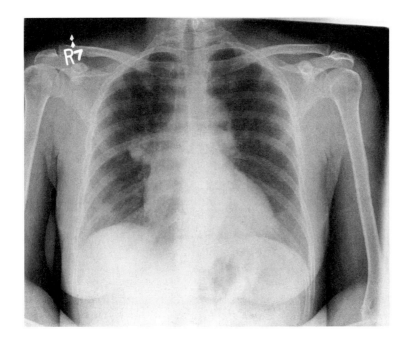

FIGURE 4-7. Chest radiograph (CXR) of patient in Case 3, showing a 3-cm right hilar mass.

CASE 4.4. ▶ Lung Mass with Possible Metastases

You are evaluating a man with a lung mass. You complete a CT scan, bronchoscopy, and mediastinoscopy of the chest. The patient has a non–small-cell carcinoma of the lung.

▶ *How would you manage the following findings?*

Case Variation 4.4.1. Ipsilateral Hilar lymph nodes positive for metastasis and no other evidence of disease (Figure 4–8)

▶ This represents a stage II lung cancer.

 QUICK CUTS   The **treatment for stage II cancer is similar to that for stage I (surgical resection).**

▶ However, the prognosis for stage II carcinoma is worse.

Case Variation 4.4.2. Mediastinal lymph nodes positive for metastasis on mediastinoscopy (Figure 4–9)

▶ This represents a stage III lung cancer, which involves a different treatment plan.

 QUICK CUTS   Chemotherapy and radiation therapy are appropriate therapy for stage III disease.

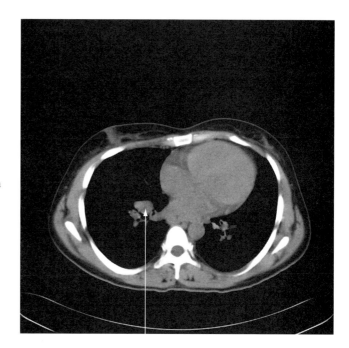

FIGURE 4-8. A computed tomography (CT) scan of the same patient showing a tumor invading a bronchus (arrow).

If the tumor became smaller and could be down-staged, then the patient could undergo resection (Table 4–4).

Case Variation 4.4.3. Positron emission tomography (PET) scan that is positive for tumor outside the lung

It appears that PET scanning is highly reliable and sensitive in detecting lung cancer metastasis. If a lesion is found outside the hilar nodes, then the patient most likely has a stage III or Stage IV (distant metastasis) cancer and should receive chemotherapy and radiation.

CASE 4.5. ▶ Symptomatic Superior Sulcus Tumor

A 45-year-old woman presents with pain in the midback and down the ulnar area of the elbow and wrist. She has little cough or shortness of breath. Cervical spine films are negative. Despite 6 months of treatment with nonsteroidal anti-inflammatory drugs (NSAIDs) and physical therapy, her symptoms have increased. On physical examination, **Horner syndrome** is evident, and on CXR, a vague haziness is visible in the **apex of the lung** (Figure 4–10A).

*What is the most likely **diagnosis?***

This patient most likely has a **Pancoast tumor,** which is a lung cancer originating in the extreme apex of the lung in the groove (superior sulcus) produced by the subclavian artery. It invades the chest wall, the lower cords of the brachial plexus, the subclavian artery and, at times, the sympathetic ganglia and produces symptoms depending on which structures are involved (Figure 4–11).

*What are the **next steps** in making a more definitive diagnosis?*

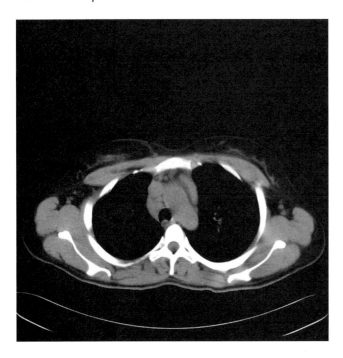

FIGURE 4-9. Computed tomography (CT) scan demonstrating mediastinal adenopathy. [From Greenfield LJ, Mulholland M, Oldham KT, et al. *Surgery: Scientific Principles and Practice.* 2nd ed. Philadelphia: Lippincott Williams & Wilkins, 1997: 1423.]

▶ A **CT scan** would be the next step, and it reveals erosion of the first and second ribs and a superior sulcus mass (Figure 4–10B). After CT, **bronchoscopy, mediastinoscopy,** and **needle biopsy** of the mass are appropriate.

Bronchoscopy reveals no lesions. Mediastinoscopy reveals no tumor in the mediastinum. Needle biopsy of the mass is positive for adenocarcinoma.

▶ *What is the **stage** of this tumor?*

▶ In Pancoast tumor, the presence of chest wall invasion makes this a T_3 tumor; this factor alone make this a stage III tumor using old staging. With newer staging, this would be a stage IIb if no nodes are present.

▶ *What is the **prognosis** in this case?*

 QUICK CUTS   Nodal involvement at surgery is the key to prognosis.

TABLE 4–4

5-Year Survival for Stages II and III Lung Cancer

Stage	5-Year Survival Rate (%)
II	44
IIIa	22
IIIb	<10

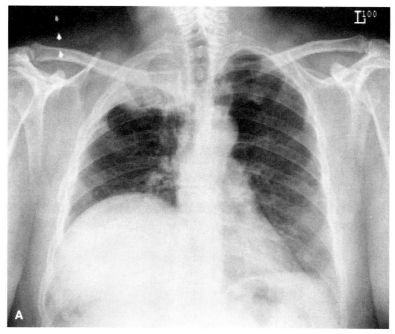

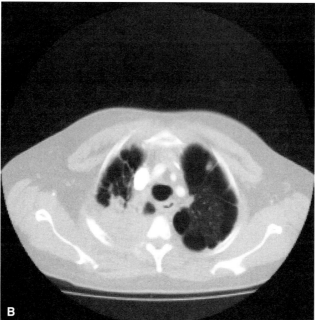

FIGURE 4-10. (*A*) Chest radiograph and (*B*) computed tomography (CT) scan of patient in Case 5, showing Pancoast tumor.

There is little hope for patient survival if lymph nodes in the mediastinum contain tumor, but the 5-year survival is 40%–50% without nodal involvement.

▷ *What is the appropriate* **treatment?**

▶ Treatment of superior sulcus tumors is carried out in **two phases.**

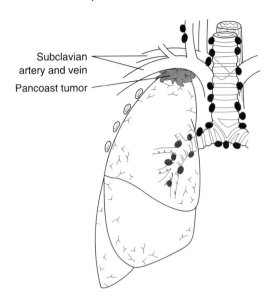

Subclavian
artery and vein
Pancoast tumor

FIGURE 4-11. Pancoast tumor and local structures. [Redrawn from Mountain CF, Libshitz HI, Hermes KE. *Lung cancer: a handbook for staging, imaging, and lymph node classification (revised international system for staging and regional lymph node classification).* Houston, TX: CF Mountain and HI Libshitz, 1999: 19.]

 Irradiation of the area occurs over a 6-week period, followed by **surgical resection** of the involved chest wall and lung.

▶ Patients do surprisingly well, considering the extent of tumor involvement and the radical treatment necessary to eradicate it. Before the development of this treatment regimen, patients died in agony because of tumor invasion of bone and nerves.

CASE 4.6. ▶ Hemoptysis and Atelectasis in a Young Patient

A 25-year-old athletic young woman presents with a recent onset of cough and shortness of breath. Not long ago, she noted that her sputum contained flecks of blood. She does not smoke. A CXR reveals partial collapse of the right upper lobe of the lung.

▶ *What is the **differential diagnosis**?*

▶ Hemoptysis has many causes, but in an otherwise healthy young woman with atelectasis, an obstructed bronchus is probably present. In such a young person, the most likely diagnosis is **bronchial adenoma.** Cancer would be unusual in a nonsmoker under 30 years of age. In addition, while one must always consider tuberculosis, atelectasis is rare with this condition.

▶ *What are bronchial adenomas?*

▶ Bronchial adenomas **arise within bronchi** and often obstruct them. The use of "adenoma" is faulty nomenclature; these tumors have considerable malignant potential. There are two main types: carcinoid tumors and adenocystic carcinomas. Carcinoid tumors arise from cells similar to those that give rise to oat-cell carcinomas. Although carcinoid tumors are usually benign when originating in the lung, they may demonstrate significant malignant potential, especially when they develop in the small bowel. Adenocystic carcinomas, which more commonly arise in the upper airway, invade locally.

What **diagnostic measures** should be undertaken to establish the diagnosis?

► A CT scan may better delineate the pulmonary anatomy and an obstructed bronchus, but bronchoscopy is required for diagnosis. This is a safe procedure in capable hands. However, **bronchial adenomas are vascular and tend to bleed when biopsied,** and the bronchoscopist must be prepared to coagulate or otherwise control any untoward bleeding.

A bronchial adenoma is visualized by bronchoscopy, and a bronchoscopic biopsy is carried out safely. A diagnosis of carcinoid tumor is made on histopathology.

 What is the next step in **treatment**?

> **QUICK CUTS** Surgery usually involves **lobectomy,** with removal of the tumor-containing bronchus.

This procedure is usually curative, but atypical carcinoid tumors may metastasize widely. Bronchial carcinoids may also produce carcinoid syndrome.

CASE 4.7. ► New-Onset Pleural Effusion without Heart Failure

A 65-year-old man, a retired shipyard worker, is admitted with **chest pain and shortness of breath** of 3 months' duration. Physical examination reveals absent breath sounds and dullness to percussion in the right lung base. The CXR reveals an **opacified right lower lung field with pleural effusion** (Figure 4–12).

 What is the **differential diagnosis**?

> **QUICK CUTS** **Pleural effusion in an older patient signifies cancer until proven otherwise.**

However, benign effusions as the result of congestive heart failure are more common. The most common cancers are bronchiogenic carcinoma and mesothelioma, particularly considering the patient's history of working in a shipyard and the strong possibility of exposure to asbestos. Benign effusion may be the residual of viral or bacterial pneumonia. Empyema and tuberculosis effusion should also be considered.

 How would you **establish a diagnosis** (assuming the effusion is not related to congestive heart failure)?

► **Thoracentesis and pleural biopsy** are indicated. Pleural biopsy detects pleural-based cancers (Figure 4–13). Culture of the pleural fluid for bacteria and tuberculosis is warranted, and examination for the presence of malignant cells is also necessary.

The pleural biopsy reveals mesothelioma.

 What **treatment options** are available?

► Mesothelioma is an aggressive malignancy that has **not been responsive to therapy,** and most patients are dead within 1 year.

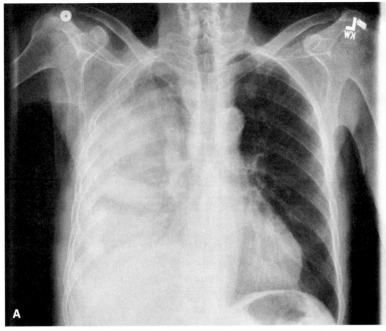

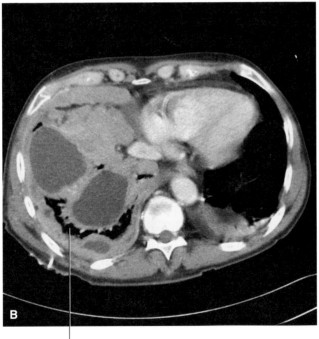

Thick-walled tumor that is pleurally based

FIGURE 4-12. A. Chest radiograph (CXR) of patient in Case 7, showing a right pleural effusion. B. CT scan of patient in Case 7, confirming the presence of a mesothelioma.

QUICK CUTS The only results that lead to cure of mesotheliomas have involved **extrapleural pneumonectomy.**

▶ In this procedure, the entire lung and the parietal and visceral pleura along with, at times, the pericardium and diaphragm are resected en bloc. This exceedingly radical procedure results in high morbidity and mortality (>10%) but offers the chance for recovery in up to 30% of patients. Irradiation and chemotherapy are ineffective.

CASE 4.8. ▶ Sudden Chest Pain and Shortness of Breath in a Young Patient

An 18-year-old female college student experiences sharp chest pain followed by shortness of breath while playing tennis. Physical examination reveals an anxious-appearing young woman who is short of breath. The trachea is shifted to the left, **and breath sounds are absent on the right** (Figure 4–14).

▶ *What is the probable **diagnosis?***

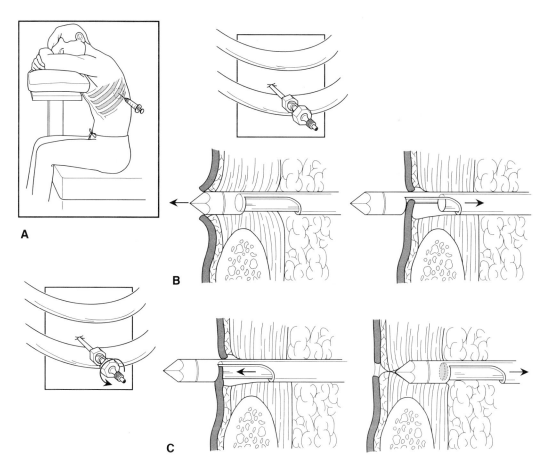

FIGURE 4-13. Pleural biopsy procedure. (Redrawn from Urschel HC Jr, Cooper JD. *Atlas of thoracic surgery.* New York: Churchill Livingstone, 1995: 91.)

▶ **Spontaneous pneumothorax** is a common condition seen in otherwise healthy young people. Its etiology is rupture of **apical blebs.** These typically small clusters of thin-walled, bubble-like structures are formed by the breakdown of the septae in the apex of the lung. Rupture may occur spontaneously or may be related to strenuous activity. **Air escapes into the pleural space, increasing the intrapleural pressure and resulting in lung collapse.** With collapse, the air leak may seal and the lung reexpand. Continued leak-age may lead to a marked increase in pleural pressure. Total lung collapse and mediasti-nal shift, as seen in this patient, are the hallmarks of tension pneumothorax, which war-rants urgent treatment.

▷ *What is the **treatment** for pneumothorax?*

▶ Air must be removed from the pleural space to allow the lung to expand and the pleural surfaces to coapt and seal the defect. The technique of simple **chest tube drainage (tube**

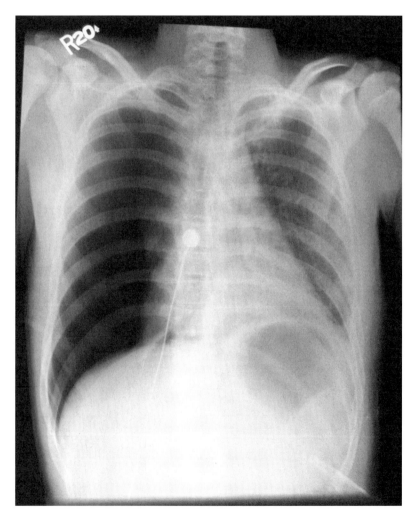

FIGURE 4-14. Chest x-ray (CXR) of the patient in Case 8.

thoracostomy) is effective in well over 90% of patients (Figure 4–15). For a first-time pneumothorax, a polyethylene tube with a one-way valve (Heimlich valve) may be sufficient. Most commonly, a small-sized no. 24 chest tube is inserted into the chest between the ribs in the lateral chest wall and directed to the apex. The tube is attached to a **water-seal–type** drainage (Figure 4–16).

How does a water seal function?

A water seal **maintains a negative pressure in the pleural space and chest tube** such that air and fluids may escape from the chest. The water seal creates a one-way valve mechanism to prevent air and fluids from reentering the cavity through the tube. Air that leaks through the injured lung parenchyma traverses through the tube and into the external container (often termed a Pleurevac). The leaking air may be seen as it bubbles through the water seal, especially when the patient coughs or performs a Valsalva maneuver. Leaking air is termed an air leak. Most air leaks are small and seal in several days.

 QUICK CUTS Properly functioning chest tubes should result in a fully inflated lung with disappearance of any residual pneumothorax and pleural effusion.

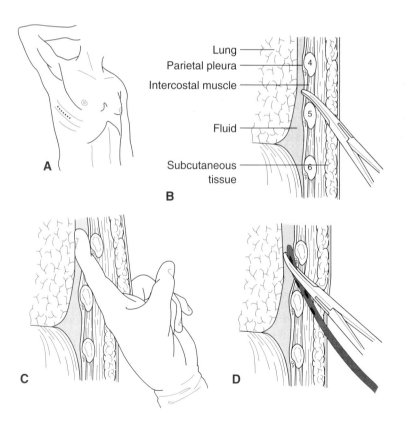

FIGURE 4-15. Insertion of chest tube. (Redrawn from Hood RM. *Thoracic surgery.* 2nd ed. Philadelphia: Lea & Febiger, 1993: 41–43.)

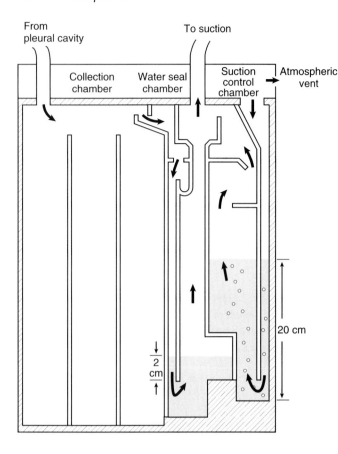

From
pleural cavity

To suction

Collection
chamber

Water seal
chamber

Suction
control
chamber

Atmospheric
vent

20 cm

2
cm

FIGURE 4-16. Apparatus for chest drainage. (From Symbas PN. *Cardiothoracic trauma.* Philadelphia: WB Saunders, 1989.)

▶ *If the lung does not expand, what is the treatment (Figure 4–17)?*

▶ It is necessary to find the cause of the problem. The most common cause is **an improperly placed chest tube or a leak at the site of entry** into the chest. **Replacement** remedies this problem. Other causes include leaks at tubing connections and large leaks from the lung parenchyma from large blebs or leaks from larger bronchi.

▶ *What is involved in the management of a **persistent air leak?***

▶ Initially, it is necessary to eliminate the causes mentioned previously. After ruling them out, the clinician would conclude that there is a parenchymal cause for the leak, and surgical intervention is necessary.

QUICK CUTS   Thoracoscopic **excision of the blebs and pleural abrasion** (pleurodesis) is highly effective in resolving persistent or recurrent pneumothorax (Figure 4–18).

▶ Pleurodesis irritates the visceral and parietal pleura, causing them to adhere, thus preventing a future pneumothorax. Pleurodesis is also used in patients with recurrent **spontaneous** pneumothorax as well as in patients **with bilateral spontaneous** pneumothoraces. Obviously, a bilateral pneumothorax is a dangerous event, and the clinician should want to eliminate any possible recurrences.

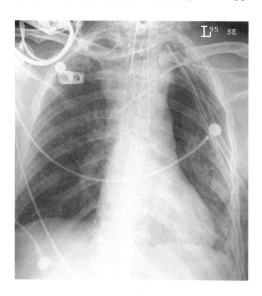

FIGURE 4-17. Chest radiograph (CXR) of a well-positioned chest tube and a persistent pneumothorax.

CASE 4.9. ▶ Pleural-Based Chest Pain, Fever, and Pleural Effusion

A 70-year-old woman develops **pneumonia** during a winter influenza outbreak. She receives antibiotics at home, and her condition improves over the next week. At that time, she notes increased pain in her chest, increased cough, and recurrent fever; she is sent to the emergency department. You are asked to evaluate her. A CXR reveals a pleural effusion in the right lung field confirmed on CT (Figure 4–19).

▶ *What is the most likely **diagnosis**?*

▶ This patient presents with a classic history of **empyema.** In the community setting, the most common causal bacteria is *Streptococcus pneumoniae.* In the hospital setting, *Staphylococcus* and gram-negative bacteria are the usual pathogens. If there is a history of alcoholism, unconsciousness, recent operation, or pulmonary aspiration, the empyema often contains anaerobic organisms. In case series of empyema, up to 35% of cultures are negative because of previous treatment.

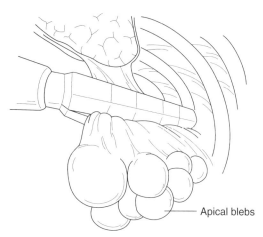

FIGURE 4-18. Excision of blebs.

Apical blebs

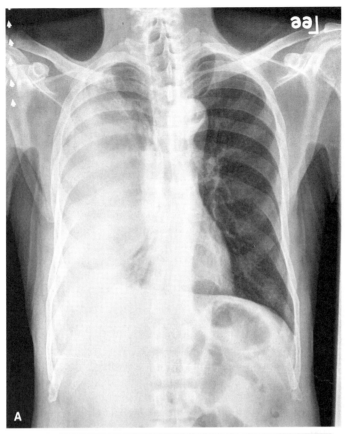

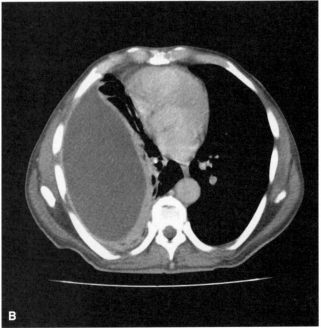

FIGURE 4-19. *A.* Chest radiograph (CXR) of the patient in Case 9.
B. Computed tomography (CT) scan of the chest of the patient in
Case 9.

> *What is the **therapeutic approach** to management?*

▶ There are three important management principles.

QUICK CUTS
1. **Initiate appropriate antibiotics** as determined by culture and sensitivity.
2. **Evacuate pus.**
3. **Reexpand the lung.**

▶ **Chest tube drainage** is the primary mode of therapy and is highly effective in draining the pus and reexpanding the lung (Figure 4–20). **Failure** to expeditiously accomplish this allows the empyema to become **loculated** by organizing fibrin. If this occurs, **thoracotomy and decortication** (removal of the thick inflammatory tissue trapping the lung) is necessary to reexpand the lung. This may be carried out through a minithoracotomy or by video-assisted thoracoscopic surgery techniques.

CASE 4.10. ▶ Progressively Increasing Substernal Chest Pain

A 53-year-old man with non–insulin-dependent diabetes (NIDDM) has experienced angina for 3 years. He has been successfully managed medically until recently. In addition to the diabetes, he has a 30–pack-year history of smoking and a history of hypercholesterolemia. He is admitted with a 2-week history of **increasingly frequent and severe chest pain** that appears to be cardiac in nature, and he now has **angina at rest.** The electrocardiogram (ECG) demonstrates an **ischemic pattern.**

> *What is the **diagnosis?***

▶ The patient suffers from unstable angina, sometimes called "**preinfarction angina.**" This is an emergency situation.

> *What are the next steps in **management?***

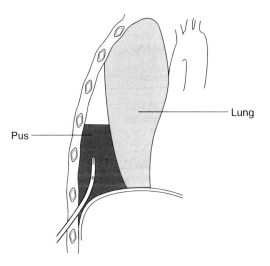

FIGURE 4–20. Empyema drainage. (Redrawn from Hood RM. *Thoracic surgery*. 2nd ed. Philadelphia: Lea & Febiger, 1993: 200.)

> **QUICK CUTS** The operative mortality is greater for high-risk patients than for low-risk patients, but they benefit from bypass surgery the most in terms of survival.

▶ The trend in the United States is to operate on higher-risk patients.

CASE 4.11. ▶ Mitral Valve Disease That Requires Surgery

A 42-year-old stockbroker with a known heart murmur of 10 years' duration is experiencing increasingly severe shortness of breath and fatigue. An echocardiogram reveals **severe mitral valve regurgitation.**

▷ *What is the likely **diagnosis** in this case?*

▶ The patient's mitral valve regurgitation most likely is due to **myxomatous degeneration** of the mitral valve. The etiology of this disorder is unknown but is thought to be due to ischemia of the myocardium, particularly the mitral valve apparatus.

▷ *How does this condition differ from **prolapse of the mitral valve and mitral stenosis?***

▶ **Prolapse** of the mitral valve (Barlow syndrome) refers to **eccentric closure** of the mitral leaflets, usually without significant mitral valve regurgitation. In young women, this is a common disorder and rarely progresses to mitral valve regurgitation. In men, the presence of prolapse may be a harbinger of severe mitral valve disease. Mitral stenosis is four times as common in young women. Although the disorder is now rare in the United States, it is still common in underdeveloped nations and in immigrants from those countries.

Usually, **mitral stenosis is caused by rheumatic fever and scarlet fever.** Inflammation occurs in connective tissues, including those in the heart. The mitral valve leaflets progressively fuse beginning at the commissures, and increasing obstruction occurs. With time, the valve leaflets and annulus undergo calcification. Pressure in the left atrium and pulmonary vessels increases, and right heart enlargement develops. Eventually, the pulmonary arterioles become scarred, and pulmonary hypertension with irreversibility develops.

▷ *What is the **treatment** for symptomatic mitral valve disease?*

▶ **Repair or replacement of the mitral valve** is warranted. In the early stages, before calcification occurs, **correction of mitral stenosis** involves **commissurotomy.** This now rarely performed procedure consists of splitting the commissures and reconstituting the lumen by mechanical dilators or under direct vision with the use of cardiopulmonary bypass. **It is possible to repair mitral regurgitation** by **excising** the insufficient or redundant portions of the **mitral leaflets** and narrowing and reinforcing the mitral annulus with an **annuloplasty** ring. If repair is not feasible, valve replacement with a prosthetic valve is necessary.

CASE 4.12. ▶ Aortic Valve Disease That Requires Surgery

An 82-year-old man who experiences **near-syncope** is brought to the hospital. History reveals a heart murmur noted at 20 years of age when he was discharged from the army. The man has had progressive shortness of breath for 2 years or more and tightness in his chest when mowing the lawn. Physical examination reveals a bright, healthy-appearing man with a systolic murmur radiating to the neck. An echocardiogram reveals **severe aortic stenosis.** Routine laboratory studies are normal.

▷ *What are the usual **causes** of aortic valve stenosis?*

▶ Aortic valve stenosis is of three main types: **congenital, arteriosclerotic,** and **deteriorative.** Congenital stenosis usually takes the form of a bicuspid valve. Over the years, the leaflets thicken, calcify, and increasingly produce a stenotic opening.

▷ *What are the **next steps** to be taken in this patient's workup?*

▶ This man has severe aortic stenosis with three major symptoms—**shortness of breath, angina,** and **syncope.** These findings signify an extremely limited life expectancy. **Without surgery, the vast majority of such patients are dead within 2 years.**
   Cardiac catheterization is indicated to determine the status of the coronary circulation. The catheterization allows for determination of the **aortic valve lumen size and pressure gradient, ventricular function,** and **presence of coronary artery disease.** Angina is common due to aortic stenosis, but intrinsic coronary artery disease may also be present. Carotid Doppler studies are indicated to rule out internal carotid artery obstruction. Syncope is a common symptom of aortic stenosis and bruits in the neck may be radiated, but identification of carotid artery stenosis is essential. If necessary, it must be corrected to avoid neurologic catastrophe.

▷ *Is this man a candidate for surgery at 82 years of age?*

▶ Aortic stenosis is generally well tolerated with good medical management, although, in some instances, congenitally stenotic valves produce symptoms of obstruction early in life (Figure 4–25).

QUICK CUTS   Symptoms do not develop in many patients until their fifth or sixth decade, at which time they are at extreme risk for sudden death. **Unfortunately, sudden death may be the first symptom.**

▶ A symptomatic patient with **a high-grade stenosis and preserved ventricular function has a good chance** for successful surgery and recovery even at 82 years of age. In this case, repair depends on the results of the catheterization, not age.

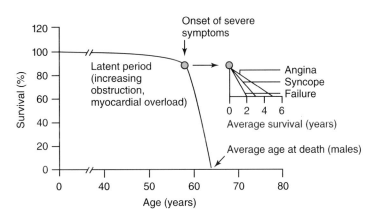

FIGURE 4-25. Natural history of aortic stenosis. (From Greenfield LJ, Mulholland M, Oldham KT, et al. [eds]. *Surgery: scientific principles and practice.* 2nd ed. Philadelphia: Lippincott Williams & Wilkins, 1997: 1519. After Ross J Jr, Braunwald E. Aortic stenosis. *Circulation.* 1968;38 [suppl 5]:61.)

The results of the catheterization indicate a high-grade aortic valve stenosis and preserved ventricular function. You decide that valve replacement is indicated.

▶ *What operation is performed?*

▶ Aortic valve replacement is usually required. Valve prostheses are of two main varieties, mechanical and tissue.

QUICK CUTS **Mechanical valves,** which are of metal and plastic construction, are extremely **durable** and mechanically efficient but require **anticoagulation** because they are thrombogenic. **Tissue valves** (human, porcine, or bovine) are **nonthrombogenic but deteriorate** in the body and require replacement beginning at about 7 years.

CASE 4.13. ▶ Congestive Heart Failure with Normal Coronary Arteries

A 45-year-old salesman who has been previously healthy and athletically active develops progressive shortness of breath and weakness 3 months following a respiratory illness. A CXR reveals a large heart shadow and congested lungs. An echocardiogram reveals an ejection fraction of 20% and moderate mitral regurgitation. Cardiac catheterization shows **normal coronary arteries** and confirms **an ejection fraction of less than 25% with poor ventricular contraction and dilatation.**

▶ *What is the likely* **diagnosis?**

▶ This patient suffers from **dilated cardiomyopathy,** probably related to the viral respiratory illness. This association is well documented, but the etiologic mechanism is unclear.

▶ *What is the* **prognosis?**

▶ Approximately one-third of patients recover, one-third will stay about the same or slightly improve with medication, and one-third worsen and die.

▶ *What is the* **treatment?**

▶ Steroids, diuretics, and immunosuppressives were the mainstays of treatment until it was discovered that **β-blockers markedly improved** heart function in these patients. Still, the condition of many patients continues to deteriorate. **Heart transplantation** may be lifesaving.

▶ *How is* **heart transplantation** *performed?*

▶ 1. A donor heart must be located from a brain-dead individual.
   2. The heart is isolated from the circulation, perfused with cardioplegia solution to protect it, and removed from the donor.
   3. The heart is transported in a cold environment.
   4. The recipient's heart is removed using cardiopulmonary bypass.
   5. The donor heart is sutured to the remnants of the recipient's atria. The aorta and pulmonary arteries are anastomosed and the circulation reestablished.

▶ *What is the* **outlook** *with a transplant?*

▶ Immediate survival is greater than 90%. A variety of immunosuppressive drugs, often including steroids and cyclosporine or tacrolimus, are useful in the achievement of immunosuppression. Survival at 1 year is 85%–90% and at 2 years is 75%.

QUICK CUTS   Most **deaths** occur from **infection** related to immunosuppressive drugs and **accelerated coronary artery atherosclerosis,** possibly as a form of chronic rejection.

CASE 4.14. ▶ Recurrent Regurgitation of Undigested Food

A 55-year-old woman, a department store salesperson, has experienced **regurgitation** of chewed but **not digested** food intermittently during the past 2 years. She has a long history of **dysphagia.** The woman complains of fetid breath, coughing, and choking but denies abdominal symptoms.

*What is the **next step?***

A careful head and neck examination is warranted, and it is important to obtain a **barium swallow** (Figure 4–26) **or upper gastrointestinal (GI) endoscopy.**

The barium swallow reveals a 4 cm × 3 cm pharyngeal diverticulum.

*What is the **etiology** of a pharyngeal diverticulum?*

A pharyngeal diverticulum, also called a **Zenker diverticulum,** is a **pulsion diverticulum** that develops in the area between the lower pharyngeal constrictor and the cricopharyngeal muscle.

QUICK CUTS   **Abnormal uncoordinated constriction of the cricopharyngeal muscle** during swallowing increases the pressure in this area of the pharynx and progressively forces out a pouch of mucosa covered by pharyngeal muscle. This action **probably results in a pharyngeal diverticulum.**

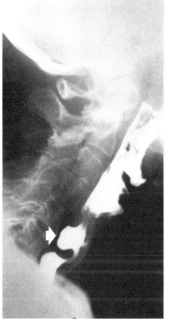
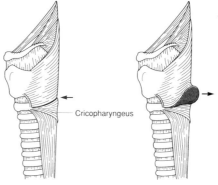
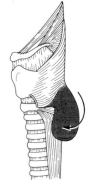

Cricopharyngeus

FIGURE 4-26. A. Barium swallow of the patient in Case 15. B. Drawing demonstrating anatomic location.

▶ A pulsion diverticulum may also occur at the distal esophageal gastric junction. It is referred to as an epiphrenic diverticulum, which fills with undigested food. The food is regurgitated and may be aspirated, resulting in severe pulmonary infection.

▷ *What is the **treatment** for an pharyngeal diverticulum?*

 The most important management principle is **transection of cricopharyngeal muscle** to relax the esophageal entrance and prevent uncontrolled contraction.

If a pharyngeal diverticulum is large, excision is appropriate at the origin from the posterior pharynx. With an epiphrenic diverticulum, excision and esophageal myotomy at the esophageal gastric junction are necessary (Figure 4–27).

CASE 4.15. ▶ Dysphagia

A 40-year-old woman complains of dysphagia and weight loss. She has had several lower respiratory infections during the past 5 years. As part of her workup, she undergoes a barium swallow (Figure 4–28).

▷ *What is the most likely **diagnosis**?*

▶ The barium swallow shows a **dilated esophagus** that ends in a "**bird's-beak**" appearance, typical of **achalasia.**

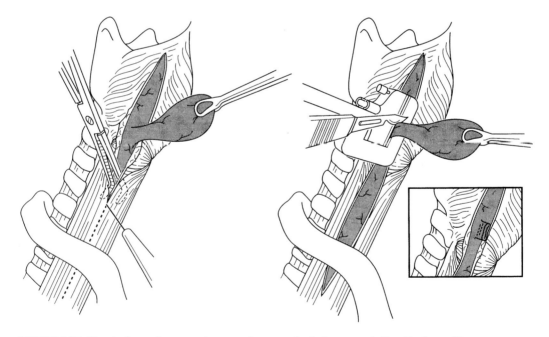

FIGURE 4-27. Cervical esophagomyotomy and removal of pharyngeal diverticulum. (From Greenfield LJ, Mulholland M, Oldham KT, et al. [eds]. *Surgery: scientific principles and practice.* 2nd ed. Philadelphia: Lippincott Williams & Wilkins, 1997: 727. After Orringer MB. Extended cervical esophagomyotomy for cricopharyngeal dysfunction. *J Thorac Cardiovasc Surg.* 1980; 80:669.)

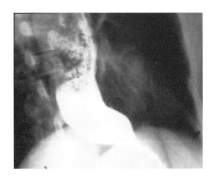

FIGURE 4-28. Barium swallow of patient in Case 15.

  A **poor peristaltic contraction** of the body of the esophagus and a failure of the lower esophageal sphincter to relax are seen on barium swallow with achalasia.

▶ If this condition is not corrected, the esophagus may greatly **dilate** and essentially become an adynamic sac.

▶ *What is the etiology?*

▶ The etiology is not clear, but histopathology usually reveals a **loss of smooth muscle ganglionic cells of Auerbach plexus and neuronal degeneration.** Achalasia is associated with severe emotional stress, physical trauma, weight loss, and Chagas disease (*Trypanosoma cruzi* infection).

▶ *What is the treatment?*

▶ Calcium channel blockers may help, but the classic treatment, which is still most effective, is disruption of the lower-esophageal high-pressure zone. Distal esophageal dilation is performed either surgically with a Heller myotomy, which improves approximately 100% of patients, or endoscopically with transesophageal pneumatic dilation, which improves 60% of patients. The Heller myotomy is an incision through the muscular layers of the lower esophagus, which allows the mucosa to bulge out and greatly enlarge the area of previous constriction. It can be performed through either an open thoracotomy or closed thoracoscopy (Figure 4–29).

CASE 4.16. ▶ Dysphagia

A 60-year-old man presents with dysphagia of 3 months' duration. A barium swallow reveals an irregular defect in the esophagus (Figure 4–30).

▶ *What is the next step in his evaluation?*

▶ Esophagoscopy and biopsy of the abnormality should occur.

▶ *What is the most likely diagnosis?*

▶ This disorder most likely represents cancer of the esophagus. Cancers in the **upper and middle third of the esophagus usually are squamous-cell carcinomas.** Tumors in the

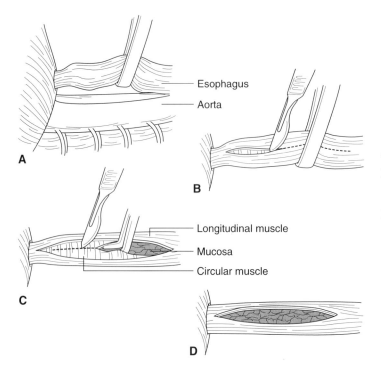

FIGURE 4-29. Distal esophagomyotomy procedure for achalasia. (Redrawn from Hood RM. *Thoracic surgery.* 2nd ed. Philadelphia: Lea & Febiger, 1993: 235.)

Esophagus

Aorta

Longitudinal muscle

Mucosa

Circular muscle

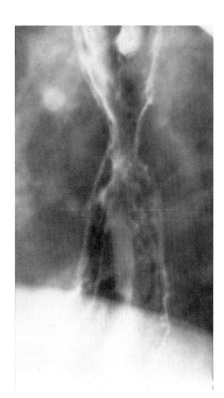

FIGURE 4-30. Mid-esophageal cancer.

lower third may be **squamous-cell carcinomas,** but increasingly they represent **adeno-carcinomas.**

▷ *What is the **etiology** of esophageal cancer?*

▶ The exact cause of this cancer is unknown but has been associated with **environmental and dietary conditions, tobacco and alcohol use, and Barrett esophagus.** In Barrett esophagus, **severe reflux esophagitis** leads to ulceration and replacement of lower esophageal squamous mucosa with columnar epithelium (Figure 4–31). A person with dysplasia of this metaplastic epithelium is at high risk of developing adenocarcinoma. **Severe dysplasia is virtually synonymous with carcinoma in situ;** the chance of developing esophageal cancer is 40 times higher in an individual with severe dysplasia than in a normal person.

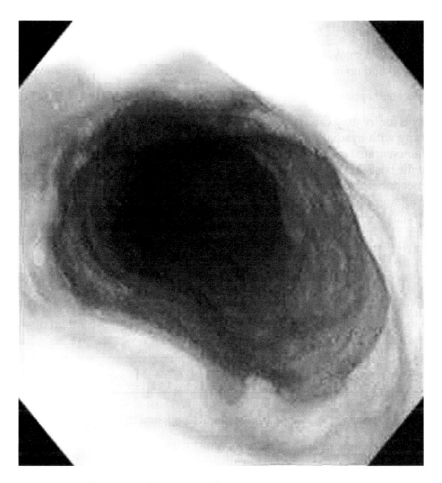

FIGURE 4-31. Barrett esophagus on endoscopy.

C H A P T E R 5

Vascular Disorders

Bruce E. Jarrell M.D., Marshall Benjamin M.D.

PERIPHERAL ARTERIAL DISEASE

CASE 5.1. ▶ Brief Neurologic Event

A 60-year-old woman presents with a single episode of weakness and numbness in her right arm. The episode lasted for 15 minutes and completely resolved in 1 hour.

▷ *What is the most likely diagnosis?*

▶ A **transient ischemic attack (TIA)** is the suspected diagnosis.

 QUICK CUTS A TIA is typified by a brief neurologic deficit such as the one described in Case 5.1, which **completely resolves within 24 hours.**

The neurologic symptoms are most likely vascular in origin because they correspond to an anatomic distribution that receives blood from the appropriate carotid artery.

In this case, the left internal carotid artery is the suspected location of the ischemic event. Current pathophysiologic thinking suggests that atherosclerotic plaques at the **carotid bifurcation or internal carotid artery region become ulcerated,** allowing cholesterol and platelet debris to break off and **form an embolism in the intracranial circulation and brain** (Figure 5-1).

▷ *If this patient is left untreated, what is the risk that she will have a repeat neurologic event?*

▶ Without treatment, this patient's chance of experiencing another TIA or stroke within 2 years is as high as 40%.

▷ *How would you evaluate this patient?*

▶ An examination for **carotid bruits, residual neurologic deficit,** and **evidence of cardiac disease,** especially murmurs that might indicate an embolic source, is necessary. If a murmur is present, an echocardiogram would be appropriate. In addition, a **duplex ultrasound study of the carotid vessels** to check for stenosis or irregular plaque morphology is essential in all patients (Figure 5-2). Both of these conditions suggest that the carotid artery may be the source of the neurologic event.

Evaluation indicates a complete resolution of the neurologic symptoms and a left carotid bruit. No cardiac murmurs are evident. Duplex examination reveals an 80% stenosis of the left internal carotid artery (Figure 5-3).

▷ *What treatment option would you select?*

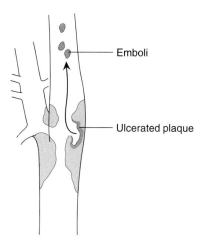

FIGURE 5-1. Emboli formation in the carotid artery.

Emboli

Ulcerated plaque

▶ Two therapeutic choices are available: medical treatment with aspirin or surgical therapy involving carotid endarterectomy. Recently, a comparison of the two treatment methods has been the subject of a large number of randomized trials (Table 5-1). Researchers have demonstrated that for a **stenosis of 70% or more in the internal carotid artery with ipsilateral symptoms** (symptoms that correspond to the carotid distribution), **surgical treatment results in a significant advantage in stroke prevention.** In a 2-year period after joining the study, the risk of major strokes was 9% for surgical patients and 26% for medical

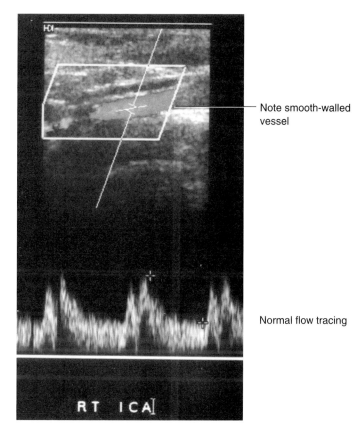

FIGURE 5-2. Duplex study of a normal carotid artery.

Note smooth-walled vessel

Normal flow tracing

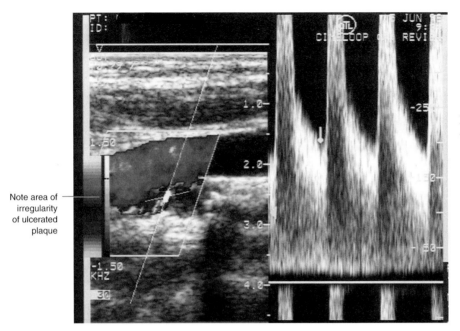

Abnormal, high-velocity flow tracing

Note area of irregularity of ulcerated plaque

FIGURE 5-3. Duplex study of an 80% stenosis of the internal carotid artery.

patients; this represents a 17% decrease in relative stroke rate. Table 5-2 gives the indications for carotid endarterectomy.

> **QUICK CUTS** Carotid endarterectomy is three times more effective than aspirin in preventing major strokes over a 2-year period.

You proceed with carotid endarterectomy.

▶ *What additional preoperative evaluation is necessary?*

▶ The recommendation for endarterectomy is dependent on the general medical condition of the patient. However, in most cases, endarterectomy can be safely performed, even

TABLE 5-1

Risk of Stroke with Medical and Surgical Therapy [from the North American Symptomatic Carotid Endarterectomy Trial (NASCET) on the Risk of Stroke for symptomatic carotid artery stenosis]

Treatment	2-year stroke risk
No treatment (estimated)	~40%
Aspirin	~26%
Carotid endarterectomy	~9%

There was a 65% reduction in relative risk of stroke in the surgical group compared to the aspirin group.

TABLE 5-2

Indications for Carotid Endarterectomy

Ipsilateral hemispheric neurological symptoms (amaurosis fugax, transient ischemic attack (TIA), completed stroke with major neurological recovery) AND >70% internal carotid stenosis
Asymptomatic carotid bruit AND >70% internal carotid stenosis

with local or regional anesthesia. Blood pressure (BP) should be well controlled preoperatively so wide intraoperative swings in BP can be avoided. An appropriate **cardiac evaluation** is necessary before surgery. In certain settings, a carotid artery angiogram is obtained to describe the anatomy of the lesion in more detail, but this procedure is no longer routine. If coronary artery bypass grafting (CABG) is indicated, it may be safely combined with carotid endarterectomy as one combined procedure in many cases.

The patient wants to know the risk of a stroke during surgery.

▶ *What do you tell her?*

▶ The **perioperative risk of a major stroke is 1%–3%** during a carotid endarterectomy performed by most experienced vascular surgeons. The operation is technically safe.

▶ *What other surgery-related complications do you discuss with the patient?*

▶ Injury to the hypoglossal nerve, vagus nerve, and the marginal branch of the facial nerve may occur if they are not identified and protected during surgery (Figure 5-4).

You proceed to the operating room to perform the carotid endarterectomy.

▶ *What are the basic steps in the endarterectomy?*

▶ Patient preparation involves establishment of invasive monitoring with an arterial line to allow careful monitoring of BP during the procedure. Either local, regional, or general anesthesia may be used.
   The endarterectomy involves the following steps (Figure 5-5):

- An incision is made along the sternocleidomastoid muscle, and dissection is performed down to the carotid sheath.
- The sheath is opened, the vagus nerve is protected, and the carotid artery is isolated, avoiding denervation of the carotid body.
- The internal carotid artery is exposed to the level of the hypoglossal nerve, which must not be injured.
- The patient is heparinized, and the vessels are clamped.
- The vessels are opened and the plaque is dissected from the underlying vessel media and adventitia, taking care to obtain a smooth distal transition back to normal artery.
- The vessel is then closed with or without a patch, and the neck is closed.

▶ *What are the important aspects of carotid endarterectomy?*

▶ **Technical perfection** is most important. The artery must be completely cleared of plaque and a smooth flow surface restored. No residual debris should be left in the lumen; it may result in the formation of an embolus to the brain. To confirm the completeness of the pro-

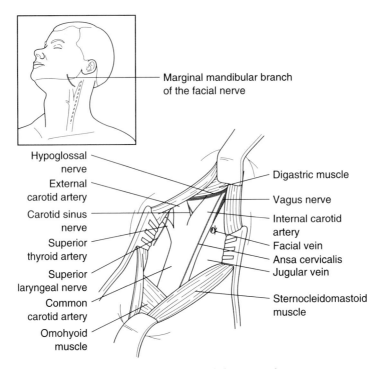

FIGURE 5-4. Nerves potentially injured during endarterectomy.

cedure, many surgeons perform an on-table angiogram or intraoperative duplex ultrasound. The most common cause of neurologic events in the immediate postoperative period is technical. If a neurologic event occurs immediately after surgery, most surgeons return to the operating room promptly and reexamine the repair.

In addition, the **monitoring and maintenance of neurologic function during carotid clamping** is important. In the conscious patient, monitoring may be performed by talking to the patient. In the patient under general anesthesia, monitoring may involve electroencephalography (EEG) or brain response to evoked potential impulses from the leg. If ischemia is evident during clamping, a temporary shunt can be inserted to maintain carotid blood flow while the carotid artery is clamped. Careful control of BP is also important during this part of the procedure.

The patient recovers from the surgery with no neurologic symptoms.

▷ *What follow-up advice would you give to the patient?*

▶ The patient should be advised that TIA or stroke may result from plaque buildup in the opposite carotid artery or may recur as a consequence of plaque recurrence on the treated side. The risk of recurrent carotid narrowing on the side of the endarterectomy is approximately 13% over 5 years. Most physicians recommend taking **aspirin** after routine endarterectomy.

▷ *What condition is most likely to cause this patient's death?*

Because atherosclerosis is a systemic disease, any patient who has had a TIA remains at risk for **myocardial infarction (MI)** in the long term.

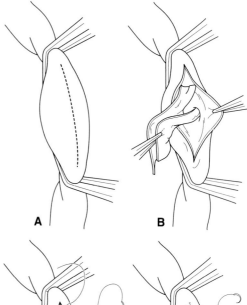

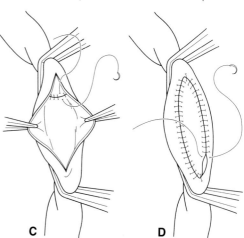

FIGURE 5-5 A,B,C,D. Carotid endarterectomy.

▶ Preventive measures in the form of lifestyle modification, including lipid control, smoking cessation, and exercise, are indicated.

CASE 5.2. ▶ Other Transient Neurologic Events

A 66-year-old woman has had a transient neurologic event. The circumstances are somewhat different from those of the patient in Case 5.1.

▷ *How would you manage the following situations?*

Case Variation 5.2.1. The patient experiences an episode of blindness in the left eye that cleared rapidly, with the occurrence of no other neurologic events.

▶ The ophthalmic artery is the first branch of the internal carotid artery.

Emboli from the carotid artery bifurcation may travel to the retina, resulting in **transient blindness,** or **amaurosis fugax.**

Patients may report either painless episodes of monocular blindness or hazy vision described as "a shade being pulled over the eye." Examination of the fundus during the episode may result in observation of a bright shiny spot in a retinal artery, or a **Hollenhorst plaque,** which is presumably a portion of the embolus. Such an episode usually resolves in 15 minutes to several hours and leaves no residua.

In this instance, the left carotid system is the suspected origin of the embolus. Evaluation and treatment are the same as in the first case—duplex scanning of the carotids and carotid endarterectomy would be appropriate if a lesion is present.

Case Variation 5.2.2. The patient, who is right-handed, relates an episode of aphasia, with the occurrence of no other neurologic events.

▶ In most right-handed patients, the speech center is most commonly in the **left hemisphere.** Therefore, the etiology of an aphasic episode most likely involves the left carotid system. The occurrence of aphasia is a TIA. Evaluation and treatment are the same as in the first case—carotid endarterectomy would be appropriate if a carotid abnormality is present.

Case Variation 5.2.3. The patient experiences marked weakness and numbness in the right arm that is not transient. The condition does not improve in 1 week.

▶ The patient's symptoms do not fit the description of a TIA. Apparently, she has had a fixed neurologic deficit (a stroke). Most physicians would not recommend endarterectomy at this time. A carotid duplex study is appropriate, followed by **observation for improvement.** When the patient has stabilized, she should be reevaluated. If recovery is favorable, and neurologic function is good, endarterectomy may be considered based on the duplex findings to prevent future neurologic events. The surgery may occur as early as 2–4 weeks after the diagnosis of stroke, or when the patient's neurologic status stabilizes.

CASE 5.3. ▶ Asymptomatic Carotid Bruit

A 55-year-old man with a bruit in his right neck is referred to you by his primary physician. You review his history and physical examination, which are both normal except for a right carotid bruit. He has no neurologic signs or symptoms.

▶ *How would you evaluate this patient?*

▶ The asymptomatic bruit may originate in the carotid artery. To determine whether an abnormality exists, a carotid **duplex** study is appropriate.

The duplex examination reveals a 65% internal carotid artery stenosis.

▶ *What is the next appropriate step?*

▶ Many surgeons would recommend a carotid endarterectomy in this patient, although this is controversial in asymptomatic patients.
▶ The most convincing data come from the Asymptomatic Carotid Artery Study (ACAS), in which patients with a 60% or greater stenosis were randomized to medical therapy with aspirin or surgical treatment with endarterectomy.

 QUICK CUTS In a 2-year period, major strokes occurred in 2.5% of individuals in the surgical group and 11% of individuals in the aspirin group, a highly significant difference.

One-half of the major strokes in the surgical group appeared preoperatively during the carotid angiogram, indicating the risk of angiography. As in the symptomatic carotid artery trials, the perioperative major stroke rate was about 1%, indicating the high skill of the surgeons. However, performance of endarterectomy is still controversial (Table 5-3).

TABLE 5-3

Results of Asymptomatic Carotid Artery Stenosis Study (ACAS)

Treatment	Rate of neurological event (%)
Aspirin	10.6
Carotid endarterectomy	4.8

There was a 55% relative reduction of stroke risk in the surgically treated group.

CASE 5.4. ▶ Acute Vascular Event in the Leg

A 65-year-old man is brought to the emergency department with a history of sudden onset of pain in his right leg and difficulty moving the leg. He says that the leg has been perfectly normal up until now. On examining his legs, you note the absence of pulses, including the femoral pulse, in the right leg. Pulses are normal in the left leg. The right leg appears cool and cyanotic, with decreased sensation throughout. All muscle groups are weak.

▷ *What is the most likely diagnosis?*

▶ This patient probably has an acute arterial embolus in his right leg. Absence of a right femoral pulse and presence of a left femoral pulse indicate that the embolus is most likely at the right iliofemoral level, a common site of occlusion due to arterial emboli (Figure 5-6). The common findings in acute arterial occlusion are described by the **"6 Ps"**: Pain, Pulselessness, Paralysis, Pallor, Paresthesias, and Poikilothermia (Table 5-4).

▷ *What is most important in terms of immediate management?*

▶ **Time is of the essence** with an acute arterial embolus, as some studies strongly indicate. The time interval between the ischemic event and clinical presentation are critical to successful limb salvage.

QUICK CUTS   The earlier the revascularization after an arterial embolus, the more complete the recovery.

Revascularization more than 6 hours after ischemia may result in a severely impaired limb or even require amputation (Tables 5-5 and 5-6).

▷ *What treatment is appropriate at this time?*

▶ **Administer heparin immediately,** and **proceed to the operating room** to allow the earliest revascularization. Generally, neither preoperative angiography nor thrombolytic

In this case, the fasciotomy should open all four compartments in the calf (Figure 5-8). Typically, the muscle bulges out at the point of excision, relieving the pressure and improving perfusion. Once the acute episode is resolved, a fasciotomy is typically closed with a split-thickness graft. During recovery, performance of physical therapy is important for maintenance of a full range of leg motion.

The patient recovers from the fasciotomy, receives physical therapy, and retains a functional leg.

▷ *What long-term management plan is appropriate?*

▶ Most surgeons would place this patient on **chronic anticoagulation therapy with warfarin.** Once the patient has recovered, echocardiography and other medical diagnostic techniques such as aortography or computed tomography (CT) of the thoracic and abdominal aorta should be used in a **search for an embolic source.** However, in many cases, no definitive diagnosis is made.

Suppose the presenting physical findings described at the beginning of Case 5.4 occur in an individual who had just undergone a coronary angiogram using the femoral artery approach.

▷ *How would your evaluation and management change?*

▶ Acute arterial ischemia, which is probably caused by a complication of the femoral arterial puncture, is still the diagnosis. **Such punctures can raise intimal flaps, dislodge atherosclerotic plaques, or initiate local thrombotic events.** The patient's condition should be managed in the same way as a spontaneous embolus.

Acute arterial ischemia may also occasionally be seen in aortic dissection. Here the false lumen extends to the femoral artery, where it finally impinges enough on the true lumen to cause inadequate blood flow.

CASE 5.5. ▶ Claudication

A 52-year-old man reports that he develops a cramp in his left calf after walking 100 yards. When he stops walking and sits down, the calf pain slowly resolves in 10 minutes. The man's history is significant for cigarette smoking (2 packs/day for 20 years) and mild hypertension.

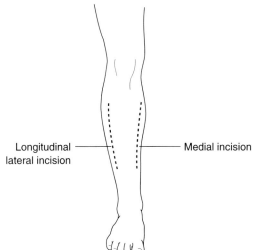

Longitudinal lateral incision — Medial incision

FIGURE 5-8. Fasciotomy of the compartments in the calf will release pressure from edema in the muscles and allow improved perfusion of the muscles. Two compartments are released through each incision.

▷ *What additional history and physical examination findings are important?*

▶ The history findings suggest intermittent claudication, which is exercise-induced ischemic pain of the calf that is relieved by rest.

   Examination of the legs is necessary to assess the peripheral arterial system for the presence of pulses, bruits, or thrills; the skin must be examined for ulcerations, and the nervous system for intact motor and sensory function (Table 5-7). Other signs such as hair loss, dependent rubor, loss of sensation, or thin, shiny skin suggest the chronic nature of the ischemia. Evidence of other cardiovascular disease related to the cardiac, cerebral, and abdominal vascular systems, as well as diabetes mellitus, may also be apparent.

▷ *What arteries in the legs are typically involved in atherosclerotic occlusions?*

▶ With intermittent claudication, popliteal and pedal pulses are often absent, indicating at least an occlusion of the **superficial femoral artery,** typically at the adductor hiatus. This is the most common location for occlusive disease of the lower extremity. If the femoral pulse is absent, significant aortoiliac disease may also be present.

You examine him and note that pulses are absent in the popliteal, dorsalis pedis, and posterior tibial arteries and present in the femoral arteries.

▷ *What examination is now appropriate?*

▶ The patient should undergo a **noninvasive vascular laboratory examination,** which involves the following steps:

   • Calculation of the ankle–brachial index (ABI), which requires measurement of the systolic arterial pressure at the ankle and at the brachial artery with a Doppler device
   • Examination of the Doppler tracing of the arterial waveform at various levels to detect stenotic arterial areas, which localizes the level of the occlusion

▷ *What are the typical Doppler findings in peripheral vascular insufficiency?*

▶ Normally, the ABI is greater than 1.0.

 QUICK CUTS In **mild claudication,** the **ABI is typically about 0.6–0.8.** Other pressure readings correlate with the severity of ischemia (Table 5-8).

TABLE 5-7

Signs of peripheral vascular insufficiency

1. Claudication: **reproducible** muscle pain cramping or weakness, typically of the **calf** muscles. It occurs during exercise and is relieved by rest.
2. Rest pain: constant, severe, burning, **forefoot** pain
3. Ischemic ulceration: painful, nonhealing ulceration, typically on the **malleoni and toes** and foot at areas of trauma
4. Gangrene: cyanotic, insensate tissue (pregangrene) progressing to black tissue (dry gangrene) or wet gangrene if infection is present

TABLE 5-8

Typical ankle/brachial systolic arterial pressures (ABI) correlate with severity of ischemia:

Normal	ABI = 1.1–0.9
Mild claudication (single lesion peripheral)	ABI = 0.8–0.6
Severe claudication (multilevel occlusive disease)	ABI <0.5
Rest pain or tissue loss	ABI <0.3

Note that in diabetics, BP measurements may be incorrect. Typically, diabetics may have calcified vessels, preventing arterial occlusion with a BP cuff. As a result, measured BP is often as high as the cuff is inflated (Table 5-9).

Normally, the Doppler waveform is triphasic, with a phase of rapid systolic flow, a brief phase of reverse flow secondary to elastic recoil of the vessel followed by a prolonged phase of diastolic outflow. **As a vessel becomes less compliant due to atherosclerosis,** the Doppler signal changes, and the reverse flow component may be lost. In severe disease, the waveform may be monophasic (Figure 5-9).

Performance of a Doppler study demonstrates that the ABI = 0.7, and clinical evidence of occlusion of the superficial femoral artery (e.g., absent popliteal and pedal pulses) is present. On the basis of these findings, you decide that the patient has peripheral vascular disease with claudication of the calf.

▶ *Would you recommend vascular reconstruction?*

▶ In this case, the principal management decision concerns **the degree to which claudication interferes with the patient's lifestyle.**

 The management for **most patients** with claudication alone is to **not perform surgery.**

TABLE 5-9

Five-Year History of Claudication:

Extremity outcome

Requires subsequent amputation	10%–15% (1%/yr) of patients
Symptoms remain stable or improve	~70% of patients
Symptoms progress, requiring revascularization	~20% of patients

Survival outcome: correlates with initial presentation and ABI, reflecting associated cardiovascular disease:

Mild claudication	97% survival
Claudication, operative	80% survival
Critical limb-threatening ischemia	48% survival

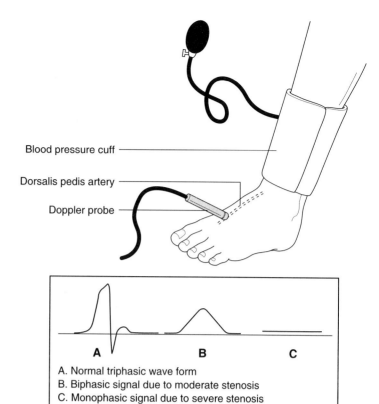

FIGURE 5-9. A. Doppler blood pressure and ankle–brachial indices, and Doppler arterial waveform.

The decision regarding surgery is based on a risk–benefit analysis, which compares the risk of an arteriogram and actual operation, including the possibility of thrombosis, infection, and amputation in the poor outcome scenario, with the benefits of increased exercise tolerance in a revascularized limb. A patient and surgeon might consider surgery if the patient's livelihood depends on a higher level of activity than currently tolerated and the patient has an otherwise good medical condition. Even so, there are good nonoperative alternatives, and most patients do not undergo surgery. The presence of an unfavorable medical condition (e.g., concomitant moderate coronary artery disease) or a multivessel disease such as that found in diabetes may detract from surgery. In this particular case, the patient is at no risk for limb loss with this level of perfusion, although the pain is bothersome.

What nonoperative therapy do you recommend?

 QUICK CUTS **Nonoperative exercise management** may prove very successful for these patients with claudication.

▶ Exercise is the plan of choice for most patients. With a carefully managed program, **the symptoms of approximately one-third of patients will improve, one-third will stabilize,** and **one-third will worsen (Figure 5-10).** Most importantly, this plan does not include an arteriogram "just to see how the vessels look" or to confirm arterial occlusions. An arteriogram has inherent risk and no benefit unless surgery is planned; it is a preoperative test.

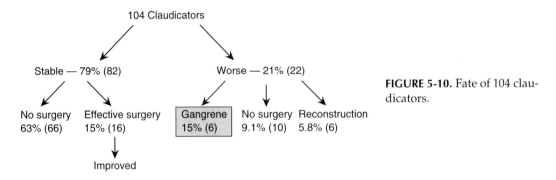

FIGURE 5-10. Fate of 104 claudicators.

Whenever possible, patients should also **modify their lifestyles.** Smoking cessation, use of lipid-lowering agents, dietary restriction of fat intake, and loss of excess weight are important. In addition, co-existing medical disorders, including hypertension, should be managed. Education about foot and skin care, as well as symptoms of worsening ischemia, should occur. Careful control of blood glucose in diabetic patients is essential. Finally, **physician monitoring of patient progress** is necessary to ensure that the long-term management continues.

CASE 5.6. ▶ Claudication and Absence of a Femoral Pulse

A 60-year-old woman has symptoms of claudication that are similar to those of the patient in Case 5.5. However, she has an absent femoral pulse on the left side.

▶ *How would your management change?*

▶ A weak or absent femoral pulse suggests poor blood flow into the leg, which is strong evidence for **aortoiliac occlusive disease.** This occlusion could be the single cause of the patient's symptoms or one of several occlusions contributing to the symptoms.

Aortoiliac occlusive disease is generally more progressive than more peripheral occlusive disease. Surgery is therefore often considered, and treatment is frequently more aggressive. Important issues are the status of the femoral pulse on the opposite side, evidence of small distal emboli, impotence in males, and claudication in other locations such as the thigh or buttock. **If this patient's disease and symptoms progress, aortoiliac reconstruction with either a balloon dilatation and/or stent placement or surgical revascularization will be necessary** (Figure 5-11).

CASE 5.7. ▶ Toe Ulceration in Peripheral Vascular Disease

You once recommended an exercise program to a 62-year-old man with claudication, who agreed to modify his lifestyle. He is apparently "lost to follow-up" but returns 1 year later, complaining of an ulcer on his big toe.

▶ *How would you evaluate this patient?*

▶ An ulceration on the big toe suggests that the **ischemia has worsened.** A vascular laboratory evaluation is appropriate.

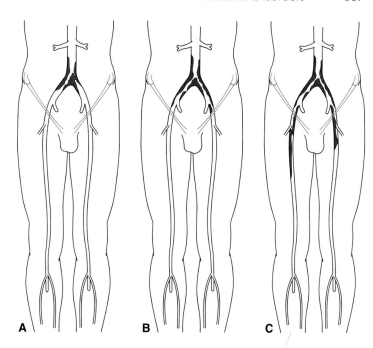

FIGURE 5-11. Patterns of arterial occlusive disease supplying the lower extremities. **A.** Limited to distal aorta and iliac arteries. **B.** Distal aortoiliac disease combined with proximal extremity disease. **C.** Lower extremity arterial disease combined with disease of the more proximal great vessels.

 ABI in a patient with rest pain (constant pain across the forefoot unrelated to exercise) is typically **0.3–0.5.**

In addition, the Doppler waveform may show further progression to a monophasic signal. Tissue loss or ulceration may be associated with even lower ABI measurements. Some patients, **especially diabetics,** have predominantly **small vessel disease,** and measuring the BP at the toe level (i.e., a toe BP) may document this condition.

The patient's ABI is 0.3.

▷ *What is the next appropriate step?*

▶ The major issue is **whether the blood supply is sufficient to allow the ulcer to heal.** In most cases it is not sufficient, and some form of **revascularization is necessary** to increase distal perfusion. This may allow healing and prevent gangrene, amputation, and generalized sepsis (Table 5-10). However, patients with limited mobility, a severely limiting

TABLE 5-10

Ankle Systolic Blood Pressure (torr) Criteria for Predicting Healing of Ischemic Foot Lesions

	Likely	Probable	Unlikely
Nondiabetics	>65	55–65	<55
Diabetics	>90	80–90	<80

cardiovascular condition, or a short life span may be best served by primary amputation. If revascularization is anticipated, assessment of the patient's **general medical status** is necessary.

Evaluation indicates that the patient's general medical condition is good, and his cardiac risk is low.

▶ *Now what is the next step?*

▶ Assessment of the patient's **vascular anatomy** is necessary to determine whether a vascular reconstruction is likely to be successful. At this point, most surgeons would perform an **arteriogram** to assess the different levels of arterial occlusion to develop a revascularization plan. Generally, results assume two patterns:

1. **Inflow disease,** or inadequate blood flow into the femoral artery, as in iliac artery occlusive disease
2. **Outflow disease,** or single or multiple occlusions of the leg arteries, especially the superficial femoral artery, the popliteal artery or the distal branches

The surgeon must decide if the occlusion(s) can be bypassed successfully to improve the blood supply to the level of the ulcer. In many cases, **the ulcer will heal with adequate debridement and wound care after revascularization.**

▶ *How would you manage the following findings seen on arteriography?*

Case Variation 5.7.1. The arteriogram shows occlusion of the superficial femoral artery with distal reconstitution.

▶ A **reversed or in situ saphenous vein** graft from the common femoral artery to the popliteal artery is typically used to bypass the obstructions (Figure 5-14).

Case Variation 5.7.2. The arteriogram shows high grade stenosis of the iliac artery but patency of the lower extremity vessels (Figure 5-13).

▶ A **surgical revascularization** using a large-diameter graft from the aorta to the femoral artery or by **balloon dilatation** and/or arterial stent placement is appropriate.

Case Variation 5.7.3. The arteriogram shows high-grade stenosis of the iliac artery and occlusion of the superficial femoral artery.

▶ This case is similar to that in Case Variation 5.7.2, but a **lower extremity revascularization in addition to the aortoiliac reconstruction** may be necessary. The patient has multilevel disease. The two procedures may be performed at the same time or sequentially; the inflow (aortoiliac occlusions) can be treated first, and this revascularization may be sufficient to relieve the symptoms. (Fig 5-12)

Case Variation 5.7.4. The arteriogram shows occlusion of the superficial femoral and popliteal arteries with distal reconstitution.

▶ **Femoropopliteal bypass** is indicated for this patient. The best artery continuous with the foot is selected as the outflow tract, with preference given to the popliteal, anterior, and posterior tibial arteries (Figure 5-15). If the tibial arteries are occluded, the peroneal artery can be chosen for bypass. It is best if it is continuous with one or two of its terminal

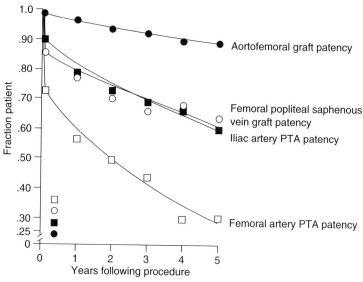

FIGURE 5-12. Five-year patency of four vascular reconstructions. Aortofemoral reconstruction is a highly successful procedure, whereas percutaneous transluminal angioplasty (PTA) of the femoral artery has poor long-term results. Iliac artery PTA in isolated iliac artery stenosis has a very acceptable long-term result.

branches; however, absence of a plantar arch and vascular calcification is not a contraindication to reconstruction, although it worsens the prognosis. When the length of the vein conduit is limited, a short bypass originating at the popliteal or even tibial artery is useful.

For more distal disease, bypass to the dorsalis pedis, plantar, or tarsal arteries is useful. Typically, diabetics predominantly have tibial disease. The more distal and more diseased the vessels, the more likely the graft is to fail and the patient is to lose his leg (Table 5-11).

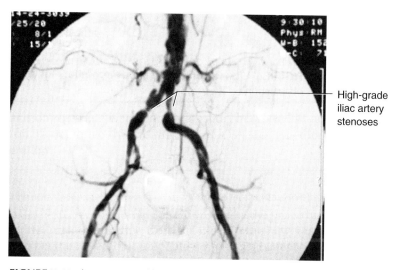

FIGURE 5-13. Aortogram of high-grade iliac artery stenosis.

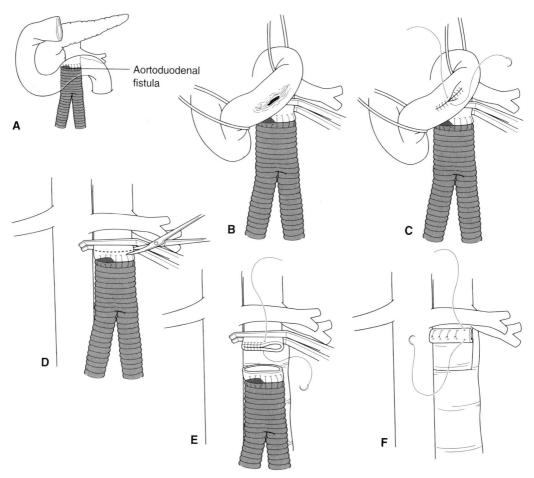

FIGURE 5-21. Anatomy and repair of aortoenteric fistula. If the aorta is grossly infected, it may require excision, closure of the proximal stump, and creation of an extra-anatomical bypass to perfuse the lower extremities. (*A*) Anatomy. (*B*) Separation of the duodenum from the aorta. (*C*) Closure of the duodenum. (*D*) Removal of the vascular graft. (*E*) Closure of the proximal aortic stump. (*F*) Reinforcement of the closure.

▶ *What is the suspected diagnosis?*

▶ The history and physical examination are typical of **chronic mesenteric ischemia,** which is usually secondary to atherosclerotic occlusion of the celiac and superior mesenteric arteries. Postprandial pain due to ischemia of the intestines causes fear of food, leading to weight loss. Heme-positive stools are usually not present. Signs and symptoms of atherosclerosis elsewhere in the body are also not unusual.

▶ *How would you evaluate and manage this patient?*

▶ If ischemia is suspected, the patient should first undergo a **mesenteric arteriogram** to establish a diagnosis and then planned revascularization, if appropriate. **Revascularization** is performed using a bypass graft from the aorta, which is reconnected to the superior mesenteric artery and celiac axis distal to the obstructions. Both prosthetic and saphenous vein grafts are used for this procedure (Figure 5-23).

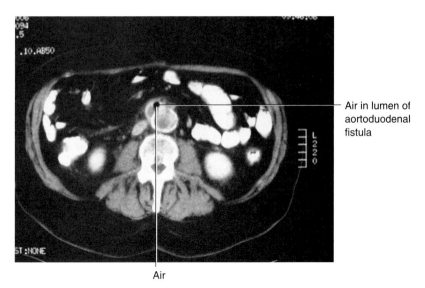

FIGURE 5-22. CT scan showing aorta at area of aortoduodenal fistula. Dye can be seen extravasating into the duodenum, which has a small bubble of air within its lumen.

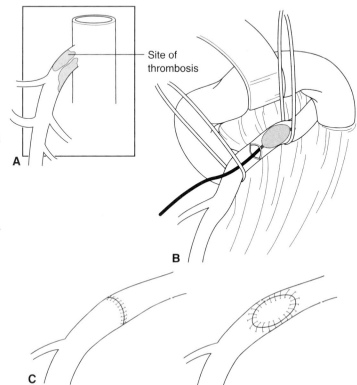

FIGURE 5-23. Revascularization of stenosis (*A*) or embolus (*B*) of the superior mesenteric artery. (*C*)The arteriotomy can be repaired by end-to-end anastomosis with or without prosthetic graft or with a patch.

CASE 5.14. ▶ Tearing Chest and Back Pain

A 58-year-old man is brought to the emergency department with diaphoresis and sudden severe chest and back pain that is tearing in nature. On physical examination, he appears pale and in acute distress, with a BP of 200/140 mm Hg and a pulse of 100 beats/min.

 What is the suspected diagnosis?

▶ The tearing chest or back pain should make you quite suspicious of **aortic dissection** as a possible diagnosis. Affected patients appear acutely ill and diaphoretic, just as in acute MI. Severe hypertension is characteristic. The pain may migrate to other areas as the dissection proceeds distally. Stroke, paraplegia, mesenteric ischemia, renal ischemia, and peripheral vascular ischemia may also occur.

▶ *How might you evaluate this patient?*

▶ **Transesophageal echocardiography, magnetic resonance imaging (MRI), spiral CT of the chest, or arteriography** will each establish the diagnosis with reliability. Most surgeons would make management decisions based upon the first test that demonstrates dissection.

You establish that the patient has a type III aortic dissection (Figure 5-24).

▶ *How would you manage this condition?*

QUICK CUTS	Standard therapy for aortic dissection is **control of the hypertension.**

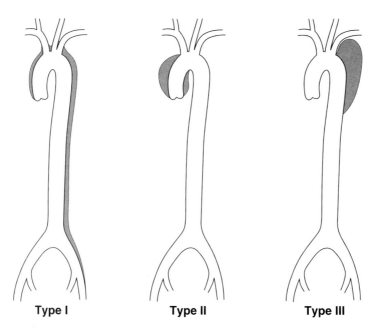

FIGURE 5-24. Diagram of types I, II, and III thoracic aortic dissections.

► Beta-blockers and other potent antihypertensive agents are effective. Conditions such as dissection of the ascending aorta, which are usually surgically repaired, are exceptions to medical management.

VENOUS DISEASE

CASE 5.15. ► Postoperative Leg Swelling

A 67-year-old woman undergoes a colectomy for a colon polyp that cannot be removed by colonoscopy. She develops some mild swelling in the left leg postoperatively, and you become concerned that this might represent deep venous thrombosis (DVT).

► *How reliable is physical examination for diagnosing DVT?*

► Findings from history and physical examination are accurate only 50% of the time as diagnostic signs of DVT. Up to 50% of patients have occult DVT (i.e., with no signs or symptoms). The most common symptom is unilateral, dull leg pain that increases with movement. The **most reliable clinical sign of DVT is new-onset, unilateral leg swelling,** which is evaluated by comparing the circumference of the calf and thigh of the affected leg with that in the contralateral limb. Calf pain on dorsiflexion of the ankle (Homans' sign), a palpable cord (often indicative of a thrombosed superficial vein), and thigh and/or calf tenderness are nonspecific (Figure 5-25).

► *How would you verify the diagnosis?*

QUICK CUTS | **Duplex ultrasound is used to confirm the diagnosis of DVT.**

► Duplex ultrasound combines B-mode ultrasound, which can visualize tissue structures, with Doppler ultrasound, which can detect flow in vessels. The sensitivity and specificity of this technique is more than 90% for the diagnosis of thrombi between the iliac vein and the knee (Figure 5-26). Venous duplex ultrasound is considered the test of choice for the detection of DVT. Contrast venography, formerly the gold standard for the diagnosis of DVT, is now used only rarely.

Duplex examination of the common femoral vein reveals that it contains a thrombus, confirming the diagnosis of DVT. There is extension into the proximal thigh but no other abnormalities.

► *How would you treat the patient?*

► **Systemic anticoagulation is achieved with IV heparin.** A 70–100 U/kg bolus is given initially, followed by a maintenance infusion of 15–25 U/kg/hr administered for 4–6 days. It should be noted that heparin has an anti-inflammatory component that dramatically reduces the discomfort associated with DVT. Bed rest (with a bedside commode) is typically recommended for the first 24–48 hours of anticoagulation therapy—until the acute thrombus becomes adherent to the vein wall.

Both **standard heparin and low-molecular-weight heparin** (LMWH) are effective in anticoagulation. LMWH, which is produced by the fractionation of heparin and possesses significant antifactor-Xa activity, does not anticoagulate to the same extent as unfraction-

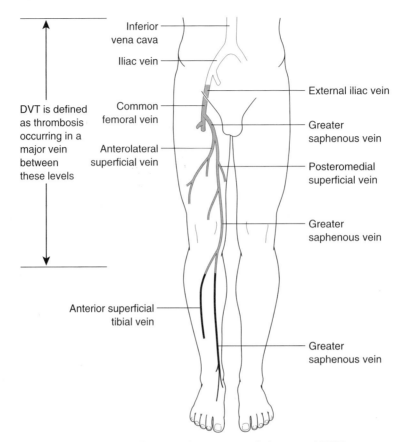

Inferior
vena cava

Iliac vein

External iliac vein

DVT is defined
as thrombosis
occurring in a
major vein
between
these levels

Common
femoral vein

Greater
saphenous vein

Anterolateral
superficial vein

Posteromedial
superficial vein

Greater
saphenous vein

Anterior superficial
tibial vein

Greater
saphenous vein

FIGURE 5-25. Drawing showing the anatomic definition of DVT.

ated heparin as measured by the partial thromboplastin time (PTT), but it has a strong therapeutic effect. LMWH may have a lower incidence of hemorrhagic side effects than unfractionated heparin.

▶ *How would you monitor the patient's treatment?*

▶ The patient's **PTT should be followed and maintained 1.5–2 times the normal value** if the heparin administration is to remain therapeutic. The half-life of heparin is approximately 90 minutes, so the PTT should be evaluated 6 hours after the initial dose, every 8 hours for the next 24 hours, and once a day thereafter. Because approximately 5% of patients taking heparin develop **thrombocytopenia,** the patient's platelet counts must be followed. Paradoxic arterial thrombosis associated with heparin-induced thrombocytopenia may also develop. If this condition develops, the heparin should be discontinued. Newer methods using LMWH in home settings to treat DVT are under study; these approaches may be as effective as inpatient treatment and reduce costs dramatically.

▶ *What long-term treatment plan is appropriate?*

▶ **After the diagnosis of DVT is made, anticoagulation therapy must be continued for 3–6 months.** Warfarin (Coumadin) may be started within the first few days of heparin administration, although the patient should receive 5–7 days of heparin therapy. Warfarin is an anticoagulant that inhibits hepatic synthesis of vitamin K–dependent clotting factors II, VII, IX, and X; it also decreases production of protein C and S. The inhibitory effect lasts

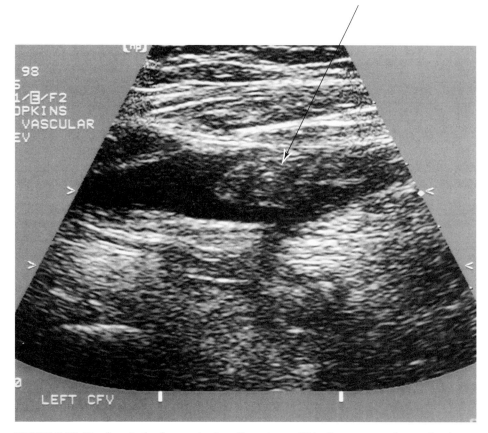

FIGURE 5-26. Duplex study demonstrating thrombus within the common femoral vein.

1–10 days, depending on coagulation factor. Goals of therapy are to achieve and maintain an international normalized ratio (INR) of 2.0–3.0 (1.3–1.5 times control prothrombin time) for 3–6 months. Warfarin can induce a protein C deficiency (a relative hypercoagulable state) early after treatment is begun, so patients must remain on heparin for several days after warfarin is started.

▷ *What do you tell the patient about the long-term morbidity of DVT?*

▶ **Recurrence** and **postthrombotic syndrome** are the two principal complications of DVT that are likely to develop. Recurrence is most common in the first several months following the initial episode (Figure 5-27). Therapy involves admission and IV heparin. Long-term treatment with warfarin should also be considered following discharge. At all future admissions, patients with a history of DVT should be considered at high risk for the development of DVT and should receive DVT prophylaxis All patients who have DVT are likely to demonstrate venous valvular insufficiency and a tendency to develop edema in the involved extremity. Chronic use of support hose will lessen the edema and easy fatigability in the leg.

Approximately 10% of DVT patients develop postthrombotic syndrome, which is characterized by chronic, marked edema; skin ulceration around the ankle areas; and occasionally venous claudication. This syndrome at least in part results from chronic venous hypertension in the lower leg, and the best treatment is prevention with chronic use of support hose. Once the syndrome has developed, therapy is aimed at healing the ulcera-

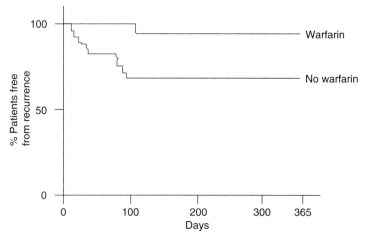

FIGURE 5-27. Graph of the incidence of recurrent DVT versus time after DVT.

tions followed by the use of fitted support hose. The physician must be cautious when using pressure-gradient support hose in DVT, because arterial insufficiency unrelated to the venous problems may also be present. Support hose could contribute to ischemic injury to the leg, which would be counterproductive.

CASE 5.16. ▶ Prevention of Deep Venous Thrombosis

A 55-year-old man has a substantial hernia, which is occasionally painful and has been enlarging. His past history is significant for a right colectomy 4 years ago for carcinoma of the colon. Physical examination reveals a moderately obese patient with a large, easily reducible, ventral hernia. No other significant physical findings are present. Your attending physician asks:

▶ *Does the patient have any risk factors for DVT or pulmonary embolism (PE)?*

▶ DVT is defined as thrombosis of the larger veins that may affect either an upper or lower extremity. **In the leg, DVT may involve thrombosis of the popliteal vein, femoral venous system, iliac veins, or the inferior vena cava.** In the arm, DVT may involve thrombosis of the axillary, subclavian, innominate, or internal jugular veins. DVT develops following 20% of general surgical procedures and in as many as 70% of major orthopedic procedures that involve the leg (Figure 5-28).

Risk factors for DVT and PE are the same: static blood flow, hypercoagulable states, and endothelial or intimal injury, which are generally known as the Virchow triad. Many conditions may lead to DVT (**Table 5-15**). In this patient, obesity, increased age, and a history of carcinoma each may contribute to an increased risk. Of these conditions, certain ones have lower or higher risks for DVT and PE (Table 5-16).

Because the patient is at increased risk for DVT, you would like to use **DVT prophylactic therapy.**

▶ *There are several options for prophylactic therapy. Which treatment would you institute?*

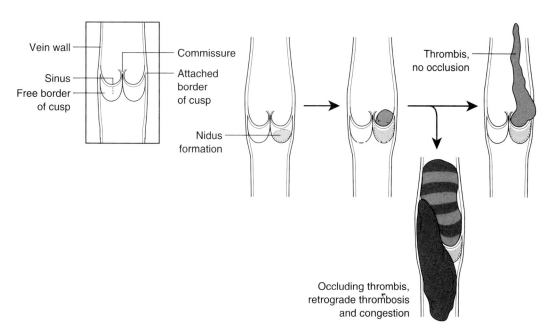

FIGURE 5-28. Drawing of the relationship between DVT and venous incompetence.

▶ Several precautions can be taken in higher-risk patients. The most commonly performed passive measures include patient positioning (knees higher than right atrium and feet higher than knees), early postoperative mobilization, and graded compression stockings.

TABLE 5-15

Risk factors for DVT

Low risk
    Healthy patient under age 40
    Short-duration surgery
    Bleeding disorders, such as chronic renal or hepatic failure
Moderate risk
    Patients over age 40
    Moderate-length procedure (2–3 hours)
    Upper abdominal and chest surgery
    Minor risk factors such as obesity, smoking
High risk
    Older patients
    Previous DVT or PE
    Long-duration surgery
    Pelvic or orthopedic surgery
    Major surgery for cancer
    Procoagulant states, such as polycythemia vera
    Hyperviscosity syndromes, such as multiple myeloma
    History of MI, congestive heart failure or COPD

TABLE 5-16

Conditions That May Lead to Deep Venous Thrombosis

Note: The terms in boldface type are often referred to as Virchow triad.
Stasis of Blood Flow
Obesity
Surgery
Trauma
Lower extremity paralysis
Cerebrovascular accident
General or spinal anesthesia
Long bone fractures
MI with congestive heart failure
Prolonged bed rest

Hypercoagulable States
Malignancy
Pregnancy
Puerperium (first 42 days postpartum)
Oral contraceptive use
Polycythemia vera
Connective tissue disease
Antithrombin III deficiency
Protein C or S deficiency
Disseminated intravascular coagulation
Heparin-associated thrombocytopenia
Thrombosis
Inflammatory bowel disease
Nephrotic syndrome
Myeloproliferative disorders
Homocystinemia
Lupus with anticardiolipin antibodies
Paroxysmal nocturnal hemoglobinuria

Intimal Injury
Surgical injury
Trauma
Indwelling catheters
Varicose veins
Advanced age
Pacemaker wires
History of DVT
Operative manipulation

QUICK CUTS Two preventive measures whose effectiveness has been clearly demonstrated are **intermittent pneumatic compression devices and low-dose or prophylactic heparin.**

Intermittent pneumatic compression devices are thought to increase venous velocity as well as increase blood fibrinolytic activity. **Prophylactic or low-dose heparin** (LDH) up-regulates antithrombin III activity, thereby increasing the natural fibrinolytic system. Intermittent compression and LDH have comparable prevention efficacy and may enhance prophylaxis even further when used concurrently.

You decide to use prophylactic LDH.

▶ *How would you administer the heparin?*

▶ Standard LDH therapy involves administration of **5,000 U subcutaneous heparin preoperatively and every 8–12 hours postoperatively** until the patient is ambulatory. LDH may not be as effective in patients with excessive activation of the coagulation system (e.g., in malignancy, with orthopedic surgery). **No blood coagulation studies are necessary for therapeutic monitoring.** When the patient is ambulatory and ready for discharge, the LDH can be discontinued.

CASE 5.17. ▶ Postoperative Shortness of Breath

A 50-year-old man, who is otherwise healthy, undergoes a laparotomy for small bowel obstruction due to adhesions. He has been doing well postoperatively. On the morning of the fourth postoperative day, he relates a brief episode of shortness of breath that occurred the previous night. No new findings are apparent on examination. The man's vital signs are all within normal limits, his lungs are clear and heart sounds are normal, his wound looks fine, and his abdomen is flat and not distended.

▶ *What potential problems could explain this episode?*

▶ The long list of potential causes includes asthma, bronchospasm, aspiration, chronic obstructive pulmonary disease (COPD), paroxysmal nocturnal dyspnea, anxiety, PE, MI, pneumothorax, and infection. The etiology of the episode is more likely to be acute, because there is no history of chronic pulmonary or cardiac problems. Because of the brief episodic nature of the incident and the absence of physical findings, **PE is suspected** and an effort should be made to rule it out.

▶ *What would be your initial steps to establish a diagnosis?*

▶ An appropriate history and physical examination should be performed. Common practice involves obtaining an ECG to investigate for MI, as well as an arterial blood gas (ABG) measurement and pulse oximetry. The most common ABG abnormality is a **decreased P_{CO_2} due to hyperventilation;** a decreased P_{O_2} is less likely. A chest x-ray (CXR) should be performed to examine for pneumonia, atelectasis, and pneumothorax. If no diagnosis is evident at this time, a perfusion lung scan should be performed.

The patient has minimal atelectasis on CXR, a normal ECG, and a wedge-shaped segmental defect on perfusion lung scan (Figure 5-29).

▶ *What would be your next step?*

▶ Confirmation of the diagnosis of PE is necessary, although some clinicians might treat the patient for PE at this point. This most commonly involves the performance of a ventilation scan. Radioactive xenon gas is inhaled, and serial scans are obtained to detect areas

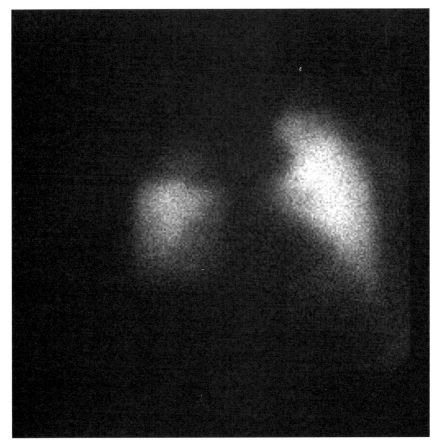

FIGURE 5-29. Segmental perfusion defect in right upper lung on lung scan.

of impaired ventilation that reflect atelectasis, pneumonia, or microatelectasis. It is well known that impaired regional alveolar ventilation results in regional pulmonary arterial vasoconstriction, which can appear as a perfusion defect on perfusion scan. Therefore, if the ventilation scan is normal in an area of segmental perfusion scan defect, the defect is highly likely to be secondary to a mechanical obstruction (i.e., PE) rather than a physiologic obstruction (i.e., vasoconstriction).

 QUICK CUTS | The combination of ventilation and perfusion scans is known as a V/Q scan.

Ventilation–perfusion mismatch occurs when perfusion is absent but ventilation is present. A mismatched segmental defect on a V/Q scan is highly likely (~ 90%) to be associated with PE (Figures 5-30 and 5-31).

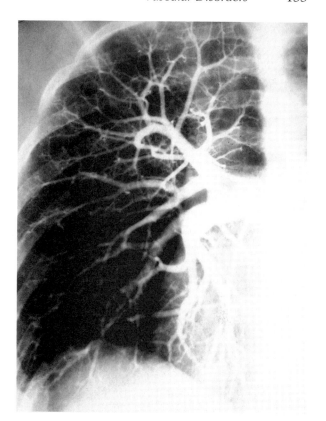

FIGURE 5-30. Normal pulmonary arteriogram.

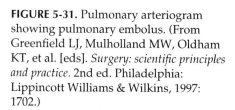

FIGURE 5-31. Pulmonary arteriogram showing pulmonary embolus. (From Greenfield LJ, Mulholland MW, Oldham KT, et al. [eds]. *Surgery: scientific principles and practice.* 2nd ed. Philadelphia: Lippincott Williams & Wilkins, 1997: 1702.)

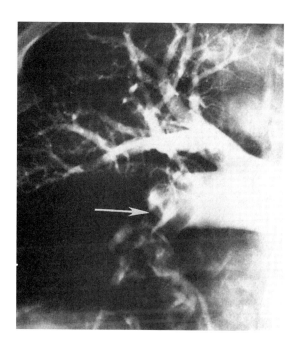

▶ *Can any other diagnostic technique be used to support the diagnosis of PE?*

▶ Further confirmation of PE may be obtained by the finding of DVT on **duplex examination of the venous system.** The combination of a mismatched segmental V/Q scan and DVT on duplex ultrasound makes the diagnosis 95% likely. If any doubt remains concerning the diagnosis of PE, or if the patient is at very high risk for a heparin complication, a **pulmonary angiogram** should be performed. It is the most accurate test to detect pulmonary embolus. This study has a higher morbidity and mortality than the duplex study or V̇/Q scan, and it is currently reserved for special instances.

A diagnosis of PE has been established.

▶ *How would you treat the patient?*

▶ **Treatment of PE, which is identical to treatment of DVT** (see Case 5.16), involves IV heparin. An initial bolus of 5,000–10,000 U of heparin IV followed by an IV heparin drip of 1,000 U/hr is appropriate. This dose would be adjusted to maintain PTT ~ 2 times the control. The patient would then be started on warfarin (Coumadin) and treated similarly to a patient with DVT.

▶ *What are the long-term complications of PE?*

▶ Most patients recover fully after anticoagulation therapy and demonstrate no evidence of pulmonary insufficiency, pulmonary hypertension, or recurrent embolism. Perfusion scans performed 1 month later have usually returned to baseline. Elderly individuals and patients with preexisting cardiopulmonary disease are exceptions.

CASE 5.18. ▶ Other Findings in Pulmonary Embolism

A 48-year-old man recently underwent a colectomy. On the third postoperative day, he develops acute shortness of breath. After examination, you suspect PE, and you initiate an evaluation.

▶ *How would you manage the patient with these findings?*

Case Variation 5.18.1. Normal ECG

▶ A normal ECG does not rule out either MI or PE, although MI is unlikely. Evaluation should continue.

Case Variation 5.18.2. Normal CXR

▶ A normal CXR rules out pathologic processes such as pneumothorax, pneumonia, and larger areas of atelectasis, but not PE or areas of microatelectasis. A normal CXR also makes a perfusion scan much more useful diagnostically. Preexisting pulmonary disease such as COPD, bronchitis, and restrictive disease can complicate interpretation of the CXR, particularly if a preexisting CXR is not available for comparison to separate old disease from new-onset disease. Evaluation should continue.

Case Variation 5.18.3. Small right pneumothorax on CXR

▶ The pneumothorax is the likely cause of the shortness of breath. This patient is symptomatic with shortness of breath and should have a tube thoracostomy chest tube inserted.

Case Variation 5.18.4. Right basilar atelectasis on CXR

▶ If this is a new finding, it may explain the patient's symptoms. If not, a lung scan is the next step; however, interpretation of the scan in the area of the atelectasis will be impossible. A pulmonary angiogram may be necessary.

Case Variation 5.18.5. Normal perfusion scan (Figure 5-32)

▶ This result virtually eliminates the possibility of PE. Several longitudinal studies have documented this finding. A rare exception is a saddle embolus, which is a large PE that has lodged at the bifurcation of the right and left pulmonary arteries and has not yet affected the smaller arteries. These are very difficult to diagnose, and pulmonary angiography is the only useful technique.

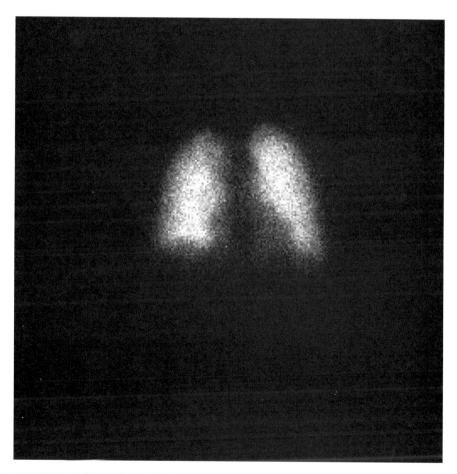

FIGURE 5-32. Normal ventilation scan. Contrast this with Figure 50–29, which shows a mismatched V/Q scan.

Case Variation 5.18.6. Multiple subsegmental defects on perfusion scan (Figure 5-33)

▶ This result is abnormal, but this scan is not diagnostic of PE. Evaluation should continue.

Case Variation 5.18.7. Wedge-shaped segmental defect on perfusion scan

▶ Assuming that this defect appears in an area of normal CXR, this is moderately suspicious for PE. The probability that this is PE is still less than 75%, and this is not reliable enough for most clinicians to proceed with treatment. Thus, the diagnosis has still not been made.

CASE 5.19. ▶ Recurrent Pulmonary Embolism on Anticoagulation Therapy

A 24-year-old man who was in an automobile crash and required a chest tube for a pneumothorax has developed shortness of breath. After an evaluation, you diagnosed a PE and began standard therapy with IV heparin. The patient has been fully heparinized for 3 days and

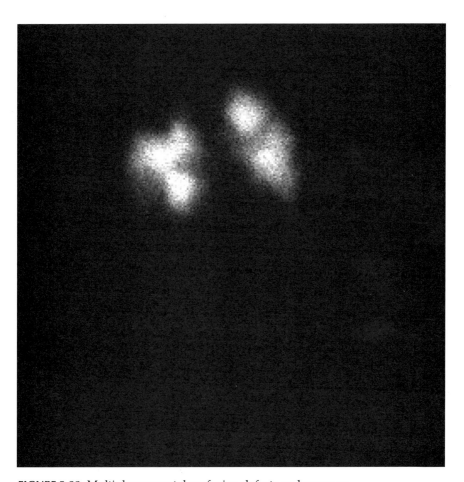

FIGURE 5-33. Multiple segmental perfusion defects on lung scan.

doing well, with a PTT consistently maintained at twice control level. Bowel function has returned to normal, and he has had no recurrent episodes of dyspnea, chest pain, or complications from the heparin treatment.

A nurse reports an acute episode in which the patient was extremely short of breath. His BP was 90/60 mm Hg for several minutes, and he appeared ashen and cyanotic. The nurse administered nasal oxygen, "turned up" his IV fluids, and is now calling you. The patient's vital signs have returned to normal, and he is feeling better. On examination, you note a heart rate of 120 beats/min, a respiratory rate of 28 breaths/min, and a normal blood pressure. The lungs are clear and heart sounds are normal. The abdomen is flat with no pain or tenderness, and the wound is healing normally.

▷ *How would you establish the correct diagnosis?*

▶ The patient, who most likely has either a recurrent PE or an acute MI, should be transferred to the intensive care unit. A rapid evaluation, including a brief history and physical examination, pulse oximetry, ECG, ABG, and CXR, is necessary. He should undergo a repeat lung perfusion scan and have a workup for MI, including evaluation of cardiac isoenzymes, serial ECGs, and cardiology consultation. In addition, his PTT should be checked again to determine the degree to which he is anticoagulated.

The lung perfusion scan reveals a new segmental perfusion defect in the lung opposite to the side of the first PE. There is no evidence of an acute MI. The patient continues to be fully anticoagulated.

▷ *How would you manage this patient?*

▶ He most likely has a **recurrent PE.** Let us assume that he has remained therapeutically anticoagulated with no lapses in treatment.

 QUICK CUTS   A PE on heparin therapy represents a **failure of anticoagulant therapy.**

Because this lung scan confirms the diagnosis of recurrent PE with reasonable certainty, a second-line method of PE prevention is necessary. The most acceptable form of additional protection is **inferior vena cava interruption** using a Greenfield filter, a metal device placed in the infrarenal inferior vena cava using a percutaneous technique (Figure 5-34). The device is safe and prevents recurrent PE in more than 95% of patients. The knowledge that more than 90% of pulmonary emboli originate from the lower extremities is the basis of the intrarenal location. The most common indications for the Greenfield filter are heparin failure to prevent PE and heparin complications such as bleeding. If no anticoagulation contraindication exists, most surgeons would maintain therapeutic anticoagulation for 3–6 months.

CASE 5.20. ▶ GI Bleeding as a Complication of Anticoagulation Therapy

A 60-year-old woman with chronic rheumatoid arthritis that has been treated with nonsteroidal anti-inflammatory drugs (NSAIDs) undergoes an elective left knee joint replacement. She develops evidence of DVT postoperatively, and duplex examination confirms the diagnosis of DVT of the left femoral vein. Accordingly, she receives an IV heparin bolus of 5000 U followed by a heparin drip infusion of 1000 U/hr, which maintains her PTT at 2 times control. On the

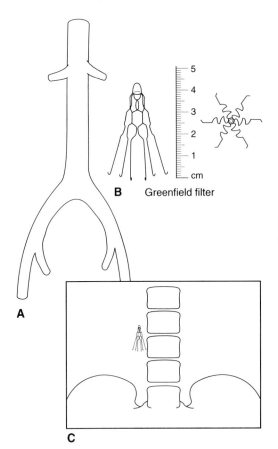

B   Greenfield filter

FIGURE 5-34. Drawing of a Greenfield filter in the inferior vena cava.

A

C

third day of heparin therapy, she vomits 100 mL of bright red blood but otherwise feels fine and has stable vital signs.

▶ *How would you evaluate and manage this patient?*

▶ Because upper GI bleeding represents a life-threatening condition, **systemic anticoagulation should be discontinued immediately. Alternate PE protection with inferior vena cava interruption** using a device such as the Greenfield filter should be provided. Appropriate antiulcer therapy should be instituted and the patient further evaluated for the source of bleeding.

CASE 5.21. ▶ Severe Deep Venous Thrombosis

A 60-year-old woman with advanced carcinoma of the cervix with extension into the left pelvic wall presents with an acute episode where her left leg became very edematous, cyanotic, and painful.

▶ *What diagnosis would you suspect?*

▶ This patient most likely has **phlegmasia cerulea dolens,** which is acute interruption of the venous outflow from obstruction secondary to her pelvic malignancy (phlegmasia means inflammation, cerulea means cyanotic, and dolens means painful). A contributing factor may be a relatively hypercoagulable state as a result of her carcinoma.

 If not treated immediately, phlegmasia cerulea dolens may lead to sensory and motor loss and possibly **venous gangrene.**

This condition is an extreme form of ileocaval DVT, with obstruction so severe that it can impair arterial inflow to the leg.

▶ *How would you manage this patient?*

▶ **Treatment involves anticoagulation and leg elevation,** with careful observation of the viability of the tissues. Once treatment is initiated, evaluation with duplex ultrasound and CT scan of the pelvis to confirm the diagnosis can proceed. Occasionally, contrast venography is necessary. The majority of patients with early phlegmasia improve with leg elevation and systemic anticoagulation. In rare instances, venous thrombectomy may be indicated.

CHAPTER 6

Upper Gastrointestinal Tract Disorders

Bruce E. Jarrell M.D., John L Flowers M.D., Molly Buzdon M.D.

CASE 6.1. ▶ Acute Epigastric Pain No. 1

A 34-year-old man presents with acute onset of sharp epigastric pain that has developed in 4 hours. He has been previously healthy. On physical examination, he appears in mild distress with moderate tenderness in the epigastrium. No masses are palpable.

▶ *What are the most likely diagnoses?*

▶ **The differential diagnosis includes pancreatitis, peptic ulcer disease (PUD), gastric ulcer, gastroenteritis, gastroesophageal reflux disease (GERD), and cholelithiasis.**

▶ *What findings on history, physical examination, and initial laboratory studies support these diagnoses?*

▶ A history of gallstones or ethanol abuse suggests pancreatitis, which should be confirmed with a serum amylase and lipase. A history of use of nonsteroidal anti-inflammatory drugs (NSAIDs) or steroids suggests PUD.

▶ *What routine screening studies are appropriate?*

▶ A complete blood count (CBC), urinalysis, amylase, lipase, and liver function tests are necessary, as well as an obstructive series, which includes a chest x-ray (radiograph) [CXR].

The CBC, amylase and lipase, and bilirubin and alkaline phosphatase are normal. Chest and abdominal radiographs are unremarkable.

▶ *What is the next step?*

▶ The management of this patient is dependent on the location of care (i.e., office versus emergency department) and the attending physician. Primary care physicians often begin diagnosis and treatment because this is the most cost-effective strategy. Most of these diagnoses are not surgical emergencies and can be electively evaluated after initiation of therapy to control the acute symptoms.

    Many physicians obtain an **abdominal ultrasound to rule out gallstones. If the ultrasound is negative, then an empirical treatment course with an H$_2$ blocker or proton pump inhibitor to treat GERD, ulcer, or gastritis** is often appropriate.

    Cases of suspected GERD warrant lifestyle modifications, including weight loss and avoiding meals before sleeping. It also means avoiding situations associated with GERD such as eating foods that decrease lower esophageal sphincter (LES) tone (e.g., chocolate, tea, coffee, alcohol) and sleeping flat in bed. This strategy results in improvement in 60%–70% of patients.

▶ *What would you do if the patient improves with this therapy?*

▶ Most physicians would simply follow such a patient and advise no further diagnostic procedures.

▶ *What would you do if the patient's symptoms persist?*

▶ If the medical management trial fails, then upper gastrointestinal (GI) endoscopy [esophagogastroduodenoscopy (EGD)] is necessary to establish a diagnosis. This approach allows visualization of the esophagus, stomach, and duodenum, as well as biopsies to rule out any malignancies and to detect *Helicobacter pylori.*

QUICK CUTS   **Many physicians perform EGD after the first episode of significant epigastric pain, especially in older individuals or those with a higher risk of tumor or infection (e.g., immunosuppressed patients).**

You perform EGD. No significant pathology is evident.

▶ *How would you manage this patient?*

▶ This patient, who most likely has nonulcer dyspepsia, should receive **symptomatic treatment with H$_2$ blockers or proton pump inhibitors, as well as treatment for** *Helicobacter* **infection, if documented.**

CASE 6.2. ▶ Acute Epigastric Pain No. 2

You are following a 45-year-old man who has had an episode of epigastric pain that did not resolve on medical therapy. He is otherwise healthy and sees you regularly. EGD is necessary.

▶ *How would you manage the following findings on EGD?*

Case Variation 6.2.1. GERD which is symptomatic even with maximal therapy

▶ Surgery is indicated in the 10%–15% of patients with GERD refractory to medical therapy. Guidelines for preoperative evaluation recommend that all patients considered for antireflux surgery should have EGD with biopsy and esophageal manometry. The manometry is critical to successful surgery (Figure 6-1). It is necessary to **demonstrate intact esophageal peristalsis before surgery** to ensure that patients are able to swallow normally postoperatively.

   If the manometry shows normal LES tone or atypical symptoms such as cough or asthma, 24-hour pH probe testing is appropriate. If the patient has dysphagia or a suspected short esophagus, a cine-esophagogram to visualize the entire esophagus is also warranted. The standard operation is a **Nissen fundoplication** (Figure 6-2). This operation restores the gastroesophageal junction and the LES (distal 5 cm of esophagus) to the normal intra-abdominal position and wraps a segment of stomach around the distal esophagus. This wrap augments LES tone while preserving LES relaxation during swallowing; therefore, it is functionally similar to a LES.

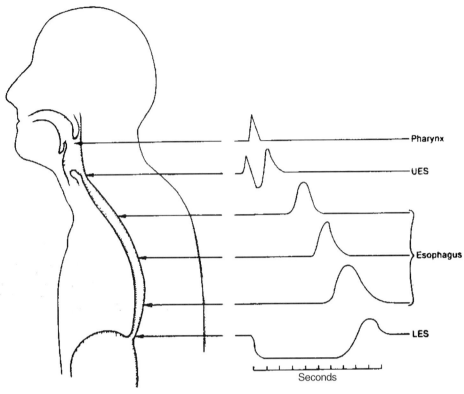

FIGURE 6-1. Intraluminal pressure of the esophagus using manometry. Swallowing is initiated as the upper and lower esophageal sphincters relax. A peristaltic contraction begins in the pharynx and travels progressively down through the esophagus. LES = lower esophageal sphincter; UES = upper esophageal sphincter. (From Castell DO, Richter JE [eds]. *The esophagus.* 3rd ed. Philadelphia: Lippincott Williams & Wilkins, 1999: 102.)

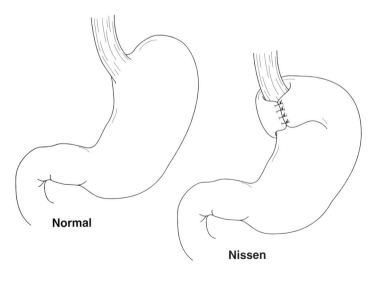

FIGURE 6-2. Nissen fundoplication. The upper stomach is wrapped around the esophagus to create a valve mechanism. (From McKenney MG, Mangonon PC, Moylan JA [eds]. *Understanding surgical disease: the Miami manual of surgery.* Philadelphia: Lippincott-Raven, 1998: 110.)

Case Variation 6.2.2. Distal esophagitis

▶ Esophagitis is a complication of GERD. It may be due to an incompetent LES, insufficient esophageal clearance of acid, or gastric dysfunction, causing increased intragastric pressure. Eighty percent of patients with GERD have a hiatal hernia (the gastroesophageal junction is in the chest). However, most patients with a hiatal hernia do not necessarily have pathologic GERD. A 24-hour pH probe can be used to document the presence of acid reflux. Manometry is also performed to measure LES pressure and the length of the LES and to characterize the amplitude and coordination of esophageal contractions. **Medical therapy usually resolves GERD; a medical approach is warranted first.** This includes propping up the head of the patient's bed at night, eating frequent small meals, and not eating a late meal before bedtime. Mild-to-moderate esophagitis usually responds to 8–12 weeks of treatment with proton pump inhibitors. This causes complete remission in 85% of patients.

QUICK CUTS   **Severe esophagitis, especially erosive esophagitis, due to reflux warrants treatment with an antireflux procedure.**

Case Variation 6.2.3. Biopsy of the distal esophagus that shows **Barrett esophagus**

▶ Barrett esophagus, which occurs in 10%–15% of patients with esophagitis, results from chronic gastroesophageal reflux. The condition involves the replacement of normal squamous epithelium of the distal esophagus by columnar epithelium, which is also termed metaplasia. It leads to an increased risk of esophageal adenocarcinoma.

A finding of Barrett esophagus warrants evaluation of biopsy for presence and **degree of dysplasia.** For minimal-to-mild dysplasia, the treatment is the same as for reflux esophagitis (e.g., H_2 blockers, bed elevation). Currently, modest data support the concept that antireflux surgery induces regression of Barrett esophagus. Nissen fundoplication is indicated for the usual indications of reflux such as intractable symptoms, severe esophagitis, and esophageal stricture, and may be recommended for the treatment of Barrett esophagus in the future.

QUICK CUTS   **Surveillance endoscopy and biopsies** are recommended every 18–24 months to determine if a Barrett esophagus progresses to dysplasia.

If a diagnosis of severe dysplasia is reached, a second pathologist experienced in this disorder should confirm the biopsy because of the implications of the diagnosis.

Case Variation 6.2.4. Biopsy of the distal esophagus that shows **Barrett esophagus with severe dysplasia**

▶ This finding is associated with a **high risk of occult adenocarcinoma in the distal esophagus. Esophageal resection is necessary.**

CASE 6.3. ▶ Acute Epigastric Pain No. 3

You are following the patient in Case 6.2, a patient who has had an episode of epigastric pain that did not resolve on medical therapy. EGD is necessary, and a hiatal hernia is apparent.

▶ *How would you manage each of the following types of hiatal hernia (Figure 6-3)?*

Case Variation 6.3.1. Type I hiatal hernia

▶ A type I hiatal hernia, or sliding hiatal hernia, which is discovered on routine evaluation, may affect patients with reflux symptoms. This common hernia usually causes no other symptoms. **These patients should receive treatment for GERD,** without surgery.

Case Variation 6.3.2. Mixed type hiatal hernia

▶ There are 2 types, a pure paraesophageal hiatal hernia, meaning that no other organs are involved and a mixed sliding and paraesophageal hiatal hernia. Both are rare but pose a risk of strangulation and necrosis of the gastric segment trapped in the chest, so repair is necessary.

Case Variation 6.3.3. Type IV hiatal hernia

▶ A type II hiatal hernia, the more common paraesophageal hiatal hernia, is a paraesophageal hernia containing other organs in addition to the stomach.

QUICK CUTS   In a type II hernia, **a portion of the stomach herniates into the chest, but the GE junction remains in the normal location.** This hernia is **extremely dangerous** because the entire stomach can necrose if it becomes involved in the hernia sac and becomes strangulated (also called a gastric volvulus).

Additional abdominal organs can also become incarcerated in the hernia sac. **If a type II hernia is found electively, it should be repaired** at this time. It may also manifest as an acute, serious illness with acidosis and hypotension and is **a surgical emergency (Figure 6-4).**

CASE 6.4. ▶ Acute Epigastric Pain No. 4

You are following the patient in Case 6.2, who has had an episode of epigastric pain that did not resolve on medical therapy. EGD is necessary.

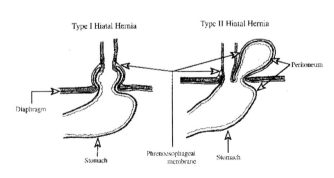

FIGURE 6-3. A type I, or sliding, hiatal hernia compared to a type II, or paraesophageal hiatal hernia. In the type I hernia, the gastroesophageal junction is in the chest as part of the sliding segment of stomach that herniates into the mediastinum. In the paraesophageal hiatal hernia, the gastroesophageal junction is in a normal location, and a segment of stomach herniates up through the phrenoesophageal membrane into the chest. (From Castell DO, Richter JE [eds]. *The esophagus.* 3rd ed. Philadelphia: Lippincott Williams & Wilkins, 1999: 385.)

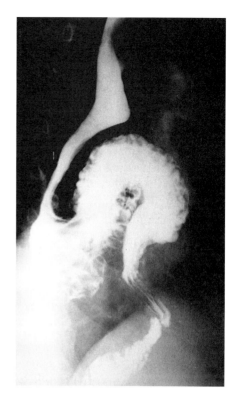

FIGURE 6-4. Contrast radiograph of a paraesophageal hernia and demonstration of gastric volvulus, which can result in necrosis of the stomach. This is a surgical emergency. (From Eubanks WS, Swanström LL, Soper NJ [eds]. *Mastery of endoscopic and laparoscopic surgery.* Philadelphia: Lippincott Williams & Wilkins, 2000: 166.)

▶ *How would you manage the following findings on EGD?*

Case Variation 6.4.1. Pyloric channel ulcer (Figure 6-5)

▶ Pyloric ulcers are associated with **increased acid production.** It is widely accepted that most peptic ulcers are associated with *H. pylori* **infection.** Elimination of *H. pylori* leads to ulcer healing and reduces the chance of ulcer recurrence.

　　A diagnosis of *H. pylori* involves the use of serum antibody testing or gastric biopsy for

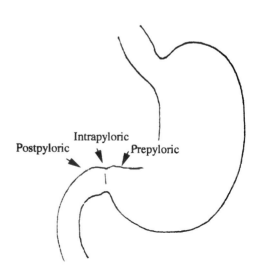

FIGURE 6-5. Location of pyloric channel ulcers in stomach and postpyloric ulcers in duodenum. (From Yamada T, Alpers DH, Laine L, et al. [eds]. *Textbook of gastroenterology.* 3rd ed. Philadelphia: Lippincott Williams & Wilkins. 1999: 1534.)

Postpyloric   Intrapyloric   Prepyloric

culture, bacterial staining (Warthin-Starry silver stain), or urease testing (CLO test). The urea breath test, which does not require a gastric biopsy, is another diagnostic tool.

Treatment of *H. pylori* involves one of several regimens. One recommended therapy includes a proton pump inhibitor such as omeprazole (20 mg bid) along with metronidazole (500 mg bid) and clarithromycin (250 mg bid). Amoxicillin may be substituted for clarithromycin. When taken for 2 weeks, these drugs have an eradication rate of 90%–96%. An alternative therapy involves bismuth, another agent that acts as an antimicrobial agent against *H. pylori*; it interferes with adhesion of the organism to the gastric epithelium and inhibits the organism's urease, phospholipase, and proteolytic activity. When taken for 2 weeks, bismuth (262 mg qid) in combination with tetracycline (500 mg qid), metronidazole (500 mg tid), and omeprazole (20 mg bid) achieves a 98% eradication rate.

Case Variation 6.4.2. Duodenal ulcer

▶ Management is the same as with the pyloric channel ulcer (see Case Variation 6.4.1).

You institute this therapy, and the test returns positive for *H. pylori*. After you treat the patient for *H. pylori*, he remains symptomatic.

▶ *What is the appropriate treatment?*

▶ **Most physicians treat mild PUD for 4–6 weeks and extend the duration of treatment to 8–12 weeks for severe disease.** If the patient remains symptomatic after treatment for *H. pylori*, upper endoscopy is necessary, with reevaluation of *H. pylori* infection.

 QUICK CUTS It is important to ask the patient about the use of ulcerogenic drugs such as **NSAIDs or steroids; discontinuation of these agents,** if possible, is warranted.

The patient completes treatment, but his symptoms persist. You repeat the EGD, and it reveals enlargement of the ulcer.

▶ *What is the next step?*

▶ If the ulcer persists after adequate treatment for *H. pylori*, **medical therapy has failed,** and surgery is a reasonable choice. Highly selective vagotomy (HSV), truncal vagotomy and pyloroplasty (V&P), or vagotomy and antrectomy (V&A) are the commonly accepted procedures (Figures 6-6 through 6-8). The best operation for PUD is a subject of debate. HSV has a low mortality rate, with the lowest rate of postoperative dumping symptoms, when compared to either V&P or V&A; however, HSV is associated with a higher rate of ulcer recurrence. In this case, most surgeons would not perform a V&A because of the high rate of complications (e.g., anastomotic leak, postoperative dumping syndrome) but would choose a **V&P or HSV,** whichever they are most comfortable with technically.

 QUICK CUTS All things being equal, HSV is the procedure of choice for uncomplicated PUD.

In this situation, it is also necessary to measure serum gastrin levels to rule out Zollinger-Ellison syndrome, because high gastrin levels are associated with recurrent peptic ulceration.

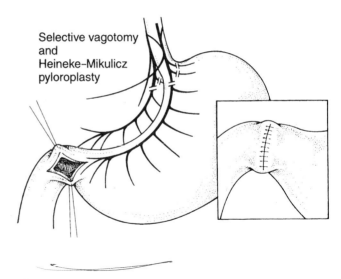

Selective vagotomy and Heineke–Mikulicz pyloroplasty

FIGURE 6-6. Truncal vagotomy and pyloroplasty. (From Lawrence PF, Bilbao M, Bell RM, et al. [eds]. *Essentials of general surgery.* Baltimore: Williams & Wilkins, 1988: 180.)

CASE 6.5. ▶ Acute Epigastric Pain No. 5

You are following the patient in Case 6.2, who has had an episode of epigastric pain that did not resolve on medical therapy. EGD is necessary, and a gastric ulcer is evident.

▷ *How does the location of the ulcer relate to gastric acid production?*

▶ There are four types of gastric ulcer (Figure 6-9). Types I and IV are associated with relatively low acid output, and types II and III are associated with relatively high acid output.

▷ *How would you manage a gastric ulcer on the lesser curvature of the body of the stomach (type I)?*

▶ **Gastric ulcers, which are related to a breakdown in the gastric mucosal protective barrier, are associated with relatively low acid production.** It is necessary to ask the patient about the use of NSAIDs or steroids; if possible, avoidance of these medications is warranted. **Because gastric ulcers are associated with a significant risk of gastric cancer,** management must be designed with this in mind. At endoscopy, it is necessary to perform 8–12 biopsies from the edge of the ulcer. If the gastric ulcer is benign, **medical treatment** with antacids, H_2 blockers, and possibly with an *H. pylori* regimen is warranted. The

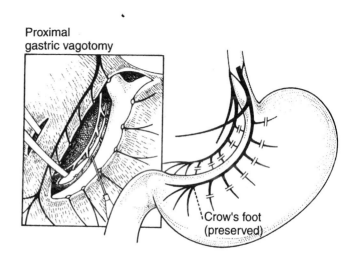

Proximal gastric vagotomy

Crow's foot (preserved)

FIGURE 6-7. Highly selective vagotomy. The gastric fundus and body are denervated, and the antrum and pylorus innervation is left intact, allowing gastric mixing and emptying to occur in a normal fashion. (From Lawrence PF, Bilbao M, Bell RM, et al. [eds]. *Essentials of general surgery.* Baltimore: Williams & Wilkins, 1988: 182.)

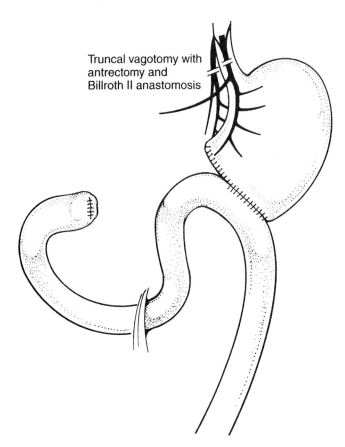

Truncal vagotomy with
antrectomy and
Billroth II anastomosis

FIGURE 6-8. Truncal vagotomy and antrectomy. Gastrointestinal continuity is restored with either Billroth I or II anastomosis. (From Lawrence PF, Bilbao M, Bell RM, et al. [eds]. *Essentials of general surgery.* Baltimore: Williams & Wilkins, 1988: 181.)

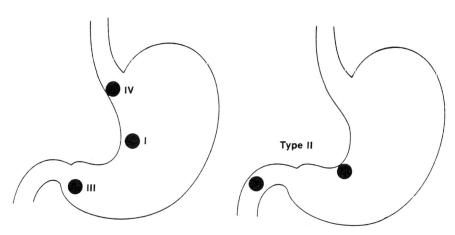

FIGURE 6-9. Types of gastric ulcer. A type I ulcer occurs at the incisura angularis on the lesser curvature, a type II ulcer is associated with a simultaneous duodenal ulcer, a type III ulcer is a prepyloric ulcer, and a type IV ulcer is a gastric cardia ulcer. (From Yamada T, Alpers DH, Laine L, et al. [eds]. *Textbook of gastroenterology.* 3rd ed. Philadelphia: Lippincott Williams & Wilkins, 1999: 1537.)

optimal duration for treatment, which has not been adequately defined, ranges from 12 to 18 weeks.

You institute this therapy, and the patient's **symptoms resolve.** The gastric biopsy demonstrates a benign pathology.

▶ *What is the next management step?*

▶ This patient can be **followed** as long as he remains free of symptoms.

You institute this therapy, and the patient's **symptoms do not resolve.** The gastric biopsy demonstrates a benign pathology.

▶ *What is the next management step?*

▶ All patients with a history of gastric ulcers who have failed to become asymptomatic on medical management should have **repeat endoscopy,** with repeat biopsies for patients with nonhealed gastric ulcers.

QUICK CUTS   Benign, nonhealed gastric ulcers may be further treated medically; however, if **after approximately 18 weeks, ulcers remain unhealed, many surgeons recommend that they be surgically resected.**

The standard operation for benign, nonhealed gastric ulcers is **partial gastrectomy,** usually described as **antrectomy;** surgeons should be certain to remove the ulcer as part of the specimen. This recommendation is based on a concern for unrecognized cancer in the ulcer. In addition, many surgeons recommend earlier surgery on giant gastric ulcers (>5 cm) because of a higher risk of bleeding as well as a higher failure rate of healing (Figure 6-10). **No vagotomy is performed.**

▶ *How would the proposed management change for a gastric ulcer at the gastroesophageal junction (type IV)?*

▶ Treatment of gastric ulcers at the gastroesophageal junction (type IV) should be similar to that just described. Again, it must be stressed that all gastric ulcers should be biopsied to rule out malignancy. If the ulcer has not healed after medical therapy, the patient should undergo

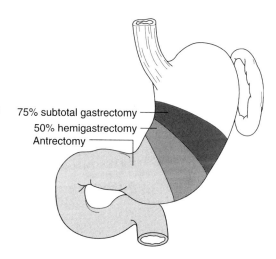

FIGURE 6-10. Various degrees of gastric resection. A total gastrectomy removes the entire stomach. (From McKenney MG, Mangonon PC, Moylan JA [eds]. *Understanding surgical disease: the Miami manual of surgery.* Philadelphia: Lippincott-Raven, 1998: 123.)

75% subtotal gastrectomy
50% hemigastrectomy
Antrectomy

repeat endoscopy at 8–16 weeks. If the ulcer is persistent but remains benign on biopsy, the clinician may continue medical therapy cautiously or refer the patient for surgery.

Surgical therapy of ulcers at the gastroesophageal junction is technically challenging. One option is a distal gastric resection with a vertical extension of the resection to include the lesser curvature of the stomach and the ulcer. The surgeon then performs a gastrojejunostomy. A more aggressive technique is a distal gastrectomy with removal of a portion of the esophageal wall and ulcer and a Roux-en-Y esophagogastrojejunostomy. **In either case, it is necessary to excise the ulcer** (Figure 6-11).

▶ *How would you manage a patient with a type II ulcer of the stomach body associated with a duodenal ulcer?*

▶ Most surgeons consider this to be an ulcer associated with excess acid production. Thus, if surgery is necessary, an acid-reducing procedure is warranted. The most common procedure is **antrectomy with removal of the ulcer.** One notable difference between the surgery for types I and IV ulcers, compared to that for types II and III ulcers, is the **addition of a truncal vagotomy;** this greatly lowers acid production.

▶ *How would you manage a patient with a prepyloric gastric ulcer (type III)?*

▶ The **management of a type III ulcer,** which is associated with increased acid production, **is similar to a type II ulcer.** A commonly performed alternative procedure is a **V&P.** The surgeon must still be certain that the ulcer does not represent cancer.

CASE 6.6. ▶ Acute Epigastric Pain No. 6

You are following the patient in Case 6.2, who has had an episode of epigastric pain that did not resolve on medical therapy. EGD is necessary.

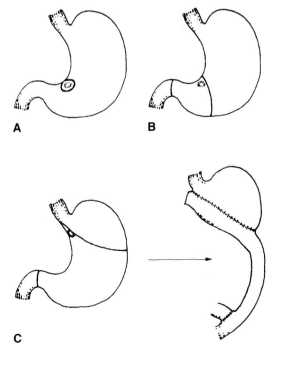

FIGURE 6-11. Three methods for resection of benign gastric ulcers. (*A*) The ulcer is excised, and the gastric walls are closed. (*B*) An antrectomy is performed, and the gastrointestinal tract is reconstructed with either a Billroth I or II reconstruction. (C) Gastric ulcer that occurs high and near the gastroesophageal junction is resected. Note that no vagotomy is performed for gastric ulcers.

A

B

C

▶ *How would you manage the following findings on EGD?*

Case Variation 6.6.1. A distal gastric ulcer, with a biopsy indicating **early gastric cancer**

▶ Before surgical resection can be performed, **it is necessary to attempt to stage gastric cancer by the use of computed tomography (CT) to assess for distant metastasis or lymph node spread (Figure 6-12). Endoscopic ultrasound (EUS) may also be useful to evaluate depth of spread or lymphatic involvement.** Laparoscopy is being used with increasing frequency for staging, but the value remains to be determined. At present, the most reliable way to stage the cancer is at abdominal exploration. For early gastric cancers of the antrum or middle stomach, the treatment of choice is a **distal subtotal gastrectomy,** including 80% of the stomach, and regional lymphadenectomy. If the tumor is confined to the mucosa and does not involve the lymph nodes, the 5-year survival is 90%.

Case Variation 6.6.2. A biopsy indicating infiltrating gastric carcinoma

▶ Several factors relate to the prognosis of gastric cancer. Histologic classifications are difficult, due to their heterogeneous morphology. In general, gastric carcinomas are described as either diffuse or intestinal. **Intestinal types** tend to form glands and have a **more favorable prognosis.** The **diffuse form** of gastric adenocarcinoma tends to extend widely in the submucosa and has a **worse prognosis.**

 Penetration of gastric cancer through the submucosa and the presence of positive lymph nodes worsens prognosis.

In general, resection usually involves resection of the stomach, omentum, and perigastric lymph nodes. There is still debate as to the extent of lymph node resection needed with

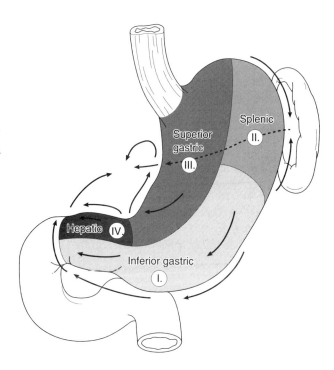

FIGURE 6-12. Lymph node drainage of the stomach as it relates to the location of the primary gastric cancer. (From McKenney MG, Mangonon PC, Moylan JA [eds]. *Understanding surgical disease: the Miami manual of surgery*. Philadelphia: Lippincott-Raven, 1998: 119.)

gastric resection. The benefits of extended lymphadenectomy, involving nodes along the aorta and esophagus, have not been proven beneficial in the United States.

Case Variation 6.6.3. A biopsy indicating infiltrating gastric carcinoma and the wall of the **stomach that appears fixed and rigid** in its entirety

▶ **Diffusely infiltrating gastric carcinoma is termed linitis plastica** and has a poor prognosis. It involves all layers of the stomach wall with a marked desmoplastic reaction. **Total gastrectomy with splenectomy** is sometimes advocated, but if the stomach is rigid and fixed throughout, **cure is rare.**

Case Variation 6.6.4. A biopsy indicating gastric carcinoma at the gastroesophageal junction

▶ The incidence of gastric cancer at the gastroesophageal junction has increased over the past 15 years. Currently, about 40% of gastric adenocarcinomas involve the proximal stomach. The prognosis for these cancers is **less favorable** than those located in the antrum. The recommendation for **gastric resection** is at least 6 cm distally beyond the tumor to prevent tumor recurrence at the anastomosis. If the cancer extends into the gastroesophageal junction, it may be necessary to perform an **esophagogastrectomy** with anastomosis in the cervical or thoracic position using either colon or a free graft small bowel as an interposition graft (Figure 6-13).

CASE 6.7. ▶ Acute Epigastric Pain No. 7

A 40-year-old man presents to the emergency department with a 4-hour history of epigastric pain that has become very severe in the past hour. He has a low-grade fever and normal blood pressure (BP). Examination is normal, except for the abdomen, which reveals marked tenderness with involuntary guarding (**rigid abdomen**) and rebound tenderness. His white blood cell (WBC) count is 18,000/mm^3 with a left shift, and the remaining laboratory studies are normal.

▷ *What study would you perform first?*

▶ An obstructive series with an upright CXR should be performed first to examine for **free air** under the diaphragm, indicating perforation of the GI tract. A rigid abdomen is typical for chemical peritonitis as usually seen in a perforated ulcer.

The patient's upright CXR demonstrates free air in the peritoneal cavity (Figure 6-14).

QUICK CUTS On an **upright abdominal radiography** or **CXR,** free air appears as air under the diaphragm. On a **left lateral decubitus film,** it is seen as air above (i.e., lateral to) the liver.

▷ *How would you use this information to make a management decision about this case?*

▶ Free air under the diaphragm is a sign of perforation; it is an indication to go to the operating room after resuscitation.

You proceed to the operating room. You find a 1-cm perforation in the anterior portion of the duodenum.

▷ *How would you interpret each of the following additional findings, and what operation would you perform?*

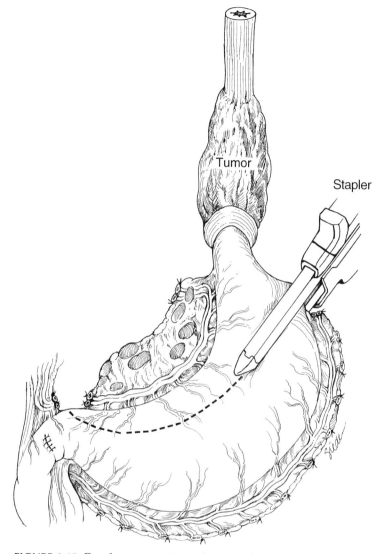

FIGURE 6-13. Esophagogastrectomy for resection of a distal esophageal cancer occurring at the gastroesophageal junction. (From Wanebo HJ [ed]. *Surgery for gastrointestinal cancer*. Philadelphia: Lippincott-Raven, 1997: 235.)

Case Variation 6.7.1. There are fresh gastric contents in the peritoneal cavity, and the perforation appears several hours old.

▶ If this patient has no prior history of ulcer disease, management of a perforation that is only several hours old involves **closure of the perforation.** This may involve use of a **Graham patch,** which consists of a piece of omentum placed over the perforation and sutured in place. Postoperative treatment to heal the ulcer and prevent recurrence is then appropriate (Figure 6-15).

Case Variation 6.7.2. There are fresh gastric contents in the peritoneal cavity, the perforation appears several hours old, and the ulcer symptoms were present for 6 months while the patient was taking H_2 blockers.

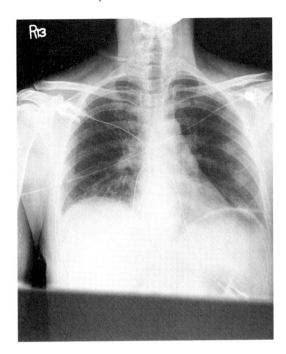

FIGURE 6-14. Upright and decubitus films of the abdomen, showing free air.

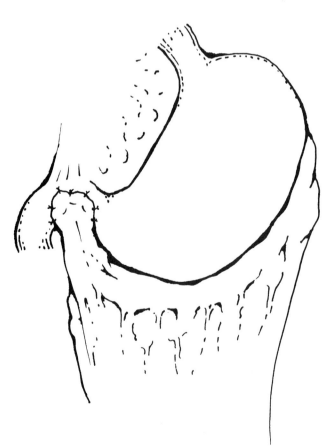

FIGURE 6-15. Repair of a perforated duodenal ulcer using an omental patch. In contrast, a gastric ulcer is not patched but resected. (From Yamada T, Alpers DH, Laine L, et al. [eds]. *Textbook of gastroenterology.* 3rd ed. Philadelphia: Lippincott Williams & Wilkins, 1999: 1541.)

▶ This information indicates that the patient has a **prior ulcer** and is at risk for future complications unless a definitive procedure is performed. **Closure of the perforation and HSV or a V&P** are suggested. Resections such as vagotomy and antrectomy or subtotal gastrectomy are not usually performed in the urgent or emergent setting.

Case Variation 6.7.3. There are fresh gastric contents in the peritoneal cavity, the perforation appears several hours old, and the patient has a history of progressive rheumatoid arthritis requiring daily NSAIDs and occasional steroids.

▶ This perforation is less likely a result of *H. pylori* and acid secretion but rather NSAIDs and steroids, which cause ulcerations due to a breakdown in the mucosal barrier. This is different than ulcerations caused by increased acid production and *H. pylori*. In this case, it would be appropriate to close the ulceration with a Graham patch and discontinue NSAIDs if possible. However, NSAIDs are most likely, necessary, and a definitive ulcer operation such as a **V&P** is warranted.

Case Variation 6.7.4. There are fresh gastric contents in the peritoneal cavity; the perforation appears several hours old; and the patient is **hypotensive** during the operation, presumably secondary to sepsis.

▶ When a patient appears septic in the operating room, the decision is usually made to **complete the operation as quickly as possible** and stabilize the patient in the intensive care unit (ICU). In this case, the perforation should be closed with a Graham patch and the operation terminated. The patient should receive intravenous (IV) antibiotics and omeprazole and return to the ICU. Definitive medical or surgical treatment may take place at a later date if ulcer problems persist.

Case Variation 6.7.5. The perforation appears 24 hours old, with fibrinous exudate and evidence for infection throughout the peritoneal cavity.

▶ If the perforation appears to have occurred 12 hours ago or more, morbidity and mortality are much higher. The **prospect of overwhelming sepsis** is greatly increased. For this reason, the **operation should be as simple as possible;** it should be restricted to **closure of the ulcer** with a Graham patch and peritoneal debridement. The patient needs close monitoring in the ICU, with adequate volume resuscitation; IV antibiotics; and ulcer prophylaxis, generally with omeprazole, due to its potent suppression of acid secretion. Definitive surgery may be planned for a later date after the patient recovers, if ulcer problems persist.

CASE 6.8. ▶ Upper Gastrointestinal Bleeding No. 1

You are caring for a 30-year-old woman with pneumonia in the ICU. She has had an ileus and has required nasogastric (NG) tube drainage. On morning rounds, you note that her NG drainage contains coffee-ground–type material and occasional blood streaks.

▷ *How would you manage this patient?*

▶ Initiation of H_2 blockade, sucralfate, or antacids with gastric pH monitoring is appropriate. If the patient is taking NSAIDs, misoprostol may also be necessary (Table 6-1). Misoprostol, a synthetic prostaglandin E_1 analog, has gastric mucosal protective properties

TABLE 6-1

Drug Therapy for Peptic Ulcer Disease

Agent	Effect	Advantages and Disadvantages
Decrease Gastric Acidity		
Antacids	Neutralize gastric acid; also may increase mucosal resistance	Inexpensive; readily available
H_2-receptor antagonists (e.g., cimetidine)	Inhibit histamine receptor on parietal cell, which decreases acid output	Excellent results; mainstay therapy; once daily evening dosing for maintenance therapy
Proton-pump inhibitors (e.g., omeprazole)	Inhibit ATPase proton pump, which is final step in acid secretion from parietal cell	Quicker healing, but more expensive than preceding agents
Increase Mucosal Defense		
Cytoprotective topical agent (e.g., sucralfate)	Binds to proteins in ulcer to form protective mucosal barrier	Not proven for gastric ulcers
Antibiotics (e.g., amoxicillin)	Eradicate *Helicobacter pylori*	Inexpensive; important in preventing recurrences in patients with *H. pylori*

ATP = adenosine triphosphate.
(From Jarrell BE, Carabasi RA, Radomski JS. *NMS surgery.* 4th edition. Philadelphia: Lippincott Williams & Wilkins, 2000: 217.)

and inhibits gastric acid secretion with coffee-ground bleeding. Upper GI endoscopy is not mandatory for this type of bleeding.

▷ *Are there patients in the hospital setting that you would manage with **"ulcer prophylaxis"**?*

▶ This patient, like many patients in an intensive care setting who are at increased risk for upper GI bleeding due to ulceration and gastritis (stress gastritis or ulceration), definitely needs ulcer prophylaxis. There are three basic approaches.

1. Wait for bleeding to occur and then treat with H_2 blockers and monitor gastric pH.
2. Treat every patient with either H_2 blockers, sucralfate, or antacids, and gastric pH monitoring.
3. Attempt to **identify patients at higher risk for upper GI bleeding and treat them prophylactically,** but do not treat the lower-risk patients (more selective approach). Most surgeons would institute selective therapy. Several conditions place patients at higher risk (Table 6-2).

You institute therapy but do not perform any diagnostic procedures. Later in the day, bright-red blood appears in the patient's NG tube.

▷ *What are the next steps in evaluation?*

▶ The first steps in evaluation of upper GI bleeding involve resuscitation. Placement of two large-bore IV lines is necessary, along with a blood draw for type and cross-match and

---

TABLE 6-2

Conditions That Put Individuals at High Risk for Upper Gastrointestinal Bleeding

Duodenal ulcer
Gastric ulcer
Diffuse erosive gastritis
Esophageal or gastric varices
Mallory-Weiss tear of the gastroesophageal junction
Gastric carcinoma
Arteriovenous malformations

(From Jarrell BE, Carabasi RA, Radomski JS. *NMS surgery.* 4ᵗʰ edition.
Philadelphia: Lippincott Williams & Wilkins, 2000: 198)

---

hematocrit. Lavage of the NG tube until blood no longer returns is essential. IV fluids are essential, and close monitoring for signs of hypotension is appropriate. The administration of H₂ blockers and monitoring of gastric pH are also necessary. Once the patient has been stabilized, **upper endoscopy** to determine the precise source of bleeding is necessary.

▶ *How would you manage the following findings?*

Case Variation 6.8.1. A duodenal ulcer with a clean, white base and no active bleeding

▶ An ulcer with a white base has not bled recently. It can be observed without endoscopic treatment. The risk of rebleeding is low.

 In all cases of duodenal ulcers, it is necessary to attempt to **maintain a gastric pH above 5** to reduce the risk of rebleeding.

An H₂ blocker or a proton pump inhibitor effectively maintains the gastric pH at 5.

Case Variation 6.8.2. A duodenal ulcer with a fresh clot adherent to the ulcer

▶ This ulcer, which exhibits evidence of recent bleeding, has a 10%–15% chance of rebleeding. Endoscopic hemostatic therapy is warranted. The commonly accepted indications for endoscopic therapy include evidence of active or recent bleeding, large initial blood loss, and a high risk of rebleeding or death with the bleed. Endoscopic therapy includes a variety of methods, including injection of epinephrine and sclerosing agents, thermal contact methods (heater probe and argon plasma coagulation), laser therapy, and newer mechanical methods such as suturing.

Case Variation 6.8.3. A duodenal ulcer with fresh clot and a visible artery at its base

▶ This type of ulcer has the **highest risk of rebleeding (as high as 40%).** A visible artery indicates that a vessel has been exposed by the ulcerative process and that rebleeding could be massive.

QUICK CUTS   Most of the time, this type of ulcer is in the posterior duodenum and involves the gastroduodenal artery.

It would be appropriate to inject the area around the artery and attempt local control. Many surgeons would electively **operate** in the next 24–48 hours if a significant bleed had occurred before endoscopy because of the concern for the need for immediate surgical intervention if another bleed occurs (Figure 6-16).

Case Variation 6.8.4. A duodenal ulcer with fresh bleeding in a patient with the onset of hypotension

▶ If the patient becomes **hypotensive** during the performance of endoscopy, immediate resuscitation with normal saline and packed red blood cells (RBCs) is necessary. The patient will most likely need to **go to the operating room.** Many surgeons recommend urgent oversewing of the vessel before exsanguinating hemorrhage occurs.

Case Variation 6.8.5. A duodenal ulcer in a patient with acute renal failure and a creatinine of 6 mg/dL

▶ This patient may have **platelet dysfunction caused by uremia,** which would make bleeding more likely. The platelet dysfunction can be lessened by dialysis and by desmopressin (ddAVP). Otherwise, the previously described treatment for upper GI bleeding is appropriate.

Case Variation 6.8.6. A duodenal ulcer in a patient with chronic alcoholic cirrhosis

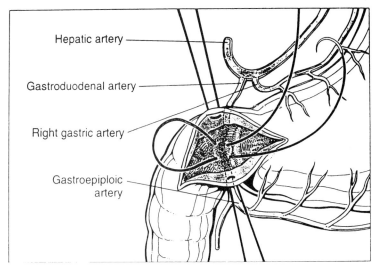

FIGURE 6-16. Suture ligature of a bleeding gastroduodenal ulcer in a posterior duodenal ulcer. Note that the stomach is opened and the artery ligated from within the lumen of the duodenum. (From Yamada T, Alpers DH, Laine L, et al. [eds]. *Textbook of gastroenterology,* 3rd ed. Philadelphia: Lippincott Williams & Wilkins, 1999: 1540.)

▶ This patient may have an **elevated prothrombin time** (PT) secondary to deficiency of factors II, VII, IX, and X, which can be temporarily corrected by fresh frozen plasma. In addition, the patient may have thrombocytopenia due to congestive splenomegaly, which can be partially corrected by platelet transfusion. Otherwise, the previously described treatment for upper GI bleeding is appropriate.

Case Variation 6.8.7. A gastric ulcer

▶ **Management of bleeding gastric ulcers is similar to that of duodenal ulcers but with one difference.** All gastric ulcers warrant biopsy, because gastric cancer may accompany ulcers. However, it is necessary to postpone biopsy for several days to weeks until the immediate bleeding has resolved and the patient has stabilized. Malignant gastric ulcers commonly appear as exophytic masses with heaped-up margins or necrotic ulcer craters, with bleeding from the edge of the craters. If the bleeding is controlled, you should plan to reevaluate the patient within 2 weeks with repeat endoscopy.

 QUICK CUTS If surgery is necessary for bleeding, **excision** rather than oversewing, as with duodenal ulcers, is warranted.

Case Variation 6.8.8. Gastritis

▶ Gastritis involves **multiple, nonulcerating erosions in the stomach,** often associated with ventilator dependence, major trauma, sepsis, severe burns, and renal failure. It is necessary to keep the gastric pH above 5 with antacids, H_2 blockers, or omeprazole. Studies have shown that sucralfate also decreases bleeding in this setting. All agents reduce the incidence of bleeding, but at present, no studies demonstrate an advantage of any single agent over another.

Most patients stop bleeding as a result of medical therapy, but on rare occasions, the bleeding does not cease. Endoscopic control of bleeding is usually unsuccessful, because of the multiplicity of bleeding sites. In that case, it is necessary to perform a subtotal gastrectomy to control the bleeding. Lesser resections fail to control the bleeding in 50% of cases. The mortality of stress gastritis remains high regardless of treatment.

Case Variation 6.8.9. Gastritis and gastric varices in a patient with a history of cirrhosis

▶ Gastritis and gastric or esophageal varices may occur with alcoholic cirrhosis (Figure 6-17). Often, the bleeding arises from gastritis and not the varices, and treatment should be instituted for gastritis.

 QUICK CUTS **Gastric varices are more difficult to treat and do not respond to banding or sclerotherapy as often as esophageal varices.**

Gastric varices may respond to injection with cyanoacrylate glue if available. If gastric variceal bleeding is severe and uncontrollable, management with **either portosystemic shunting (surgical or transjugular intrahepatic portosystemic shunt [TIPS]) or splenectomy** is necessary (Figures 6-18 and 6-19).

Case Variation 6.8.10. Gastritis and gastric varices with a history of chronic pancreatitis

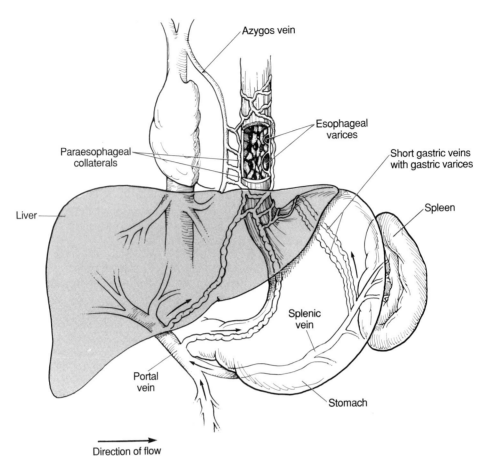

FIGURE 6-17. Vessels and blood flow involved in esophageal and gastric varices. (From Kaplowitz N. *Liver and biliary diseases.* 2nd ed. Baltimore: Williams and Wilkins, 1996: 551.)

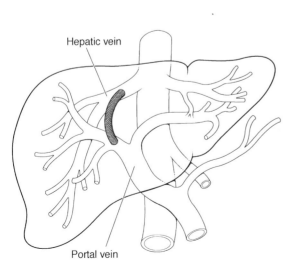

FIGURE 6-18. Transjugular intrahepatic portosystemic shunt (TIPS), in which an intrahepatic portion of a hepatic vein is cannulated percutaneously followed by the creation of an artificial tunnel between the hepatic vein and the portal vein. The tunnel is then dilated and held open with an expandable stent. (From Yamada T, Alpers DH, Laine L, et al. [eds]. *Textbook of gastroenterology.* 3rd ed. Philadelphia: Lippincott Williams & Wilkins, 1999: 723.)

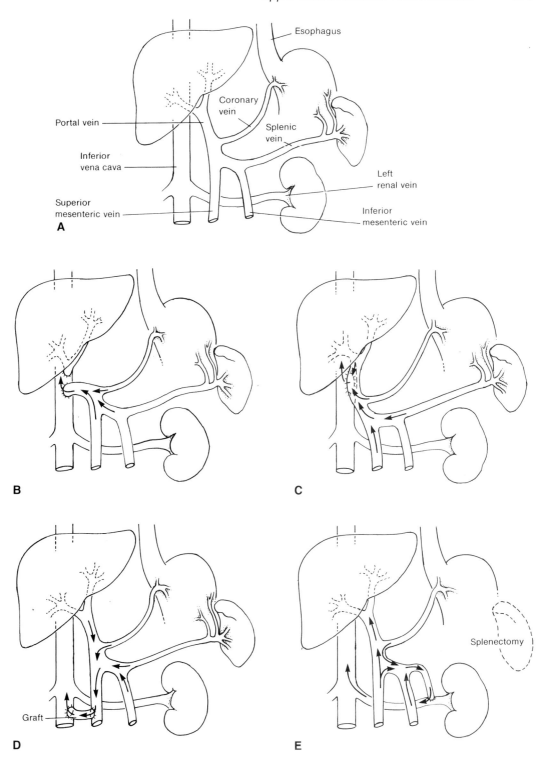

FIGURE 6-19. Portosystemic shunts commonly used in the surgical treatment of portal hypertension. (*A*) Normal arrangement. (*B*) End-to-side portacaval shunt. (*C*) Side-to-side portacaval shunt. (*D*) Side-to-side mesocaval shunt. (*E*) End-to-side splenorenal shunt. (*continued*)

Pancreatic and Hepatic Disorders

Bruce E. Jarrell M.D.

COMMON PANCREATICOBILIARY DISORDERS

CASE 7.1. ▶ Asymptomatic Gallstones

A 24-year-old woman with a family history of polycystic kidney disease is being screened by ultrasound to determine if she has the disease. She does not have the disease, but ultrasound examination shows several small gallstones (Figure 7-1). Further history and review of symptoms find no evidence of symptomatic gallstone disease.

▶ *How would you manage this patient?*

 QUICK CUTS Studies have found that the **natural history of asymptomatic gallstones is benign.**

▶ Generally, less than 10% of patients with asymptomatic gallstones develop symptoms requiring surgery over a 5-year period. For this reason, **cholecystectomy is not generally recommended** in asymptomatic patients except in certain individuals. Exceptions may include immunocompromised patients, because they are prone to more serious complications of gallstone disease; patients with a porcelain gallbladder (calcified gallbladder); and patients with gallstones larger than 3 cm, which are associated with the development of gallbladder carcinoma. Experts once believed that it was necessary to remove gallstones in asymptomatic diabetic persons because of high complication rates; however, this practice is no longer performed.

CASE 7.2. ▶ Right Upper Quadrant Pain No. 1

A 24-year-old woman presents to the emergency department with a 12-hour history of pain in her upper right abdomen, nausea, vomiting, and anorexia. Physical examination shows guarding and tenderness in the right upper quadrant (RUQ).

▶ *What are the most likely diagnoses?*

▶ The most likely diagnosis is one of three conditions: symptomatic **cholelithiasis, biliary colic, or acute cholecystitis.** Without fever, acute cholecystitis is unlikely. In a young woman, the differential diagnosis of RUQ pain includes gastroenteritis, peptic ulcer disease (PUD), acute hepatitis, renal colic, pleural-based pneumonia, and pyelonephritis.

▶ *What specific items in the history or physical examination would you look for to support these diagnoses?*

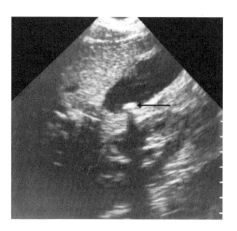

FIGURE 7-1. Ultrasound study shows a sonolucent density in the gallbladder.

▶ The factors that predispose to gallstone formation include increasing age, family history of gallstones, female sex, obesity, history of recent pregnancy, and previous diagnosis of gallstones. As a result of the 1992 National Institutes of Health consensus conference, diabetes is no longer associated with gallstones.

Symptoms of gallstone disease include fever, pain or guarding in the RUQ, and biliary colic. Examination of the abdomen may elicit the **Murphy sign,** which is inspiratory arrest during deep palpation of the RUQ due to pain (Figure 7-2). The pain may also originate in the epigastrium or radiate to the back or scapula.

▶ *What would make you suspicious that another diagnosis is more likely?*

▶ A history of indigestion, long-term nonsteroidal anti-inflammatory drug (NSAID) use, antacid use, tarry stools, or ethanol abuse prompt consideration of **PUD or gastritis.**

The patient has no suspicious history or physical examination findings that suggest a diagnosis other than gallstone disease.

▶ *How would you establish the diagnosis?*

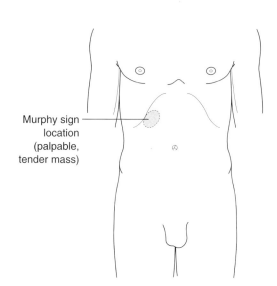

Murphy sign location (palpable, tender mass)

FIGURE 7-2. Location of Murphy sign. While the patient is taking a breath, there is an arrest of inspiration due to pain on palpation of the right upper abdomen.

▶ The most efficient method of diagnosis is an **ultrasound** of the RUQ. Findings on ultrasound suggestive of gallbladder disease include thickening of the gallbladder wall, pericholecystic fluid, and presence of gallstones (Figure 7-3).

▷ *What blood chemistries would you expect to be abnormal with a diagnosis of cholelithiasis?*

▶ Blood tests should include a complete blood count (CBC) with differential, amylase, lipase, and liver function tests. **Mild leukocytosis** is present in most patients who have a white blood count (WBC) of 12,000–15,000/mm³ and uncomplicated cholelithiasis. **Mild jaundice** with a bilirubin as high as 2–3 mg/dl may be present in 20% of patients; it is secondary to inflammation and cholestasis, not common bile duct obstruction. **Alkaline phosphatase and transaminase** levels may also be elevated.

The patient's blood studies return normal except for a mild elevation of her alkaline phosphatase.

▷ *What would be your next step?*

 Once symptomatic cholelithiasis is established, the treatment is **cholecystectomy.**

▷ *Should the patient receive antibiotics?*

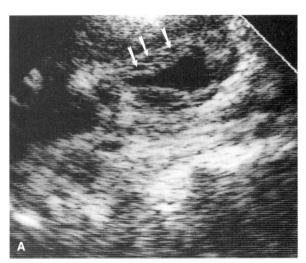

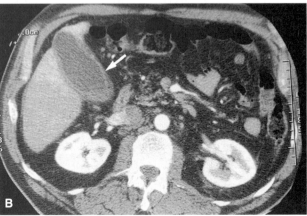

FIGURE 7-3. A. Ultrasound of the abdomen showing edema of the wall of the gallbladder. (From Kaplowitz N. *Liver and biliary diseases.* 2nd ed. Baltimore: Williams and Wilkins, 1996: 257.) **B.** CT scan showing edema in acute cholecystitis. (From Yamada T, Alpers DH, Owyang C, et al. *Textbook of gastroenterology.* 3rd ed. Philadelphia: Lippincott Williams & Wilkins, 1999: 3037.) Arrows point to edematous gallbladder wall.

▶ Most patients with uncomplicated, symptomatic cholelithiasis **do not need antibiotics** at presentation. A cholecystectomy is considered to be a clean-contaminated situation, and a single, preoperative dose of a first-generation cephalosporin is recommended. Antibiotics may be appropriate for longer-term use in patients who have a high risk of developing septic complications following cholecystectomy. This typically includes patients over 70 years of age, patients with acute cholecystitis, and patients with a history of obstructive jaundice, common duct stones, or jaundice. Patients who have undergone preoperative endoscopic retrograde cholangiopancreatography (ERCP) also warrant treatment with preoperative antibiotics.

The patient decides to proceed with a cholecystectomy.

▷ *What type of cholecystectomy would you recommend?*

▶ The commonly accepted standard procedure is **laparoscopic cholecystectomy.** Open cholecystectomy is only occasionally performed today.

▷ *What are the basic steps in a cholecystectomy?*

▶ Entry to the abdomen occurs through an incision or through trocars for the laparoscopic procedure. After exploration of the abdomen, the surgeon removes the gallbladder from the fundus to the junction of the cystic and common duct (retrograde cholecystectomy), or vice versa. The important parts of the procedure include removing the fundus from the bed of the liver, identifying and ligating the cystic duct without injury to the common duct, and ligating the cystic artery. Many surgeons believe that an operative cholangiogram to visualize the biliary tree and rule out other disease such as common duct stones is also important (Figure 7-4).

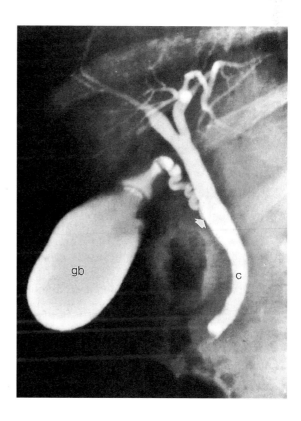

FIGURE 7-4. Intraoperative cholangiogram showing a normal common duct and filling of the duodenum. (From Yamada T, Alpers DH, Owyang C, et al. *Textbook of gastroenterology.* 3rd ed. Philadelphia: Lippincott Williams & Wilkins, 1999: 2721.)
gb = gallbladder
c = common bile duct
arrow-junction of cystic duct with common bile duct

▷ *What are the major complications of a cholecystectomy?*

▶ **Injury to the common duct** is a serious complication that may result in chronic biliary strictures, infection, and even cirrhosis. Injury to the hepatic artery is also a serious concern that may lead to hepatic ischemic injury or bile duct ischemia and stricture.

You perform a laparoscopic cholecystectomy.

▷ *What is your postoperative management plan?*

▶ Observe the patient for recovery from general anesthesia. Within 7–24 hours, most patients are ready for discharge, and they can be seen in the office in 7–10 days.

CASE 7.3. ▶ Right Upper Quadrant Pain No. 2

You see a 30-year-old woman in the emergency department with RUQ pain, nausea, vomiting, and a temperature of 102°F. An ultrasound study reveals gallstones and a thickened, edematous gallbladder wall. Blood work indicates a WBC count of 19,000/mm^3 and an elevated alkaline phosphatase; the remaining studies are normal.

▷ *What is the most likely diagnosis?*

▶ The patient most likely has **acute cholecystitis with cholelithiasis** (acute calculus cholecystitis).

▷ *What is the next step?*

▶ It is necessary to start **antibiotics** after obtaining blood cultures. Generally, antibiotics that cover **gram-negative rods and anaerobes** are warranted preoperatively and for 24 hours postoperatively in patients undergoing cholecystectomy. The most frequent organism cultured from patients is *Escherichia coli*, followed by *Enterobacter, Klebsiella*, and *Enterococcus*. A second-generation cephalosporin is adequate for most high-risk cases. Most patients need intravenous (IV) resuscitation and are placed on nothing-by-mouth (NPO) feeding. A nasogastric (NG) tube is necessary if they have nausea or vomiting.

▷ *What course do you expect the patient to follow over the next 1–2 days?*

▶ With antibiotics and fluids, the patient's temperature will most likely return to normal. Her condition will improve.

▷ *What is your management plan?*

▶ The patient should have a **laparoscopic cholecystectomy in the next 48–72 hours.**

CASE 7.4. ▶ Right Upper Quadrant Pain No. 3

You admit a woman with symptomatic cholelithiasis. In addition to an elevated alkaline phosphatase and gallstones on ultrasound, her bilirubin is elevated at 4 mg/dL.

▷ *How does this finding change the proposed management plan?*

▶ You should suspect common bile duct obstruction when a patient presents with jaundice or has elevated liver enzymes. It is also necessary to determine whether the ultrasound shows dilated bile ducts, which is evidence for obstruction of the common bile duct.

QUICK CUTS   **It is essential to clear the common duct of stones** if they are present.

Management may involve several approaches. In the past, an open cholecystectomy with exploration of the common bile duct was more common. Currently, either of the following treatment plans is recommended: **ERCP followed by laparoscopic cholecystectomy** *or* **laparoscopic cholecystectomy, with intraoperative cholangiogram, and common duct exploration** *or* **laparoscopic cholecystectomy and postoperative ERCP (Figure 7-5).**

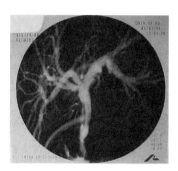

FIGURE 7-5. A T-tube cholangiogram, following a common duct exploration, showing free flow of dye into the duodenum.

Removal of common duct stones is not always necessary if the stones are smaller than 3 mm in diameter. Some surgeons advocate observing these stones, because up to one-half pass spontaneously.

CASE 7.5. ▶ Right Upper Quadrant Pain No. 4

A woman who is 6 months pregnant is admitted with symptomatic cholelithiasis.

▷ *What is the appropriate management plan?*

▶ Gallstones are present in 3%–11% of pregnant women, and in most cases, are asymptomatic.

QUICK CUTS   Symptomatic cholelithiasis and gallstone **pancreatitis can be managed nonoperatively in the majority of pregnant patients** with hydration and pain management.

If the patient has recurrent episodes of pain or an episode of biliary colic, acute cholecystitis, obstructive jaundice, or peritonitis, surgery or ERCP is justifiable. If possible, cholecystectomy is safest during the second trimester. In selected cases, ERCP and sphincterotomy are usually safe. After delivery, the gallbladder is removed.

CASE 7.6. ▶ Right Upper Quadrant Pain No. 5

A 35-year-old woman is admitted with symptomatic cholelithiasis and gallstones visible on ultrasound. Blood studies show that she an elevated amylase.

▷ *How does this laboratory finding influence management?*

▶ Most patients with an elevated amylase have mild pancreatitis, which is probably irrelevant unless significant signs and symptoms of the condition are present. The pancreatitis may result from either edema and inflammation of the distal bile duct and pancreas due to the gallbladder inflammation or a common duct stone. Usually, the amylase returns to normal quickly, and the patient improves by the next day. **Cholecystectomy and operative cholangiography may then be performed (Figure 7-6).**

 QUICK CUTS A cholangiogram is mandatory with biliary pancreatitis.

▶ *How would the proposed management change if the patient appears ill secondary to acute pancreatitis?*

▶ If the patient has significant complications from the pancreatitis, such as high fluid requirements, hypocalcemia, oliguria, hypotension, or pulmonary complications, **it is necessary to delay the cholecystectomy.** If she also has a dilated common bile duct or a stone in her distal duct, then consideration of ERCP is appropriate because of the probability of distal bile duct obstruction. Relieving the obstruction is important for rapid recovery.

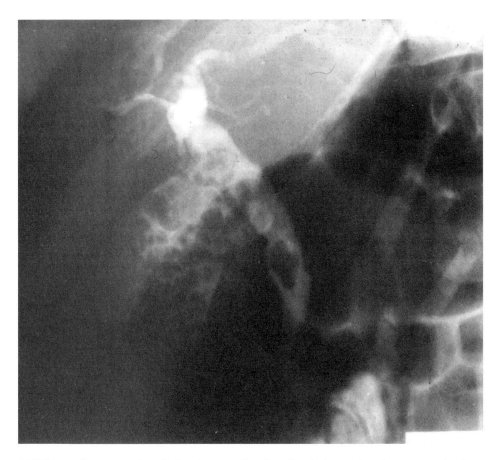

FIGURE 7-6. Intraoperative cholangiogram showing distal obstruction due to a retained stone.

CASE 7.7. ▶ **Right Upper Quadrant Pain No. 6**

A 60-year-old man has marked RUQ pain and gallstones on ultrasound examination. He has a temperature of 104°F and a blood pressure (BP) of 100/60 mm Hg.

▷ *What is the most likely diagnosis?*

▶ The high fever may indicate **acute cholecystitis or a complication** of gallbladder disease such as cholangitis, empyema of the gallbladder, or a pericholecystic abscess.

You begin resuscitation with IV fluids and antibiotics.

▷ *What studies would you perform to establish a diagnosis?*

▶ An **ultrasound examination** would still be the first study.

You perform an ultrasound and find that the gallbladder is distended with fluid that has internal echoes and gallstones.

▷ *What is the next step?*

▶ This is most likely an empyema of the gallbladder. This condition generally requires IV antibiotics and **emergent exploration** with cholecystectomy, depending on the prior health of the patient. When the patient's general health is poor, percutaneous cholecystostomy to drain the gallbladder is an option with a lower operative risk (Figure 7-7).

How would the proposed management change if the ultrasound study showed previous removal of the gallbladder, a dilated common bile duct, and air in the biliary system?

▶ This suggests a serious complication such as **suppurative cholangitis,** which results when bacterial infection occurs with bile duct obstruction. In this case, the bacteria are gasforming organisms. Patients commonly demonstrate jaundice and require urgent decompression of the bile duct. Quick stabilization with IV fluids and antibiotics is essential.

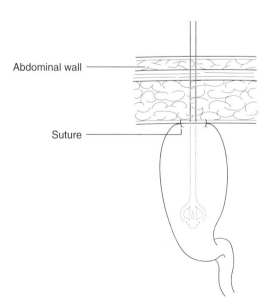

FIGURE 7-7. Percutaneous cholecystostomy for temporary drainage of an infected gallbladder.

> **QUICK CUTS** In cases of **suppurative cholangitis,** the best treatment is emergent **ERCP with sphincterotomy, decompression** of the biliary tree, and stone removal if feasible (Figure 7-8).

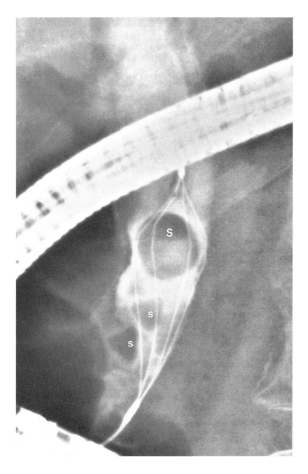

FIGURE 7-8. Endoscopic retrograde cholangiopancreatograph (ERCP) showing a distal common bile duct obstruction due to a stone and extraction of stone. (From Yamada T, Alpers DH, Owyang C, et al. *Textbook of gastroenterology.* 3rd ed. Philadelphia: Lippincott Williams & Wilkins, 1999: 2723.)

If this is not successful, there are two options.

1. A transhepatic cholangiogram and stone extraction, which may be performed by an interventional radiologist *OR*
2. If this procedure is not successful, cholecystectomy and common bile duct drainage

Many surgeons do not perform cholangiography in this situation because it may worsen the patient's sepsis and potentially cause injury to the common duct due to poor visualization of the common duct due to inflammation.

CASE 7.8. ▶ Right Upper Quadrant Pain No. 7

A 78-year-old man who presented to the emergency department with a 12-hour history of RUQ pain and tenderness has been admitted. He appears quite ill.

▷ *How would you evaluate and manage the following situations?*

Case Variation 7.8.1. A temperature of 104°F, a BP of 90/60 mm Hg, and a WBC count of 20,000/mm³

▶ This patient has acute biliary sepsis and needs emergent evaluation, antibiotics, and resuscitation. It is necessary to establish a diagnosis and institute definitive therapy. If the cause is biliary in nature, urgent surgery is essential in most cases.

Case Variation 7.8.2. A temperature of 96°F and a WBC count of 3900/mm³

▶ The patient should be treated in a similar manner as previously described (see Case Variation 7.8.1).

QUICK CUTS	Elderly patients may manifest signs of sepsis with hypothermia and leukopenia.

Case Variation 7.8.3. A tender 3-cm–diameter, palpable mass in the RUQ, a temperature of 103°F, and mental obtundation

▶ This mass is most likely an **inflamed gallbladder** with omentum attached to the gallbladder that "walls it off." When the gallbladder is palpable, typically in sick elderly patients, many surgeons term the condition a "palpable gallbladder." The implication is that an emergent cholecystectomy is necessary as soon as resuscitation occurs because there is a high risk of gallbladder rupture, which carries a high mortality. The mental obtundation is a sign of sepsis.

    Some similar older patients have air in the wall of the gallbladder, which indicates that a gas-forming organism has invaded the tissues. This is obviously a serious complication and requires urgent surgery. It is termed an **emphysematous gallbladder.**

CASE 7.9. ▶ **Right Upper Quadrant Pain No. 8**

You are asked to see a 51-year-old man who presented to the emergency department with recent onset of jaundice (bilirubin, 9 mg/dL), fever, and RUQ pain and tenderness.

 What is the most likely diagnosis?

▶ The condition most likely is **acute cholangitis.**

 What are the basic steps in the patient's initial evaluation?

▶ The basic steps are **resuscitation, antibiotics, and an urgent ultrasound study of the biliary tree.** If obstruction or dilation of the common bile duct is seen, then **ERCP and biliary decompression** are warranted.

 What is the likelihood that this patient has pancreatic cancer with distal bile duct obstruction?

▶ This cancer is very unlikely. Biliary sepsis does not usually develop in patients with pancreatic cancer, even after instrumentation. Patients present with abdominal or back pain, weight loss, and jaundice.

 How do the following situations influence the proposed management?

Case Variation 7.9.1. Previous cholecystectomy

▶ If the patient has had a recent cholecystectomy, there is a possibility that he has a **retained stone in the common bile duct.**

> **QUICK CUTS**   A common duct stone occurring within **2 years** after a cholecystectomy is termed a **retained stone,** whereas a stone appearing after 2 years is termed a **primary common bile duct stone.**

An RUQ ultrasound is appropriate, and if it is positive, attempted ERCP or percutaneous transhepatic cholangiography with stone extraction is necessary. If this procedure is not successful, the patient should return to the operating room, where bile duct exploration can be performed.

The patient may also have a diagnosis of **biliary stricture** resulting from an injury that occurred during cholecystectomy. The evaluation is the same, but the treatment is surgical exploration and bypass of the stricture, usually with a choledochojejunostomy (Figures 7-9 and 7-10). Endoscopic dilatation is another option for treatment, although studies have found that it is less beneficial.

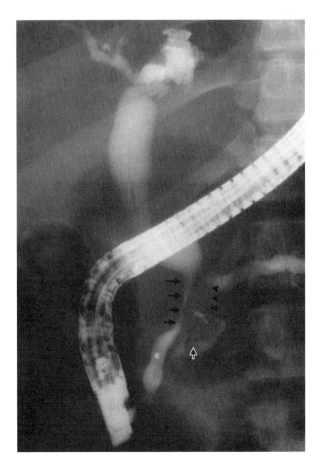

FIGURE 7-9. Cholangiogram of a distal bile duct stricture.

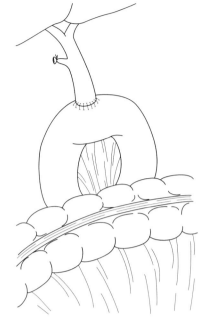

FIGURE 7-10. Choledochojejunostomy.

Case Variation 7.9.2. No previous cholecystectomy

▶ The most likely diagnosis is a **common duct stone with biliary obstruction.** An RUQ ultrasound evaluation to examine the gallbladder and the common bile duct is appropriate. An ultrasound is good for detecting gallstones and bile duct dilation but not as good at visualizing distal bile duct stones. If the patient is found to have gallstones, IV antibiotics are warranted, followed by ERCP with stone extraction. A cholecystectomy is necessary afterward.

CASE 7.10. ▶ Complications of Laparoscopic Cholecystectomy

You perform a laparoscopic cholecystectomy for cholelithiasis in a 40-year-old man.

▷ *What is the appropriate management in each of the following postoperative situations?*

Case Variation 7.10.1. Postoperative fever and abdominal pain

▶ Most patients have an uneventful recovery after laparoscopic cholecystectomy, although they may have significant **fever or pain, which may indicate an infection or biliary leak.**
   The two most useful tests are an **abdominal ultrasound study and hepatobiliary nuclide scan** (HIDA scan). This scan involves the IV injection of hepatoiminodiacetic acid. The dye is excreted into the biliary tract as long as the serum bilirubin is below 8–10 mg/dL. A HIDA scan is a particularly good test for detecting biliary leaks, as well as acute cholecystitis (the gallbladder fails to visualize in acute cholecystitis) [Figure 7-11]. If no biliary leak or collection is evident on ultrasound, and the scan reveals normal hepatic excretion, then it is appropriate to follow the patient. If a collection is found and it is of significant size, it should be drained completely. If a biliary leak or obstruction is seen, the patient should undergo an ERCP to define the biliary anatomy. Some surgeons also obtain a computed tomography (CT) scan to rule out a hepatic abscess proximal to hepatic duct obstruction.

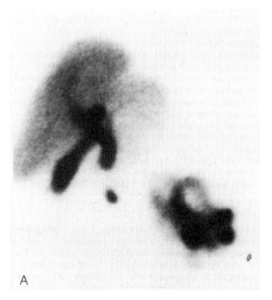
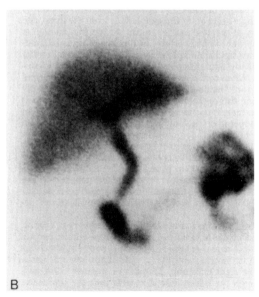

FIGURE 7-11. HIDA scans **A.** With gallbladder visualization. **B.** Without gallbladder filling but good filling of the duodenum. The HIDA scan is useful for detecting biliary leaks, obstructed cystic ducts, and common bile duct obstructions. (From Lawrence PF, Bilbao M, Bell RM, et al. [eds]. *Essentials of general surgery.* Baltimore: Williams & Wilkins, 1988: 236.)

Case Variation 7.10.2. Jaundice

▶ The workup is similar to that previously described (see Case Variation 7.10.1).

Case Variation 7.10.3. A leak on HIDA scan and a cystic duct stump leak on ERCP (Figure 7-12)

▶ Management usually involves **biliary drainage with a temporary stent** placed during ERCP (see Figure 7-21 later in this chapter). Exploration is necessary in the patient who fails to improve rapidly.

▶ *How would the proposed management change if both the HIDA scan and the ERCP demonstrate complete obstruction of the bile duct?*

▶ Reexploration and some sort of **biliary drainage procedure** are necessary. Occasionally, primary repair of the ductal injury is possible, but more often, a new anastomosis with the gastrointestinal (GI) tract is essential. The typical operation is a choledochojejunostomy.

CASE 7.11. ▶ Painless Jaundice

You are asked to evaluate and manage a 55-year-old man with jaundice of recent onset. He denies pain but has marked pruritus. Blood studies reveal a direct bilirubin of 6 mg/dL, normal aspartate aminotransferase (AST) [SGOT] and alanine aminotransferase (ALT) [SGPT], and an alkaline phosphatase of six times normal.

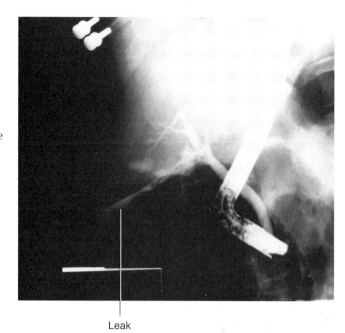

FIGURE 7-12. Endoscopic retrograde cholangiopancreatograph (ERCP) and cholangiogram showing extravasion of dye near the cystic duct remnant and along the undersurface of the liver.

Leak

▷ *What are the most common diagnoses?*

▶ The pattern indicates an **obstructive process to the biliary tree.** The differential diagnosis is **cancer of the head of the pancreas; periampullary carcinoma; cholangiocarcinoma (Klatskin tumor); stricture of the common bile duct; and, occasionally, a common bile duct stone impacted in the ampulla.** Pancreatic adenocarcinoma and cholangiocarcinoma, which may be associated with tobacco use, are usually accompanied by weight loss. In addition, these cancers may be accompanied by vague abdominal or back pain. Strictures of the common bile duct typically occur in chronic alcoholics who have chronic pancreatitis or patients who have had prior biliary surgery. **Common bile duct stones that are impacted in the ampulla typically result in intermittent symptoms of abdominal pain, jaundice, fever, and chills; thus, they do not fit this picture.** However, on occasion, presenting features may be similar to those of patients with carcinoma.

▷ *How would you further define the problem?*

▶ An **abdominal ultrasound study** is a good initial step to visualize the common bile duct, as well as stones in the gallbladder or duct.

An ultrasound study indicates a dilated common bile duct and no gallstones or pancreatic masses.

▷ *What is the next management step?*

▶ If distal common duct obstruction is present but no mass is seen on ultrasound, contrast-enhanced **CT of the abdomen** is appropriate. CT is better than ultrasound at visualizing the distal common duct area.

Transcutaneous abdominal ultrasound is not the best method for visualizing the distal bile duct and pancreatic head area, because **intestinal gas obscures the view.**

It may be possible to visualize the mass further with finer CT cuts of the pancreas, (Figure 7-13) but often, the pathology can still not be elucidated. If a mass can be visualized, ERCP may further define the lesion and allow the gathering of brushings for cytology.

You perform a CT scan of the abdomen and see no mass in the pancreas.

▷ *What is the next management step?*

▶ In this setting, upper GI endoscopy and **endoscopic ultrasound** performed through the duodenal wall commonly allow an excellent assessment of the pancreatic head. It is possible to combine ERCP with EUS if further information is necessary. CT and EUS also both allow **assessment of the tumor to discover whether local metastasis, positive lymph nodes, portal vein involvement, or liver metastases are present (Figure 7-14).**

An EUS allows you to visualize a 2-cm mass in the head of the pancreas (Figure 7-15).

▷ *Is biopsy of the mass appropriate?*

▶ **Most experienced pancreatic surgeons are comfortable proceeding with pancreatic exploration without a preoperative pathologic diagnosis.** The advisability of a percutaneous, preoperative biopsy is a matter of debate because of concern about cancer spread and conceivable prevention of a curable resection. Regardless, some surgeons prefer to biopsy the lesion and have a definitive diagnosis prior to surgery. It is important to have or establish a tissue diagnosis at surgery but prior to pancreatic resection, because the operation is extensive and the risk of significant complications is high.

Establishing a tissue diagnosis is particularly difficult in patients with **chronic pancreatitis,** where a thickened, scarred pancreatic head can feel like cancer. In contrast, pancreatic cancer can be associated with adjacent pancreatic areas with chronic scarring due to a local inflammatory process, making the biopsy look similar to chronic pancreatitis and misleading the surgeon into thinking the process is benign.

Final evaluation using an endoscopic transduodenal biopsy reveals a definitive diagnosis of pancreatic adenocarcinoma involving the head of the pancreas.

▷ *What preoperative findings would make the patient inoperable?*

▶ To tolerate this procedure, the patient must have an **acceptable general medical condition, with no evidence of distant metastasis** and a normal chest x-ray (CXR) and no neurologic symptoms or bone pain. Further evaluation is necessary if any of these conditions is present. The CT scan and EUS require careful evaluation to check for evidence of **local invasion** of the portal vein, nearby structures, or local lymph nodes (Figure 7-16). The **liver**

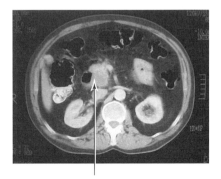

FIGURE 7-13. Computed tomography (CT) scan showing a mass in the head of the pancreas.

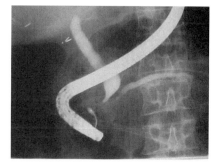

FIGURE 7-14. Endoscopic retrograde cholangiopancreato-graph (ERCP) showing a narrowing of the distal common bile duct and a "double duct" sign, which is a dilated common bile duct and pancreatic duct.

must be free of metastatic lesions (Figure 7-17). The use of laparoscopy assists in staging the patient. This allows direct visualization of some of these structures and confirms any metastases by biopsy. Confirmed metastases are a sign of incurable disease. In essence, the best chance for resectability is a small lesion that is limited to the pancreas.

There are no obvious metastases on CT scan or EUS, and you determine that the patient is operable.

▷ *What operative decisions are necessary?*

▶ It is often difficult to determine the resectability of pancreatic cancer preoperatively. Local invasion of visceral vessels may not always be apparent on CT or EUS. A CT scan may miss liver lesions smaller than 2 cm and peritoneal and omental metastases. Therefore, the **first phase of surgery involves assessing for distant metastasis** by examining the liver and peritoneal surfaces, with biopsy of suspicious lesions for frozen section diagnosis. Lymph node metastases in the periaortic or celiac region indicate the tumor is beyond the limits of resection and should be confirmed with biopsy.

Other determinations of unresectability include tumor involvement of the inferior vena

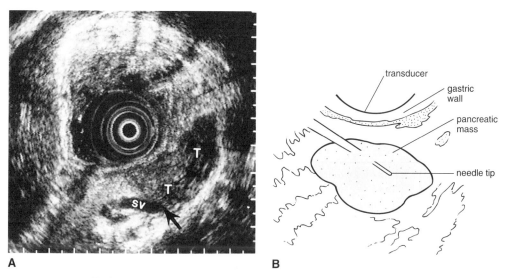

A   B

FIGURE 7-15. A. Endoscopic ultrasound (EUS) showing a mass in the pancreas. **B.** Needle biopsy under EUS guidance. (From Yamada T, Alpers DH, Owyang C, et al. *Textbook of gastroenterology.* 3rd ed. Philadelphia: Lippincott Williams & Wilkins, 1999: 3012, 3016.) Arrow is pointing to obstruction of the splenic vein by the tumor.

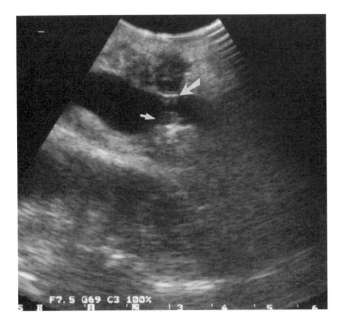

FIGURE 7-16. Ultrasound showing superior mesenteric vein involvement with pancreatic cancer. (From Wanebo HJ [ed]. *Surgery for gastrointestinal cancer.* Philadelphia: Lippincott-Raven, 1997: 179.) Arrows point to tumor. Dark space is vein.

cava, aorta, superior mesenteric artery or vein, or portal vein. The determination of involvement of the portal vein often cannot be determined until later in the procedure after structures have been mobilized. **If these findings indicate no metastasis and no local invasion, pancreaticoduodenectomy may proceed.**

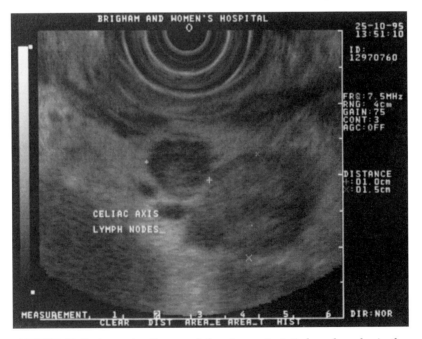

FIGURE 7-17. Endoscopic ultrasound showing metastatic lymph nodes in the celiac axis region. (From Wanebo HJ [ed]. *Surgery for gastrointestinal cancer.* Philadelphia: Lippincott-Raven, 1997: 213.)

▷ *What are the basic steps in pancreaticoduodenectomy?*

▶ After evaluation for metastasis and resectability, the head of the pancreas is mobilized from the retroperitoneum and superior mesenteric vein and portal vein. The common bile duct and the first portion of the duodenum are transected in order to preserve the pylorus. The pancreatic neck is transected, followed by detachment of the head and uncinate process from the posterior structures. The jejunum at the ligament of Treitz is transected, the specimen removed, and the GI tract reconstructed (Figure 7-18).

Tumor resection is successful. The pathology returns with complete removal of the primary adenocarcinoma of the pancreas with negative margins and no local or metastatic disease. The patient asks about his prognosis.

▷ *How would you respond?*

▶ Most surgeons believe that the **cure rate at 5 years is very low,** in the range of 5%–10%. However, in some studies, the reported 5-year survival rate for resected pancreatic adenocarcinomas in the head of the pancreas has been as high as 35%–48% in patients with negative nodes. Several factors favor long-term survival, such as tumor diameter less than 3 cm, negative nodal status, diploid tumor DNA content, tumor S-phase fraction less than 19%, negative resection margins, and the use of postoperative adjuvant chemotherapy and radiotherapy.

▷ *How would your response change if you had performed a palliative biliary and gastric bypass after finding unresectable pancreatic adenocarcinoma with local spread (Figure 7-19)?*

▶ Surgical palliation with biliary and gastric bypass may prevent gastric outlet or duodenal obstruction and bile duct obstruction. Abdominal and back pain can be decreased by celiac axis injection with alcohol to ablate the nerves. **The mean survival in patients undergoing surgical palliation is less than 8 months.**

CASE 7.12. ▶ Painless Jaundice due to Obstruction at the Common Bile Duct Bifurcation

You are asked to evaluate a 60-year-old man with painless jaundice. An abdominal ultrasound shows dilated intrahepatic ducts but no dilation of the common bile duct.

▷ *What is the next step?*

▶ If intrahepatic biliary obstruction but no extrahepatic biliary obstruction is present, this may represent a cholangiocarcinoma, or Klatskin tumor. Klatskin tumors are tumors of the biliary tree at the bifurcation of the hepatic ducts. Because they are not always seen as a mass on CT, the next best step is either **ERCP or percutaneous transhepatic cholangiography** to demonstrate the level of obstruction. For lesions higher in the bile duct, percutaneous transhepatic cholangiography is preferable, because it visualizes the proximal hepatic ducts better than ERCP. **Biopsies and cytology** may also be performed during these procedures to make the diagnosis of cancer.

On percutaneous transhepatic cholangiography, you find a constricting lesion typical of a Klatskin tumor. The biopsy returns cholangiocarcinoma.

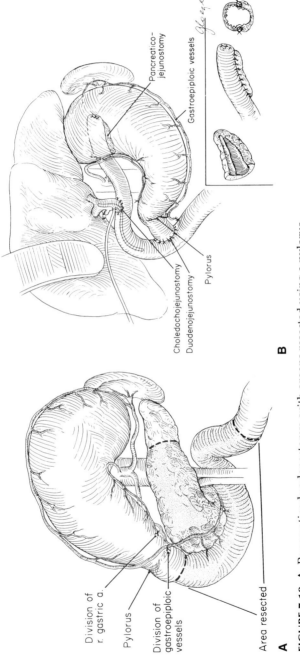

Division of
r. gastric a.

Pylorus

Division of
gastroepiploic
vessels

Area resected

A

Pancreatico-
jejunostomy

Gastroepiploic vessels

Choledochojejunostomy

Duodenojejunostomy

Pylorus

B

FIGURE 7-18. A. Pancreaticoduodenectomy, with organs resected using a pylorus-preserving method. **B.** Reconstruction of the gastrointestinal tract connecting the pancreas, bile duct, and proximal duodenum to the bowel. (From Wanebo HJ [ed]. *Surgery for gastrointestinal cancer.* Philadelphia: Lippincott-Raven, 1997: 395.)

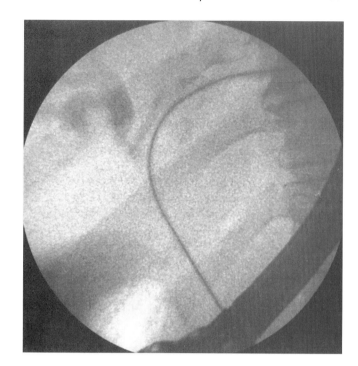

FIGURE 7-19. Biliary stent in a patient with a distal bile duct obstruction due to unresectable cancer. (From Kaplowitz N. *Liver and biliary diseases*. 2nd ed. Baltimore: Williams & Wilkins, 1996: 721.)

▶ *What is the next step?*

▶ Klatskin tumors are associated with a poor prognosis because of the high rate of vascular invasion, unresectability, and metastatic disease. If **no evidence for unresectability or metastasis** is evident on CT, **exploration with resection** of the bile ducts and gallbladder is appropriate. Tumors may extend into the left or right hepatic duct, in which case a hepatic lobectomy or trisegmentectomy may be necessary. **However, most tumors are unresectable.**

On exploration, no local metastatic disease is present. You perform a complete resection of the primary cholangiocarcinoma at the hepatic duct bifurcation. The patient recovers and asks about his prognosis.

▶ *What is your response?*

▶ The survival rate for patients with Klatskin tumors is poor; most tumors are unresectable at the time of diagnosis. Although recent improvements have been made in the treatment of these tumors, **the 5-year survival rate is still 15%** for patients undergoing curative resection.

▶ *How would your response change if you performed only palliative stenting of the hepatic duct strictures after finding unresectable cholangiocarcinoma with local spread?*

▶The 5-year survival rate in patients undergoing palliative stenting for cholangiocarcinoma is **less than 5%.** The most common cause of death is locally invasive disease. Neither radiation nor chemotherapy has any proven long-term benefit in the treatment of cholangiocarcinoma.

CASE 7.13. ▶ Other Biliary Tract Cancers

You are evaluating a 50-year-old woman for jaundice.

▶ *How would you manage the following situations?*

Case Variation 7.13.1. Diagnosis of ampullary adenocarcinoma

▶ The patient should have a complete evaluation similar to the preceding patient (see Case 7.12). If no metastases are present, exploration is necessary. Most ampullary cancers require a pancreatoduodenectomy (Whipple procedure) to remove the lesion. In contrast to pancreatic cancer, ampullary cancer has a higher cure rate, with reported survival at 5 years as high as 65% (much higher than that for any other biliary cancer).

Case Variation 7.13.2. Diagnosis of duodenal adenocarcinoma

▶ The management of duodenal tumors depends on the size and location of the lesion. If the tumor involves the ampulla, it is necessary to perform a pancreatoduodenectomy. Removal of a lesion in the first or fourth part of the duodenum may be possible with segmental resection. Patients with duodenal cancers have a worse prognosis because their carcinomas usually involve nearby structures.

Case Variation 7.13.3. A mass in the gallbladder fossa visible on ultrasound

▶ A mass in the gallbladder fossa is usually a malignant gallbladder adenocarcinoma. These tumors may cause symptoms similar to gallstones. CT is appropriate to evaluate the mass further and look for evidence of metastasis (Figure 7-20).

   If CT reveals an infiltrating mass in the gallbladder with no evidence of metastatic disease, it is advisable, if possible, to perform **an open cholecystectomy, a wide resection of the surrounding liver and a hilar lymph node resection.** Most surgeons advocate a wedge resection of the liver with a 2–3-cm margin around the gallbladder. Laparoscopic cholecystectomy is probably not appropriate because of the inability to remove hepatic tissue.

   Recurrent cancer may occur at the trocar sites. The most common means of spread in carcinoma of the gallbladder is by direct extension into the liver. Unfortunately, **the dis-**

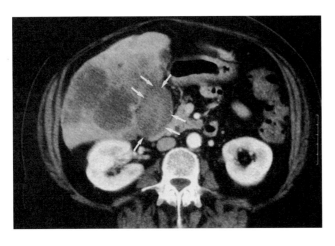

FIGURE 7-20. Computed tomography scan of a gallbladder cancer. (From Yamada T, Alpers DH, Owyang C, et al. *Textbook of gastroenterology.* 3rd ed. Philadelphia: Lippincott Williams & Wilkins, 1999: 3037.)

covery of most of these cancers occurs late in their course, when they involve a large portion of the liver, making them unresectable.

Case Variation 7.13.4. A 3-cm polyp in the gallbladder

▶ Observation of small polyps is usually appropriate. Cholecystectomy is warranted for removal of larger polyps (>2 cm) because of the 7%–10% risk of developing adenocarcinoma of the gallbladder.

Case Variation 7.13.5. A calcified gallbladder

▶ A calcified gallbladder, also called a porcelain gallbladder, has a 50% association with adenocarcinoma and should be removed.

CASE 7.14. ▶ Acute Epigastric Pain No. 10

You are following a 29-year-old man who had an episode of epigastric pain. His serum amylase and lipase are three times normal, and no gallstones are visible on ultrasound examination of the abdomen.

▷ *What management is appropriate?*

▶ This patient most likely has pancreatitis based on initial assessment. To be certain that you are not missing other possible diagnoses, an obstructive abdominal series is necessary to rule out other common disorders such as a perforated ulcer with free air. Findings in pancreatitis include a generalized ileus (usual), as well as a localized ileus of the second and third portions of duodenum secondary to a localized inflammatory process. CT of the abdomen is not mandatory for patients with uncomplicated pancreatitis.

 The usual treatment for pancreatitis involves **NPO feeding, IV hydration, pain control, and observation.**

Many patients recover quickly as a consequence of this therapy. If a particular patient does not improve rapidly, it may be necessary to administer total parenteral nutrition (TPN) to maintain good nutrition.

▷ *How would the presence of gallstones influence the proposed management?*

▶ Gallstone pancreatitis is generally managed in a similar way. The serum amylase level is monitored over the next 24–48 hours. When the amylase decreases and the patient improves, **laparoscopic cholecystectomy** is warranted.

CASE 7.15. ▶ Acute Epigastric Pain No. 11

A 34-year-old man has severe abdominal pain that has been progressively increasing over the past several hours. His amylase value is elevated. You admit him and begin therapy. Over the next hour, you note that he appears severely ill; hypotension, hypoxemia, and multiorgan failure develop rapidly.

▷ *What is the most likely diagnosis?*

▶ The patient most likely has **severe necrotizing pancreatitis** with massive third-space fluid loss due to local pancreatic inflammation. In addition, he has systemic inflammatory response syndrome, resulting in multiorgan system failure. It is hypothesized that this syndrome is mediated by cytokine release, resulting in acute respiratory distress syndrome (ARDS), multiorgan system failure, and hemodynamic instability.

▷ *What steps are necessary next?*

▶ Major **fluid resuscitation in a critical care unit** is essential. CT of the abdomen is useful to assess the extent of local inflammation and to search for additional causes of decompensation, including bowel necrosis and perforation, abscess formation, and biliary obstruction with infection (Figure 7-21).

▷ *How would you assess the patient's mortality?*

▶ Most physicians use the **Ranson criteria (Table 7-1)**. These criteria were developed for alcoholic pancreatitis. **If patients meet three of the Ranson criteria, the mortality rate is 28%; with five or six, mortality is 40%; and with seven or eight, mortality is 100%.** Other scores such as the Acute Physiology, Age, and Chronic Health Evaluation (APACHE) 2 score may be more appropriate for pancreatitis from other causes.

After receiving 6 L of normal saline over 12 hours, the patient remains hypotensive with a very low urine output—10 mL/hr in the past 4 hours.

▷ *What is your plan for fluid resuscitation?*

▶ The adequacy of resuscitation should still be a concern. The patient may need a **pulmonary artery catheter** if his hemodynamic status cannot be resolved using the central venous pressure (CVP) as a guide.

The patient has labored breathing and a pulse oximeter reading of 90%.

▷ *What is the best way to assess the patient's pulmonary status and manage his ventilation?*

▶ This patient warrants immediate physical examination with chest auscultation, an arterial blood gas (ABG), and a CXR. Supplemental oxygen and continuous pulse oximeter monitoring are necessary during this examination. This patient's problems may be due to **pulmonary edema from overhydration, ARDS from a systemic response to the pancreatitis, atelectasis, or pneumonia,** which are often difficult to distinguish by CXR. An

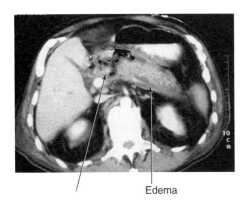

Edema

FIGURE 7-21. Computed tomography scan of the abdomen showing the head and body of the pancreas severely edematous and inflamed.

TABLE 7-1

Ranson Prognostic Signs Associated with Acute Pancreatitis

On admission
Age >55 years
White blood cell (WBC) count >16,000 cells/mm^3
Glucose >200 mg/dL
Lactate dehydrogenase (LDH) >350 IU/L
Aspartate aminotransferase (AST) >250 IU/L

After 48 hours
Hematocrit decrease = 10%
Blood urea nitrogen (BUN) increase = 5 mg/dL
Ca^{2+} level <8 mg/dL
PaO$_2$ <60 mm Hg
Base deficit >4 mEq/L
Fluid sequestration >6 L

ABG provides important information on oxygenation (PO$_2$) as well as adequacy of ventilation (PCO$_2$), which help decide the need for mechanical ventilation. Experienced clinicians usually intubate before the patient's condition becomes serious. The decision to intubate is usually made based on a combination of ABGs and clinical status.

Your resident student wants to know the correlation between serum amylase and severity of the pancreatitis.

▶ *What would you say?*

▶ **Amylase levels do *not* correlate with the severity of pancreatitis** or the prognosis.

You decide that the pulmonary failure in this patient requires intubation and ventilation. Over the next 2 days, **signs and symptoms of sepsis** develop, with fever, leukocytosis, and septic shock.

▶ *What is the next step?*

▶ You should be most concerned about **pancreatic abscess,** although other sources of sepsis such as pneumonia, IV access infection, and urinary tract infection (UTI) warrant investigation. To evaluate for pancreatic abscess, a dynamic CT scan is the most reliable examination (Figure 7-22). This CT scan includes the use of radiographic contrast material timed to determine the vascularity of the pancreas.

A CT scan shows a peripancreatic collection.

▶ *What is the next step?*

QUICK CUTS For a peripancreatic collection with internal loculation or debris, **sampling by a percutaneous route** under CT scan or ultrasound guidance is necessary, if possible. For a large number **of WBCs or bacteria,** the **diagnosis of an abscess** is appropriate, and **abscess drainage** is essential. **Drainage may occur either surgically or percutaneously** with a catheter.

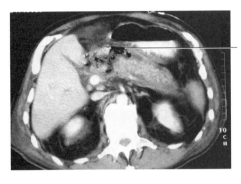

— Abscess

FIGURE 7-22. Computed tomography scan of a pancreatic abscess with air in the cavity.

▶ An experienced clinician should decide which type of drainage to use, because some collections contain a large amount of debris and cannot be drained with a catheter. Appropriate antibiotics, usually for gram-negative and anaerobic coverage, are necessary. If adequate percutaneous drainage is not possible, open surgical drainage is required.

The patient is recovering from percutaneous pancreatic abscess drainage when he suddenly becomes hypotensive, and the drainage becomes bloody.

▷ *What condition do you suspect, and how do you manage it?*

▶ The most likely diagnosis is **erosion of the catheter or abscess into a major artery** such as the splenic, gastroduodenal, or superior mesenteric arteries, or a pancreatic vessel. Diagnosis involves **angiography; control consists of embolization** in most cases.

Suppose a severe case of pancreatitis occurred in a 70-year-old patient.

▷ *Would you change your approach?*

▶ In older patients with abdominal pain and increased amylase levels, it is necessary to consider diagnoses other than pancreatitis. Abdominal catastrophes such as **mesenteric ischemia and volvulus** could manifest similarly. The pain pattern of mesenteric ischemia may be less localized to the epigastric region, but in obtunded patients, this could be difficult to determine. A serum amylase elevation by itself is not a reliable enough marker of pancreatitis in severely ill patients. CT is very useful in assessing the intra-abdominal process.

In practice, any patient who is severely ill with suspected pancreatitis warrants close examination to rule out some other cause. CT is one good way to reassure oneself of the presence of pancreatitis, because it shows edema of the pancreas and surrounding tissue. If that is not present, then one should be suspicious of the diagnosis. If after the CT, the diagnosis remains uncertain, exploratory laparotomy may be appropriate.

▷ *What is the expected course of a patient with severe pancreatitis?*

▶ The sicker the patient, the more likely the development of serious complications. The mortality of severe pancreatitis remains high.

CASE 7.16. ▶ Acute Epigastric Pain No. 12

A 34-year-old alcoholic man who has developed acute pancreatitis initially improves, but his symptoms fail to resolve completely. Instead, he **continues to have moderate abdominal pain, anorexia, persistent elevation of serum amylase, and inability to eat due to early satiety.**

▶ *What is the suspected diagnosis?*

▶ The presumptive diagnosis is a **pancreatic pseudocyst,** which is a collection of fluid near the pancreas presumably due to leakage of pancreatic fluid and edema. It can cause pain due to a local compressive effect, especially on the posterior wall of the stomach, which causes the early satiety.

▶ *How would you confirm this diagnosis?*

▶ This is best visualized by **CT of the abdomen,** although an abdominal ultrasound study can also be useful (Figure 7-23). Small pseudocysts are common with pancreatitis and do not usually cause this picture.

The CT shows a pseudocyst in the lesser sac that is 8 cm in diameter.

▶ *What is the next step?*

▶ The common practice would be **NPO feeding, TPN, and observation,** as long as no signs of infection are present.

You institute this therapy, and the patient improves over the next 10 days. The pain resolves, the amylase returns to normal, and the pseudocyst shrinks to 2 cm.

▶ *What is the next step?*

▶ Treatment involves beginning feeding and following the patient's symptoms and serum amylase. If these are stable, the **pseudocyst is resolving,** and the patient feels better and can be discharged.

▶ *How would you manage the patient if the pain and other symptoms continued or recurred and the serum amylase remained elevated?*

 If a pseudocyst is present on CT and the patient **fails to improve by 6 weeks, surgical intervention is appropriate.**

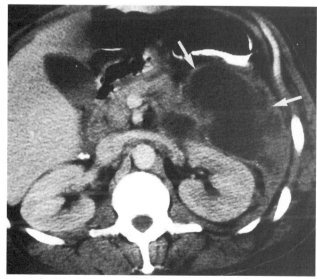

FIGURE 7-23. Computed tomography scan of the abdomen showing a pancreatic pseudocyst.

▶ The 7-week waiting period is observed for two reasons: Many pseudocysts resolve in 6 weeks, and the cyst wall must contain enough fibrous tissue to allow surgical suturing to occur. The procedure of choice involves drainage of the fluid collection into the GI tract, most commonly with a **cystogastrostomy** (Figure 7-24). The surgeon opens the stomach anteriorly and locates the cyst with a needle and syringe through the posterior stomach. Because the cyst is contiguous with the posterior stomach wall in most cases, it is necessary to make a communication with the cyst through the posterior wall. This procedure is very effective in resolving the pseudocyst. A **biopsy** is always taken to ensure that the cyst is inflammatory in origin rather than **cystadenoma or cystadenocarcinoma of the pancreas.** Surgeons are increasingly using alternative methods to drain pseudocysts, including endoscopically and radiologically guided procedures, which should only be performed under the guidance of an experienced clinician.

COMMON HEPATIC DISORDERS

CASE 7.17. ▶ Hepatic Mass

A 37-year-old woman is seen for vague RUQ pain. Laboratory studies are normal. An RUQ ultrasound study reveals no gallstones but does show a 3 x 4-cm mass in the right lobe of the liver.

▷ *What are the common diagnoses?*

▶ **Most likely, this lesion is benign.** If **cystic** on ultrasound, it is probably a **simple cyst.** If **solid,** it is most likely a **hemangioma.** Other likely tumors include focal nodular hyperplasia and hepatic adenoma. In older individuals, **metastatic carcinoma, primary hepatocellular carcinoma, and cholangiocarcinoma** are potential diagnoses.

▷ *What special history features or physical findings are appropriate?*

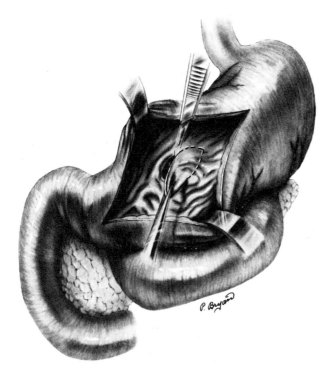

FIGURE 7-24. Cystogastrostomy for pancreatic pseudocyst. (From Howard JM, Idezuki Y, Ihse I, et al. [eds]. *Surgical diseases of the pancreas.* 3rd ed. Baltimore: Williams & Wilkins, 1998: 428. After Bradley EL III, Zeppa R. The pancreas. In *Davis-Christopher textbook of surgery.* 13th ed. Sabiston DC [ed]. Philadelphia: WB Saunders, 1986.)

▶ Inquiries regarding history of use of oral birth control pills, exposure to environmental toxins, hepatitis B and C, previous injury to the liver, and known primary tumors are necessary. On physical examination, signs of chronic liver disease, including cirrhosis, polycystic kidney disease, and primary kidney tumors, should be sought.

▶ *How would you evaluate and manage the following types of lesions?*

Case Variation 7.17.1. Cystic lesion with no internal echoes suggestive of a simple cyst (Figure 7-25)

▶ Although a simple cyst can cause symptoms of RUQ discomfort, it is **asymptomatic** in most cases. Rarely, a hepatic cyst may cause hemorrhage, secondary bacterial infection, and obstructive jaundice. Generally, a simple cyst needs **no further management.** If symptoms persist, treatment of the cyst with aspiration followed by a sclerosant or by simple excision is warranted. If multiple cysts are present in the liver in a patient who also has polycystic kidney disease, the patient has polycystic liver disease. Treatment is similar to that for simple cysts of the liver.

Case Variation 7.17.2. Multilocular cyst with **calcifications in the wall** and internal echoes (Figure 7-26)

▶ A suspected **echinococcal cyst,** which results from *Echinococcus granulosus,* a GI parasite, may be present. The serologic test for *Echinococcus* is usually positive. Treatment is aimed at **operative sterilization** of the cyst by injecting the cyst under controlled operative conditions using hypertonic saline (a scolocidal agent), followed by **excision of the cyst.** It is necessary to take care not to spill the cyst contents into the peritoneum, which could allow them to infect the peritoneal cavity.

Case Variation 7.17.3. Cystic lesion suggestive of an abscess

▶ A hepatic abscess usually presents with fever, elevated WBC count, and abdominal tenderness. Treatment of a pyogenic abscess should consist of **IV antibiotics and CT-guided drainage.** In most cases, resection can be avoided. An **amebic abscess** may be treated with **metronidazole alone** and no surgery.

Case Variation 7.17.4. Solid-appearing lesion (Figure 7-27)

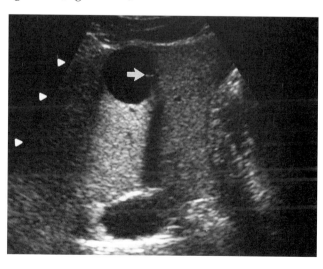

FIGURE 7-25. Ultrasound of the liver showing a hepatic cyst. (From Yamada T, Alpers DH, Owyang C, et al. *Textbook of gastroenterology.* 3rd ed. Philadelphia: Lippincott Williams & Wilkins, 1999: 2978.)

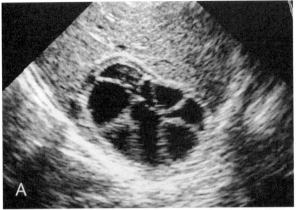
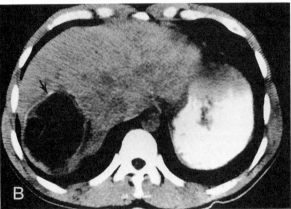

FIGURE 7-26. Computed tomography scan of the liver showing *Echinococcus* cyst. **A.** Ultrasound study of ecchinococcal cyst showing a multiseptated cystic structure. **B.** CT scan without contrast shows a cystic structure with internal walls and calcification of the fibrotic wall. (From Kaplowitz N. *Liver and biliary diseases.* 2nd ed. Baltimore: Williams & Wilkins, 1996: 241.)

▶ The differential diagnosis for a solid liver lesion includes **hemangioma, focal nodular hyperplasia, hepatic adenoma, metastatic cancer, and hepatocellular carcinoma.** The history is important. Pertinent findings include oral contraceptive use, which is present in a high percentage (as high as 90%) of patients with hepatic adenoma and occurs less frequently in patients with focal nodular hyperplasia. A history of hepatitis (B or C) or cirrhosis may suggest hepatocellular carcinoma.

   Note that liver function tests may be unremarkable in individuals with any one of these three conditions. α-fetoprotein, as well as hepatitis B surface antigen, may be positive in patients with hepatocellular carcinoma.

The lesion is solid. You suspect a hemangioma.

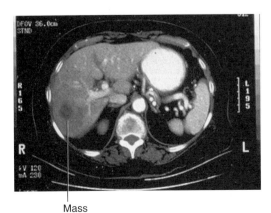

FIGURE 7-27. Computed tomography scan of solid liver lesion.

Mass

How would you establish the diagnosis?

▶ A **labeled RBC scan** is highly reliable in making the diagnosis of hemangioma, which is the most likely diagnosis (Figure 7-28). This lesion is a collection of ectatic vascular cavernous spaces lined by endothelium. A bolus-enhanced dynamic CT or magnetic resonance imaging (MRI) scan may also confirm the diagnosis of a hemangioma, which has a characteristic appearance of a vascular lesion that fills from the periphery to the center (Figure 7-29).

The discovery of most hemangiomas is incidental; it occurs during an ultrasound examination to check for gallstones. Hemangiomas are usually asymptomatic and almost never present with spontaneous hemorrhage. Thus, removal is not warranted. Most surgeons use the following as a general **guideline for surgical removal of benign hepatic masses.**

QUICK CUTS **Symptomatic** lesions, lesions with a **risk of spontaneous rupture,** and lesions with **uncertainty as to the diagnosis** warrant removal.

Biopsy of a hepatic lesion should only be performed after it is certain that the lesion is not a hemangioma, because of a high risk of bleeding. Hepatic adenoma also has a high bleeding risk with biopsy. Thus, biopsy is only performed selectively to confirm a diagnosis.

You obtain a labeled RBC scan. It is negative for hemangioma.

What is the next step?

▶ CT is an appropriate test to differentiate between the other possible diagnoses. Patients with **focal nodular hyperplasia** occasionally demonstrate **a central stellate scar on CT scan** but require a liver biopsy to establish a diagnosis (Figure 7-30). **No treatment for focal nodular hyperplasia** is indicated. It is often difficult to distinguish from hepatocellular carcinoma and hepatic adenoma, but it is not considered premalignant. **Hepatic adenomas** may regress after discontinuation of oral contraceptives. **It is necessary to resect persistent or large lesions** for two reasons: (1) they have been known to develop into hepatocellular carcinoma, and (2) they are associated with a **risk of rupture.** Hepatic ade-

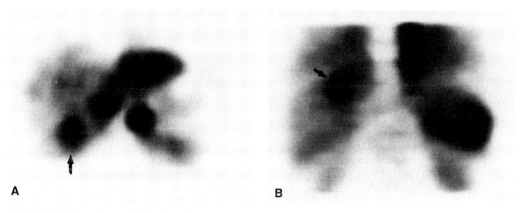

A   **B**

FIGURE 7-28. Labeled red blood cell scan showing a hemangioma. (From Yamada T, Alpers DH, Owyang C, et al. *Textbook of gastroenterology.* 3rd ed. Philadelphia: Lippincott Williams & Wilkins, 1999: 3084.)

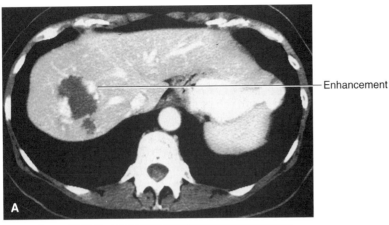

— Enhancement

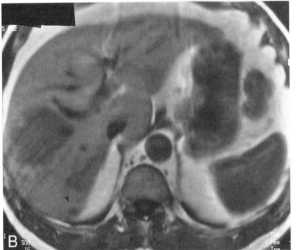

FIGURE 7-29. A. Computed tomography scan showing peripheral enhancing hepatic lesion. (From Yamada T, Alpers DH, Owyang C, et al. *Textbook of gastroenterology.* 3rd ed. Philadelphia: Lippincott Williams & Wilkins, 1999: 3031.) **B.** MRI on T-1 weighted image shows minimal signal from the lesion. **C.** MRI on T-2 weighted image shows an intense signal typical of hemangioma. (Parts B and C from Kaplowitz N. *Liver and biliary diseases.* 2nd ed. Baltimore: Williams & Wilkins, 1996: 245.)

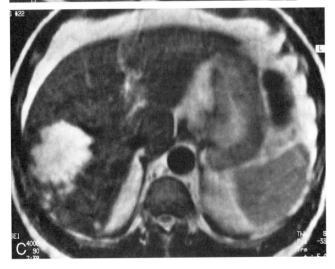

nomas are thought to have an especially high risk of rupture during pregnancy and therefore should be treated prior to pregnancy.

The CT scan suggests hepatocellular carcinoma. You perform a biopsy, and the pathology returns hepatocellular carcinoma.

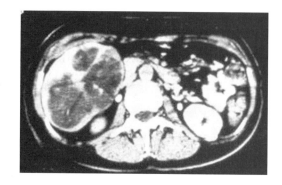

FIGURE 7-30. Computed tomography scan of the liver showing focal nodular hyperplasia.

▷ *What management is appropriate?*

▶ The first step is to **determine whether metastatic disease exists,** usually with a **CT scan of the chest and abdomen** to examine for lung metastasis and other abnormalities. Abdominal metastases are typically in the hepatic hilar lymph nodes and celiac nodes, and they extend locally into the diaphragm and other structures. **If no metastases exist, then a surgical assessment** of the hepatic lesions is appropriate.

The prognosis is favorable for patients with lesions that are **resectable with a 1-cm margin, solitary, less than 5 cm in diameter, in noncirrhotic livers, without vascular invasion, and of low-grade malignancy.** If lesions are multiple or involve a critical structure such as the portal vein or hepatic veins, resection is not warranted. However, when **resection** is appropriate, surgeons should perform it aggressively, because it offers the patient the **highest rate for cure similar factors are shown for colorectal metastasis to the liver (Table 7-2).**

You decide to remove the mass.

▷ *What are the basic principles of hepatic resection?*

▶ The basic principles of hepatic resection are **complete removal of the lesion without patient death** (Figure 7-31). The hepatic inflow and outflow are isolated and occluded to the resected segment. Liver tissue is then transected in a location where a 1-cm margin is obtained, maintaining hemostasis while crossing the liver. In the hands of experienced surgeons, otherwise healthy patients tolerate the procedure well.

CASE 7.18. ▶ Fever and Pain in the Right Upper Quadrant

A 37-year-old man with a history of IV drug abuse is hospitalized for an extensive upper extremity abscess. He receives treatment incision and drainage and IV antibiotics. Despite 3 days of IV antibiotics, he remains febrile (temperature to 103°F).

▷ *What are the possible causes of this patient's fever?*

▶ It is necessary to drain the wound adequately and treat it properly. Other processes that may cause fever in IV drug abusers are endocarditis, intra-abdominal abscess, pancreatitis, pneumonia, UTI, or infected indwelling catheters. Human immunodeficiency virus (HIV)-related infections are also a possibility in IV drug users who share needles. You should examine the patient for these possibilities and send blood cultures.

On examination, the patient's abdomen is tender in the RUQ. Laboratory studies reveal that his WBC count is 24,000/mm³ and his alkaline phosphatase is elevated.

TABLE 7-2

Prognostic Factors in Resectable Colorectal Metastasis to the Liver

Factors That Influence Resectability of Liver Tumors

	Positively	Negatively
Number of lobes	Single lobe	Bilobar
Extrahepatic metastasis	No	Yes
Medical condition	Good	Poor
Cirrhosis	No	Yes

Factors That Influence the Prognosis of Resected Liver Lesions

	Positively	Negatively
Number	Solitary	Multiple
Size of lesions	Small (≤5 cm)	Large (>5 cm)
Chronicity	Metachronous with primary tumor	Synchronous with primary tumor
Surgical margin	>1 cm	<1 cm
Stage (primary tumor)	I or II	III
Location of primary tumor	Colon primary	Rectal primary

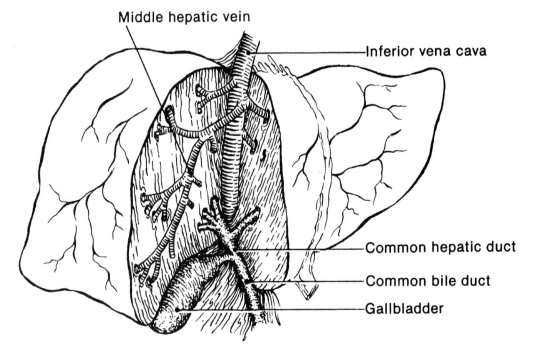

FIGURE 7-31. Planes of resection of the liver. (From Jarrell BE, Carabasi RA III, Radomski JS. *NMS Surgery.* 4th ed. Philadelphia: Lippincott Williams & Wilkins, 2000: 261.)

▶ *How would you work up this patient?*

▶ Findings of RUQ tenderness and fever with leukocytosis point to a hepatobiliary condition. This could include **complications of gallstones or infectious processes** such as cholangitis or liver abscess. Appropriate tests include ultrasound or spiral CT. An ultrasound demonstrates many hepatobiliary processes, including liver abscesses and biliary obstruction or stones, whereas CT may be better at identifying hepatic abscesses near the dome of the liver and visualizing other lesions such as intra-abdominal abscesses or diverticulitis (Figure 7-32).

A CT scan reveals multiple low-density lesions within both lobes of the liver with peripheral rim enhancement indicative of liver abscesses.

▶ *What treatment is appropriate?*

▶ Liver abscesses may be either **pyogenic (caused by bacterial spread) or amebic (caused by *Entamoeba histolytica*).** Typically, liver abscesses result from a partial or complete obstruction of the biliary system with spread of bacteria up the biliary tree. Bacterial translocation from a perforated abdominal viscus into the portal vein or arterial embolization of bacteria via the hepatic artery due to IV drug abuse is also likely in this case. Abscesses can be small and multiple or large and singular.

QUICK CUTS

The preferred treatment of multiple, small pyogenic abscesses is broad-spectrum IV antibiotics for 4–6 weeks. Generally, initial therapy of large, single pyogenic liver abscesses is percutaneous drainage via radiologic guidance.

For proper treatment with antibiotics, it is necessary to obtain a sample culture. Larger abscesses are treated by percutaneous drainage. It is appropriate to leave the catheter in place for 2–3 weeks and give IV antibiotics simultaneously. **If coexisting biliary pathology ex-**

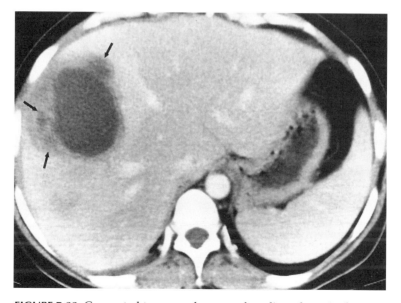

FIGURE 7-32. Computed tomography scan of a solitary hepatic abscess.

ists, the drained abscess fails to improve, or surgery is necessary for any other reason, open drainage is warranted.

▶ *If the patient has a large, single liver abscess and serologies positive for* **E. histolytica,** *how does this alter the proposed treatment plan?*

▶ The treatment for **amebic abscesses is metronidazole** alone; bacterial superinfection may occur with aspiration of uncomplicated amebic abscesses.

CHAPTER 8

Lower Gastrointestinal Disorders

Bruce E. Jarrell M.D., John L. Flowers M.D.

SMALL INTESTINAL DISORDERS

CASE 8.1. ▶ Crampy Abdominal Pain No. 1

A 45-year-old woman has a 3-day history of **nausea and crampy abdominal pain** followed by vomiting and **abdominal distention**. She has had **no bowel movements** in the past 3 days. She has no other significant history except for a previous appendectomy.

On physical examination, mild tachycardia and mild orthostatic hypotension are present. The patient is otherwise normal, **except for the abdomen, which is distended, tympanitic, and mildly tender throughout but without rebound or localized tenderness.** The bowel sounds have a crescendo–decrescendo quality with periods of hyperactivity and periods of silence. There is no stool in the rectum. White blood cell (WBC) count is 14,000/mm³, and hematocrit is 44%.

▶ *What is the most likely diagnosis?*

▶ A small bowel obstruction is the most likely possibility, although a number of other problems such as ileus could have a similar clinical picture.

The next step is to obtain an abdominal radiograph.

▶ *What abdominal radiograph is warranted?*

▶ An obstructive series, which usually includes an **upright posterior–anterior and lateral chest radiograph (CXR) and a flat and upright abdominal radiograph,** is necessary.

▶ *How should you interpret this series (Figures 8-1 and 8-2)?*

▶ This radiograph, which is most typical of small bowel obstruction, shows multiple air fluid levels in the small bowel and no evidence of air in the colon or rectum. There is no evidence of a complication such as perforation or necrosis of the bowel (Figures 8-1 and 8-2).

▶ *What is the patient's predicted fluid and electrolyte status?*

▶ Dehydration due to vomiting and poor oral intake is expected. In addition, the usual metabolic picture involves a contraction alkalosis with hypokalemia, which develops as a result of a multistep process. When H^+ is secreted into the stomach, HCO_3^- is secreted into the plasma. To maintain neutrality, Cl^- is also secreted into the stomach. With vomiting, there is loss of H^+, Na^+, Cl^-, and water, which leads to alkalosis and volume contraction. In response to this state, the kidney preferentially retains Na^+ and H^+ at the expense of K^+, which is lost in the urine.

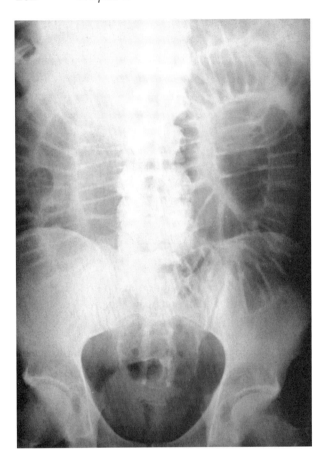

FIGURE 8-1. Plain radiograph of the flat abdomen, showing bowel obstructive. Note the large amounts of air in the supine position. (From McKenney MG, Mangonon PC, Moylan JA [eds]. *Understanding surgical disease: the Miami manual of surgery.* Philadelphia: Lippincott-Raven, 1998: 139.)

▶ *How would you correct this metabolic problem?*

▶ Correction of this deficit requires rehydration with sodium and potassium-containing intravenous (IV) fluids. The alkalosis usually corrects itself after rehydration.

▶ *What is the overall management plan?*

▶ Rehydration and assessment of the patient's overall condition are necessary. It is **usually safe to manage small bowel obstructions with nasogastric (NG) drainage and IV fluids.** This management strategy may last for several days in the majority of cases **in the absence of marked leukocytosis, fever, acidosis, or localized tenderness** and no radiographic findings suggestive of ischemia closed loop obstruction or perforation. **Serial physical examination, laboratory studies, and abdominal radiography** are important parts of the observation plan.

The patient improves over the next several days. Her pain and distention resolve, and her appetite returns.

▶ *What would be the management plan at this point?*

▶ Removal of the NG tube and feeding should begin. If the patient tolerates the food, then discharge is appropriate. No further radiographs or other evaluation is necessary.

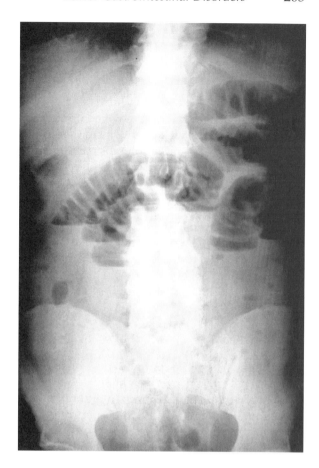

FIGURE 8-2. Upright abdominal radiograph showing bowel obstruction. Note the air fluid levels. Together, Figures 8-1 and 8-2 make up an "obstructive series." (From McKenney MG, Mangonon PC, Moylan JA [eds]. *Understanding surgical disease: the Miami manual of surgery*. Philadelphia: Lippincott-Raven, 1998: 139.)

 QUICK CUTS Many small bowel obstructions **resolve with nonoperative management.**

The final diagnosis is adhesions secondary to the prior appendectomy; this diagnosis is presumptive in that there is no way to prove this specific diagnosis except at laparotomy. The patient should return if symptoms recur.

▶ *Does the initial assessment and management change in any way as a result of the following findings?*

Case Variation 8.1.1. 1-day duration of present illness

▶ You would be more suspicious of a more proximal obstruction in the gastrointestinal (GI) tract. Proximal obstructions tend to have less abdominal distention on physical examination. The management remains unchanged.

Case Variation 8.1.2. No previous abdominal surgery

▶ Adhesions may develop with no prior surgery, but other causes such as a **hernia, small or large bowel tumors, tumors metastatic to the bowel, or inflammatory processes** should also be suspected.

Case Variation 8.1.3. Heme-positive stool in rectum

▶ Increased suspicion of an **obstructing tumor or ischemic bowel** is warranted.

Case Variation 8.1.4. No bowel movements but still passage of flatus

▶ If the patient has no bowel movements but continues to have flatus, this is termed a **partial small bowel obstruction.** The radiographic picture may show the usual findings but also may show air in the colon or rectum. Partial small bowel obstruction is more likely to resolve without surgery and is less likely to have a complication such as ischemia or perforation.

Case Variation 8.1.5. Small amount of diarrhea

▶ This finding is also typical of a **partial obstruction.** You should also suspect a fecal impaction and severe constipation as a cause of the diarrhea. Gastroenteritis is another possible explanation, although the overall picture is not typical of this diagnosis. Examination for fecal impaction is appropriate. You should otherwise manage the patient for a partial small bowel obstruction.

Case Variation 8.1.6. Presence of an inguinal hernia

▶ An inguinal hernia, a common cause of obstruction, may go unrecognized preoperatively in patients who are overweight or have altered consciousness (Figure 8-3). If present, this condition requires **urgent repair and relief of the bowel obstruction** because of the risk of strangulation. Typically, this is performed through a midline laparotomy incision to allow complete evaluation of the bowel and its viability.

Case Variation 8.1.7. A Clark level 4 melanoma that was excised 2 years ago

 Melanoma is the **most common tumor that metastasizes to the intestine.**

Melanoma frequently manifests as a bowel obstruction and can present many years or even decades later. Tumor-related obstructions often **do not resolve with nonoperative management,** and surgery is indicated. Even so, the tumor is often extensive, and surgical resection is not possible. The patient should be explored to establish a diagnosis and to relieve the obstruction.

Even a patient with known tumor may have an obstruction due to another cause such as adhesions. However, if it is an unresectable tumor, the prognosis is poor.

Case Variation 8.1.8. Ovarian cancer that had been previously excised

▶ Ovarian cancer can **recur locally or as peritoneal studding,** resulting in obstruction. Treatment is similar to melanoma (see Case Variation 8.1.7). **Debulking incurable ovarian tumors may improve survival** and warrants consideration.

Case Variation 8.1.9. Metastatic breast cancer treated with chemotherapy 1 year ago

▶ Metastatic breast cancer can also manifest as bowel obstruction. Treatment is similar to that used in Case Variation 8.1.7.

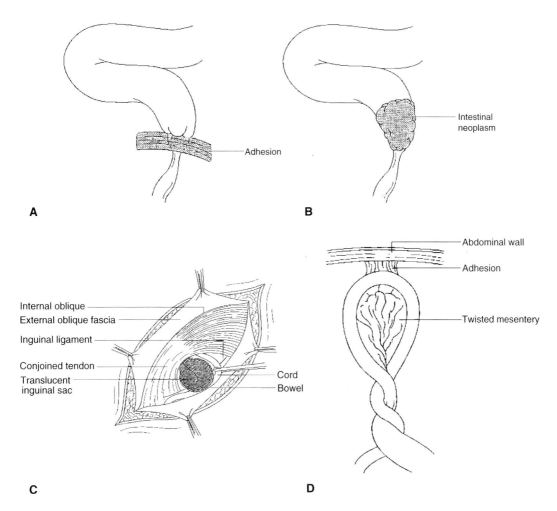

FIGURE 8-3. Common causes of bowel obstruction. **A.** Adhesion, **B.** neoplasm represent the types of simple obstruction that occur most often, and **C.** groin hernia. **D.** Closed loop obstruction. (From Greenfield LJ, Mulholland MW, Oldham KT, et al. [eds]. *Surgery: scientific principles and practice.* 2nd ed. Philadelphia: Lippincott Williams & Wilkins, 1997: 818, 820.)

Case Variation 8.1.10. Localized abdominal tenderness with rebound

▶ **Localized tenderness** with other signs and symptoms of bowel obstruction should alert the clinician that a **potential serious complication** such as a closed loop obstruction, perforation, ischemia, or an abscess is present. Localized tenderness is an **indication that surgical exploration** rather than observation is necessary.

Case Variation 8.1.11. WBC count of 24,000/mm^3

▶ Marked leukocytosis is another indicator of a serious complication and warrants exploration.

Case Variation 8.1.12. Moderate metabolic acidosis

▶ Metabolic acidosis with no other obvious cause warrants suspicion of **ischemic or necrotic bowel.** Depending on the patient's overall status and the radiographic findings, there are two options: (1) urgent exploration, or (2) mesenteric arteriography to check for an arterial occlusive lesion before exploration.

Case Variation 8.1.13. Temperature of 103°F

▶ This degree of temperature, which indicates a bowel perforation or ischemic process with sepsis, warrants exploration.

CASE 8.2. ▶ Crampy Abdominal Pain No. 2

You admit a 38-year-old woman with abdominal findings similar to the patient in Case 8.1. You decide that your new patient has a small bowel obstruction and no evidence of complications. You place an NG tube, correct fluid and electrolyte abnormalities, and plan to follow the progress of the obstruction. With observation and serial examinations, you note that the woman has **partial improvement** with some flatus and one small bowel movement. You decide to remove the NG tube because she has made progress. When you do, she becomes nauseated and distended over the next 6 hours, and it appears that her obstruction has recurred.

▶ *What is the next step?*

▶ The patient, who has failed nonoperative management, should go to the operating room for exploratory laparotomy.

You decide to explore this patient.

▶ *What is the most likely **operative finding**?*

 The most likely finding is an **adhesive band** of scar tissue from the earlier procedure that is occluding a segment of bowel.

▶ This band can be single, affecting a small amount of bowel, or multiple, affecting a large amount of the bowel.

▶ *What operation would you perform?*

▶ Lysis of adhesions to free up the entire section of involved bowel would be appropriate. Typically, you find one band that is highly obstructing, with distended bowel proximally and empty bowel distally. This definitively confirms the diagnosis of small bowel obstruction.

▶ *What is your postoperative plan?*

▶ The patient remains nothing-by-mouth (NPO) with an NG tube for several days until bowel function returns. After she resumes eating, you may discharge her. Most patients who have undergone a lysis of adhesions are cured of obstruction in the short term. Follow-up primarily consists of wound observation to check for any signs of infection. No currently known therapy prevents recurrence of the adhesions or obstruction over the long term.

CASE 8.3. ▶ **Crampy Abdominal Pain No. 3**

You are asked to see a 46-year-old woman in the emergency department who has the signs and symptoms of a small bowel obstruction.

▷ *How would each of the following radiographs influence your decision making?*

Case Variation 8.3.1. Closed loop obstruction (Figure 8-3)

▶ Typically, an adhesive band occludes the inlet and outlet of a loop of bowel, allowing secretions and air to accumulate in the loop and distend it. The loop can become ischemic due to blood flow obstruction from either twisting the blood supply or the adhesive band obstructing the blood supply. The loop can also perforate. The patient should be urgently explored after resuscitation.

On exploring the patient in case variation 8.3.1, you find a single loop of bowel that has twisted around an adhesion, causing an obstruction of the loop. You untwist the loop and cut the adhesion. On reinspection of the previously twisted segment of bowel, you note that it appears viable but edematous and obviously injured.

▷ *What options would you consider in the management of this patient?*

QUICK CUTS

The primary issue is whether the bowel is viable. If observation does not provide a definitive indication, **either resection and reanastomosis or a "second look" operation is necessary.** A "second look" operation is a **planned reexploration 24 hours later** to inspect the questionable bowel. Resection of any ischemic or necrotic bowel followed by anastomosis reestablishes bowel continuity.

▶ Many surgeons prefer this "second look" operation, a proven, safe method of patient management. The major pitfall in management is delaying the second operation. Clinicians may convince themselves that patients are doing well after the first operation and do not need the second surgery. If in fact, ischemic bowel is present, it may not make patients sick for several days, and by the time it is evident, they are much sicker. Thus, the delay significantly jeopardizes patients.

Case Variation 8.3.2. Crampy abdominal pain and free air in the peritoneal cavity

▶ Exploration is necessary to resolve this problem. If the free air occurred during observation for a small bowel obstruction, it is most likely due to either an ischemic perforation or perforation due to overexpansion of the bowel. Thus, part of the process of observation includes monitoring the degree of intestinal distention on the radiographs.

▷ *How might the operative findings differ in the same patient, with free air on abdominal radiograph?*

▶ The operative findings in this patient might be similar to the previous patient with the additional finding of a perforation in the distended loop of bowel. This would most likely require resection.

Case Variation 8.3.3. Crampy abdominal pain and an inguinal hernia

▶ This patient has evidence of a small bowel obstruction and bowel within a hernia sac. Urgent exploration is necessary after resuscitation.

You decide to explore a patient with an incarcerated inguinal hernia and a small bowel obstruction.

▷ *What are the options for operative management?*

▶ Management may differ depending on how sick the patient appears.

- In a relatively stable patient with no signs of systemic illness, exploration through a hernia incision in the groin is appropriate. The surgeon can explore the hernia, inspect the bowel and return it to the peritoneal cavity if viable, and repair the hernia.
- In a patient who appears ill, exploration through a midline abdominal incision is preferred. This allows a more thorough inspection of the entire bowel. If the bowel is questionable or necrotic, either observation until it is viable or resection and reanastomosis are possible. The surgeon may repair the hernia entirely or partially (to prevent immediate recurrence followed by formal repair at a later date when the patient has recovered).

CASE 8.4. ▶ Injury to the Bowel during Lysis of Adhesions

You are exploring a 60-year-old man with a small bowel obstruction that involves particularly dense adhesions. In the process of lysing one, you enter the bowel lumen.

▷ *What are the management options?*

▶ An unplanned enterotomy is an undesirable event when it occurs during lysis of adhesions. If holes are small, primary repair is appropriate. If holes are large, multiple, or involve densely adherent bowel, the segment of affected bowel may require resection.

▷ *What problems might you anticipate in the postoperative period?*

▶ The greatest risk of an enterotomy is a postoperative leak and development of a **small bowel fistula.**

CASE 8.5. ▶ Crampy Abdominal Pain No. 4

You are asked to see a 49-year-old man on the medical service who is recovering from pneumonia. Abdominal distention, nausea, and crampy abdominal pain have recently developed.

▷ *What might be causing the distention?*

▶ Inpatients with multiple other diseases such as heart failure, sepsis, or chronic obstructive pulmonary disease (COPD) may look as if they have a bowel obstruction. This man could have a small bowel obstruction; if this is present, treatment as described in the previous cases is warranted. However, distention has many additional causes, including **paralytic ileus, air swallowing, and constipation.** An ileus is a paralytic state in which the bowel fails to maintain peristalsis. Nausea, vomiting, and abdominal distention develop, and, from a functional standpoint, nothing can pass through the bowel.

*If you are uncertain of the diagnosis of bowel obstruction in a complex situation such as this, is there any way you can **confirm the diagnosis** of a small bowel obstruction without an operation?*

▶ If you are uncertain of the diagnosis or if NG drainage leads to only partial improvement, **an upper GI series with small bowel follow-through prior to the decision to explore the patient** is warranted. If the bowel is obstructed, the barium stops at the obstruction, and this establishes the diagnosis.

Severe constipation should also be evident with this study, although a colon full of stool is usually visible on a plain radiograph of the abdomen. If the barium finds its way to the colon and eventually to the rectum, there is no mechanical bowel obstruction, and surgery will not help. Treatment of constipation involves enemas and disimpaction, not surgery. Paralytic ileus from many causes may also produce obstructive symptoms. It may lead to poor peristalsis and a slow transit time as seen on the small bowel follow-through.

CASE 8.6. ▶ Abdominal Pain No. 5

A 70-year-old woman presents to the emergency department with a 1-day history of nausea, vomiting, and increasingly severe abdominal pain. She has a low-grade fever as well as mild distention of the abdomen, which is nontympanitic and mildly tender. Her pain seems much more severe than her abdominal findings. Her abdominal radiograph shows a nonspecific ileus.

On initial evaluation, the patient is stable, with a blood pressure (BP) of 140/85 mm Hg (her baseline). She has a WBC count of 15,000/mm^3 and no acidosis.

▷ *What is the next step?*

▶ Based on the initial findings, a suspicion of **ischemic bowel** is appropriate. Two approaches are possible.

1. Proceed to the operating room if you think the patient has necrotic bowel.
2. Perform further evaluation prior to a management decision.

In this case, because the patient appears stable and has no strong evidence for necrosis, further evaluation is most likely safe. After **hydration, it is necessary to ensure that the patient is well oxygenated and perfused. Sigmoidoscopy** to establish the diagnosis of colon ischemia and the depth of ischemia if present may be warranted. A negative sigmoidoscopy does not rule out ischemia, and evaluation should continue if ischemia is suspected. The patient could then safely undergo a **mesenteric angiogram** to allow the clinician to diagnose a vascular problem and decide whether surgical revascularization was an option.

The patient undergoes sigmoidoscopy, which reveals a segment of ischemic but not necrotic sigmoid colon, and an angiogram (Figure 8-4). Clinically, she improves after antibiotics and hydration.

▷ *What is the next step?*

▶ She has most likely had an ischemic event that has resolved for the time being but is **likely to recur.** The next episode could be worse, resulting in colon necrosis. You have established an anatomic abnormality on angiogram. Repair of this defect would most likely prevent a recurrence of ischemia. She should undergo semielective **revascularization** of her mesenteric circulation.

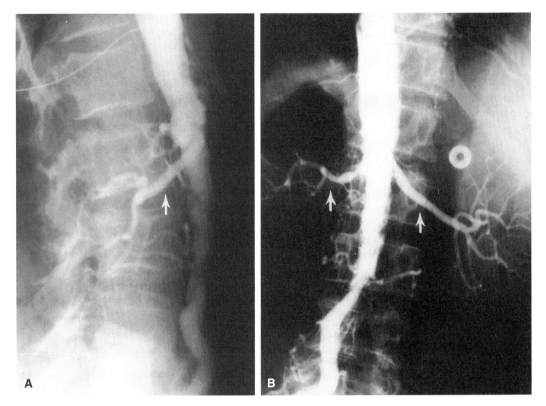

FIGURE 8-4. Superior mesenteric artery occlusion as shown on a mesenteric arteriogram, with (*A*) lateral view and (*B*) anteroposterior view. Note that the lateral view best demonstrates the defect. (From Yamada T, Alpers DH, Laine L, et al. [eds]. *Textbook of gastroenterology.* 3rd ed. Philadelphia: Lippincott Williams & Wilkins, 1999: 837.) The arrows point to the left renal artery and the common hepatic artery, but no SMA is seen.

The patient undergoes revascularization successfully. (Fig 5.23)

▷ *What long-term management plan is appropriate?*

▶ Most surgeons would place the patient on antiplatelet therapy with **aspirin.** In addition, evaluation for the presence of cardiac and peripheral vascular disease is warranted, because it is probably present and will affect her survival. (Case 5.13)

CASE 8.7. ▶ Abdominal Pain No. 6

A 75-year-old woman similar to the patient in Case 8.6 presents to the emergency department. Based on the history and physical examination, mesenteric ischemia is a possibility.

▷ *How would the following findings influence your evaluation?*

Case Variation 8.7.1. Significantly worsening pain over the next hour

▶ Concern that the patient has necrotic bowel should prompt you to proceed to the operating room.

Case Variation 8.7.2. WBC count of 24,000/mm³

▶ Ischemia, necrosis, or perforation with infection should be suspected. Most surgeons would view this as an indication to proceed to the operating room.

Case Variation 8.7.3. WBC count of 2500/mm^3

▶ Your concerns should be similar to those in Case Variation 8.7.2. Elderly individuals, in particular, sometimes respond to overwhelming sepsis with leukopenia, often with a marked left shift.

Case Variation 8.7.4. Moderate-to-severe metabolic acidosis

▶ Your concerns should be similar to those of a patient who has a WBC count of 24,000/mm^3 (see Case Variation 8.7.2).

Case Variation 8.7.5. Atrial fibrillation

▶ **Embolization** to the bowel from a thrombus in the left atrium associated with atrial fibrillation should be suspected. Depending on the patient's overall status, an angiogram of the mesenteric circulation before exploration is a possibility; exploration is most likely necessary.

Case Variation 8.7.6. History of abdominal bruit

▶ A bruit may suggest **stenosis of the coeliac and mesenteric vessels** and consequent ischemia. An angiogram preoperatively could be helpful in the operative planning. By itself, a bruit is not an indication for surgery. In addition, most patients with bowel ischemia do not have bruits.

Case Variation 8.7.7. A hematocrit of 55%

▶ Polycythemia is most likely to be **secondary to severe dehydration,** which could be corrected by rehydration. Treatment involves rehydration. Although polycythemia vera is less common in older patients, it may also occur. It is a **hypercoagulable state,** and like other hypercoagulable conditions, can cause stasis, low flow, and thrombosis in the mesenteric vascular beds. Treatment of primary polycythemia consists of phlebotomy, and hydration. Angiography should still be performed for operative planning. Polycythemia as a secondary event may also be associated with COPD, and depending on the state of the patient, a pulmonary evaluation would be appropriate.

Case Variation 8.7.8. History of congestive heart failure

▶ Congestive heart failure can be associated with low flow states in the mesenteric circulation. An angiogram can confirm a **low flow nonocclusive state** in a suspected combination of congestive heart failure and mesenteric ischemia. Treatment of this condition involves direct mesenteric infusion of a vasodilator such as papaverine and efforts to improve cardiac output.

Case Variation 8.7.9. History of thoracic aortic dissection

▶ Aortic dissection can occlude any vessel orifice in the aorta. The combination of dissection and mesenteric ischemia suggests an occlusion related to the dissection. Angiography allows for diagnosis and the planning of surgical correction.

Case Variation 8.7.10. BP of 90/60 mm Hg (in the emergency department)

▶ The combination of suspected mesenteric ischemia and hypotension may indicate ischemia, causing sepsis and hypotension, or hypotension, causing nonocclusive ischemia due to low flow. Overall patient assessment, measurement of hemodynamics, angiography, or surgery may be necessary to diagnose the problem correctly.

Case Variation 8.7.11. Bloody diarrhea

▶ This suggests an **ischemic segment of colon with necrosis of at least the mucosa** and subsequent sloughing. The next step in evaluation is **sigmoidoscopy** to assess the colon. If full-thickness necrosis is present, **exploration** and resection are necessary. If only **mucosal ischemia** is present, it is possible to avoid resection by **optimizing hemodynamics, antibiotic administration, and close observation.**

Laboratory studies reveal that the patient is acidotic, with a blood pH of 7.14, and a WBC count of 25,000/mm³. You decide that she may have necrotic bowel and that abdominal exploration is warranted.

▶ *How should you manage the following operative situations?*

Case Variation 8.7.12. Necrosis of the left colon

▶ Resection of the colon back to well-perfused edges is necessary. If the patient is stable and conditions are favorable, reanastomosis of the colon is appropriate. If not, a colostomy and Hartmann pouch operation (stapling the distal colon closed and placement back into the abdomen) are warranted (Figure 8-5).

Case Variation 8.7.13. Necrosis of the intestines from the ligament of Treitz to the transverse colon

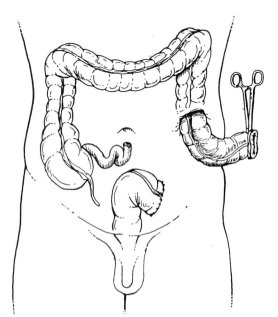

FIGURE 8-5. Hartmann procedure. The proximal bowel is brought out as a colostomy, and the distal bowel is stapled closed and left in the abdomen. (From Lawrence PF, Bilbao M, Bell RM, et al. [eds]. *Essentials of general surgery.* Baltimore: Williams & Wilkins, 1988: 214.)

▶ In the majority of cases, this is a hopeless situation. Management should probably not involve resection, with closure of the abdomen, thus allowing patients to succumb to the illness. Surgical resection and reanastomosis may be appropriate in younger individuals with no other illnesses. Resection of the majority of bowel is appropriate, leaving patients with a short bowel syndrome and the need for chronic total parenteral nutrition (TPN) or small bowel transplantation.

Case Variation 8.7.14. Necrosis of 2 feet of jejunum and ischemia of adjacent bowel

▶ Resection of the necrotic bowel back to healthy edge is necessary, with reanastomosis performed under favorable conditions. If there is doubt as to the viability of the remaining bowel, a "second look" procedure should be performed the next day. In seriously ill patients, another alternative is an ileostomy, which allows direct observation of the viability of the bowel. Because there is no intestinal anastomosis, there is no risk of anastomotic breakdown. Patients may also benefit from postoperative mesenteric angiography to allow assessment of the vasculature.

Case Variation 8.7.15. Ischemia but no necrosis of the intestines and acute occlusion of the origin of the superior mesenteric artery

▶ In this situation, it is desirable to revascularize the bowel. The superior mesenteric artery should be exposed and the occlusion either removed or bypassed. The bowel can then be inspected for viability and managed accordingly. In addition, these patients are ideal subjects for preoperative mesenteric angiography.

Case Variation 8.7.16. Ischemia of the intestines with multiple small punctate areas of necrosis throughout the jejunum and ileum in a patient with a pulse in the superior mesenteric artery and mild chronic congestive heart failure

▶ This suggests either multiple small emboli or a low flow state. Obviously, necrotic areas warrant resection. Postoperative optimization of hemodynamics and a "second look" operation are a reasonable management scheme, although the outlook is poor. Angiography may demonstrate a low mesenteric flow rate.

Case Variation 8.7.17. Viable but ischemic intestines in a patient with a pulse in the superior mesenteric artery but evidence of a low flow rate

▶ The hemodynamic status of this patient should be optimized. Preoperative angiography and recognition of the low flow state would be better treated by optimizing vascular perfusion than with surgery. This would avoid an unnecessary operation.

INFLAMMATORY BOWEL DISEASE

CASE 8.8. ▶ Abdominal Pain No. 7

You are asked to see a 24-year-old woman in the emergency department with crampy abdominal pain, nausea, and vomiting. Past history is significant for a 2-year history of Crohn's disease of the terminal ileum. She initially received treatment with steroids and has been in remission on no steroids for 6 months.

The patient's abdomen is distended, and her obstructive series is compatible with a **small**

bowel obstruction. She has no fever or localized pain and no signs of complications, including no acidosis and only a mild leukocytosis (WBC count = 13,000/mm^3).

▶ *What is the most likely diagnosis?*

▶ The suspected diagnosis is **a small bowel obstruction secondary to a stricture of the bowel involved with Crohn's disease.** Crohn's disease shares some similarities with ulcerative colitis (Table 8-1).

▶ *How could you confirm the diagnosis?*

TABLE 8-1

Inflammatory Disease of the Colon: Ulcerative Colitis and Crohn's Disease

Characteristics	Crohn's Disease	Ulcerative Colitis
Usual location	Any segment of colon; ileocolic disease is most common	Rectum, left colon or entire colon
Anatomic and clinical features	Segmental distribution, skip areas Inflammation with deep fissures Thickened bowel wall, fibrous strictures Abscesses, fistulas Common, continuous rectal bleeding Noncaseating granulomas Mesenteric lymphadenopathy Focal aphthous ulcers Deep ulceration with cobble-stone appearance Strictures	Continuous disease: ~50% involves rectum only, half is pancolitis, 10%–20% involve terminal ileum Mucosal disease: epithelial ulceration and crypt abscesses Rectal bleeding Bowel stricture rate; should raise suspicion of cancer
Radiologic features	Upper gastrointestinal series with small bowel follow-through Enteroclysis study shows "String sign"-narrowing of terminal ileum from edema	Mucosal ulcerations with islands of intact mucosa (pseudopolyps)
Medical management	Steroids for acute flare-ups Immunosuppressive drugs Metronidazole for perianal disease	Steroids for acute disease 5-aminosalicylic acid for prevention of relapse
Natural history	Rarely goes into complete remission Tends toward obstruction, local infection, and fistulas Poor nutrition Increased incidence of carcinoma, but less than with ulcerative colitis	Increased incidence of carcinoma that progressively increases with duration

▶ **Computed tomography (CT) of the abdomen** would be useful because it might demonstrate the area of stenotic bowel in the terminal ileum. It could also help determine the existence of any complications such as perforation or formation of an abscess or fistula. In addition, it might suggest another diagnosis (e.g., tumor).

A CT scan of the abdomen reveals a stenotic segment of bowel in the terminal ileum region and no other suggestions of complications.

▶ *What is the management plan?*

▶ Most surgeons would manage this patient nonoperatively with TPN, bowel rest, and careful observation.

▶ *How would the management change if the CT scan demonstrated an internal fistula between two segments of small bowel?*

▶ The management would remain unchanged. **Management is based on patient symptoms and active problems, not radiologic findings.**

The patient improves over the next week and has return of flatus and bowel movements.

▶ *What is the next management step?*

▶ It is appropriate to begin feeding the patient and discharge her if oral intake is tolerated.

CASE 8.9. ▶ Abdominal Pain No. 8

You are caring for a patient similar to the woman described in the previous case (see Case 8.8). She receives treatment for small bowel obstruction due to Crohn's disease for 3 weeks but shows no signs of resolution of the obstruction.

▶ *What is the next step?*

▶ If an obstruction fails to resolve or recurs after nonsurgical management, consideration of **surgical therapy** is necessary.

▶ *What basic principles should you follow for this procedure?*

▶ It is necessary to observe the following principles:

- **Relieve the obstruction.** This will most likely mean resecting a segment of involved bowel.
- **Preserve as much normal bowel** as possible.

The standard practice is **to resect strictures and involved bowel back to grossly normal-appearing bowel.** In cases of multiple strictures or recurrent exploration for obstruction, an alternative approach involves performance of **stricturoplasties,** which opens a strictured area by cutting the stricture axially and repairing it transversely to dilate the lumen.

You resect a short stricture of the terminal ileum and reconnect the bowel. The patient recovers from the surgery and is discharged.

▶ *What problems should you anticipate in future years?*

▶ Reoperation may be necessary; in some series, the rate of reoperation is as high as 50% for additional problems related to Crohn's disease. Resection of the terminal ileum may also lead to problems, because it is responsible for the reabsorption of bile acids and vitamin B_{12}. Impaired bile acid absorption can **cause diarrhea, depletion of the bile salt pool, and malabsorption as well as oxalate stones.** Gallstones are more common, and vitamin B_{12} deficiency may occur.

CASE 8.10. ▶ Perianal Disease in a Patient with Crohn's Disease

You are asked to care for a 20-year-old woman with Crohn's disease and perianal disease. On examination, you note a tender perineum and inflammation.

▷ *What management is appropriate?*

▶ This patient's condition poses a difficult problem, and surgery is generally indicated only to drain perirectal abscesses, if present. Management of superficial fistulas involves opening the tract. It is more useful to insert setons, which are plastic tubes placed through the fistula that slowly allow the fistula to close for deeper tracts. **Metronidazole** is useful in the management of the majority of patients with perianal problems.

CASE 8.11. ▶ Management of Crohn's Colitis

You are caring for a 19-year-old woman with Crohn's disease that involves the colon.

▷ *How does Crohn's disease in the colon differ from Crohn's disease in the small bowel?*

▶ Crohn's disease of the rectum is an unfavorable, unrelenting problem that often leads to fecal diversion. When the disease is limited to the colon, 5-acetylsalicylic acid compounds have some effect in addition to steroids. When the disease is limited to the small bowel, 5-acetylsalicylic acid compounds have little effect. If surgical complications are present, the most common procedure is a subtotal colectomy and ileostomy if the rectum is involved. If not, then the ileum can be anastomosed to the sigmoid colon or rectum and continence retained.

CASE 8.12. ▶ Complications of Long-Standing Ulcerative Colitis

A 36-year-old woman with a long-standing diagnosis of ulcerative colitis that has been managed medically consults you for advice on long-term prognosis and management.

▷ *What recommendations would you make?*

> **QUICK CUTS**   Individuals with ulcerative colitis are at an **increased risk of developing colorectal cancer,** which is related to the **duration of their illness and the extent of disease.**

▶ The risk for developing cancer is generally low for the first 10 years of the ulcerative colitis (2%–3%), but then increases by 1%–2% a year. Thus, the risk of colon cancer may be as high as 20% in a patient who has had ulcerative colitis for 20 years. The American Gastroenterological Association recommends that patients with pancolitis undergo colonoscopy every 1–2 years beginning after 8 years of the disease. For patients with colitis involving only the left colon, screening colonoscopy performed every 1–2 years beginning after 10 years of the disease is usually sufficient. Suspicious lesions such as strictures, polypoid lesions, and mucosal plaques warrant biopsy. Random biopsies are also necessary, because the colon cancer of ulcerative colitis does not always follow the sequence of polyp to cancer; it may also develop on a flat mucosal surface. If **severe dysplasia** is identified on biopsy, **removal of the colon and rectum is indicated.**

Severe dysplasia is evident on several biopsies taken during a recent colonoscopy.

▷ *What surgical principles are important in dealing with the risk of cancer?*

▶ Procedures that **remove the entire colonic and rectal mucosa are curative,** eliminating the risk of cancer. It is also important to **restore anal continence** and **establish a reservoir function** to allow defecation to occur at convenient times for the patient. In addition, it is necessary to use a procedure that accomplishes these goals in a highly **reliable fashion with low operative risk.**

▷ *What are the newer procedures?*

▶ Treatment of ulcerative colitis has involved several procedures. In the past, total proctocolectomy and ileostomy was the approach of choice. Regardless of whether the patient had a continent ileostomy, no ileostomy was desirable, and normal defecation was preferable. Subtotal colectomy, mucosectomy (removal of the rectal mucosa) and ileorectal anastomosis, which is still sometimes indicated for older patients, then became the procedure of choice. Its failure rate is as high as 20%–50% after 5–10 years.

 Newer procedures, which preserve anal continence but remove the entire colon and rectum, are now in use. Currently, the **most acceptable procedure is total proctocolectomy, which removes the mucosa and thus the risk of cancer, with the creation of an ileal pouch (reservoir) and anastomosis of the pouch to the anus (restores continence) [Figure 8-6].** The reoperative rate is 15%–25%, with an overall failure rate of 5%–15% after 8 years.

▷ *After the patient recovers from surgery, what long-term follow-up is appropriate?*

▶ If all of the patient's colon and rectum are removed, then no further cancer surveillance is necessary, because the risk of colon cancer is eliminated. If residual rectal mucosa is present, proctoscopy at 6-month to 1-year intervals is necessary as surveillance for colon carcinoma. (Any of the usual problems that may occur after complicated surgery could also develop, and she should receive education about these problems.)

She recovers from her total proctocolectomy and ileal pouch–anal anastomosis. She returns 6 months later with fever, blood-tinged diarrhea, and pain on defecation.

▷ *What is the most likely diagnosis?*

▶ The suspected diagnosis is "**pouchitis,**" which is an inflammation of the reservoir from an unknown cause. On endoscopy, a hemorrhagic mucosa with edema and small ulcerations is seen. This problem develops in up to one-third of patients with an ileal pouch.

▷ *What treatment is appropriate?*

▶ Treatment is with **metronidazole,** which resolves the problem in the majority of patients.

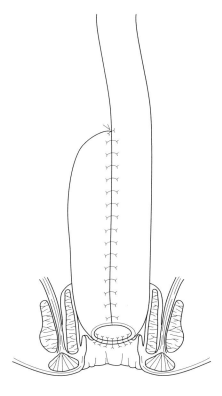

FIGURE 8-6. After total proctocolectomy for ulcerative colitis, gastrointestinal reconstruction is accomplished by creation of an ileal pouch and anastomosis of the pouch to the anus.

CASE 8.13. ▶ Complications of Acute Colitis

A 29-year-old woman presents with a several-month history of abdominal cramps, diarrhea, and a 5-lb weight loss of several months' duration. Bloody diarrhea began this morning. Except for the diarrhea, the history and physical examination are unremarkable.

▶ *What evaluation and management are appropriate?*

▶ The patient may have inflammatory bowel disease. A **colonoscopy** or barium enema is necessary to determine if the pathologic disease is ulcerative colitis, Crohn's colitis, or some other process. Ulcerative colitis typically affects young individuals. This disease usually begins in the distal colon and rectum and can extend proximally to involve the entire colon in about 50% of patients. Typically, it involves only the mucosa initially. It is characterized by crypt abscesses and raised ulcerations.

Crohn's colitis, an inflammatory disorder, may affect any part of the GI tract from the mouth to the anus. It typically occurs as skip lesions and involves all layers of the bowel wall. Severe perineal disease, including fistula, may occur. Treatment for both diseases includes corticosteroids, sulfasalazine, immunosuppressive drugs, and antibiotics.

After institution of therapy, the patient stabilizes and is placed on chronic therapy and followed clinically with a diagnosis of ulcerative colitis. Two months later, she returns to the emergency department acutely ill, with recurrence of bloody diarrhea, abdominal pain, and distention. Her temperature is 101°F, her BP is stable and normal, and her heart rate is 120 beats/min. Her abdomen is distended and acutely tender.

▶ *What is the suspected diagnosis?*

▶ You would be concerned about **toxic megacolon** in a patient with ulcerative colitis and abdominal pain, distention, fever, and bloody diarrhea.

▶ *What is the initial evaluation?*

▶ Routine blood studies and an abdominal obstructive series to rule out bowel perforation are necessary. Many physicians would also perform CT of the abdomen to be certain that there is not an abdominal process such as an abscess or perforation. **A typical appearance on abdominal radiography usually establishes the diagnosis (Figure 8-7).** Sigmoidoscopy may also be helpful but should be performed cautiously.

Her radiographs show a very dilated colon with mucosal edema, and no signs of abscess or perforation.

▶ *How would you initially manage this patient?*

▶ **Provided that the patient is stable, a trial of medical therapy is indicated.** Treatment consists of placement of an NG tube, NPO feeding, TPN, and IV fluids and broad-spectrum antibiotics. Most physicians would also use high-dose **IV steroids.** The acute problem resolves in 50% or more patients with this therapy. **Close observation for worsening signs and symptoms,** with frequent abdominal examinations and radiographs, is necessary, because the mortality of patients who have a bowel perforation from toxic megacolon ranges from 27% to 44%.

▶ *How would you manage the following findings?*

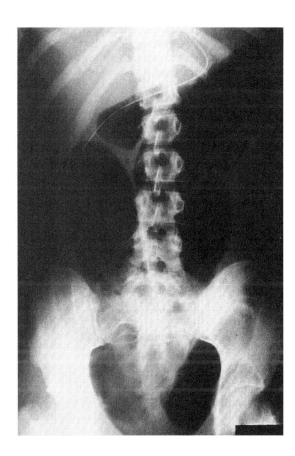

FIGURE 8-7. Plain film of the abdomen showing acute toxic megacolon. (From Greenfield LJ, Mulholland MW, Oldham KT, et al. [eds]. *Surgery: scientific principles and practice.* 2nd ed. Philadelphia: Lippincott Williams & Wilkins, 1997: 1097.)

Case Variation 8.13.1. Free air on upright CXR

▶ The patient should be taken immediately **to the operating room;** this is evidence of perforation. The mortality rate is extremely high when perforation has occurred. The procedure of choice is **ileostomy with** formation of a **Hartmann pouch of the rectum and total abdominal colectomy** (see Figure 8-5). This procedure, which leaves the rectum intact, may not cure the patient or remove the risk of cancer. Therefore, further discussion of management and subsequent definitive surgery is necessary once the patient recovers.

Case Variation 8.13.2. Air in the wall of the colon

▶ This also is a sign of impending perforation, and the patient may require operative intervention. The Hartmann procedure is used (see Case Variation 8.13.1).

Case Variation 8.13.3. Significant improvement over the next several days

▶ With improvement in the patient's condition, emergent surgery can be avoided.

Case Variation 8.13.4. No changes over the next several days

▶ If the patient fails to improve over 3–6 days, surgery is appropriate.

Case Variation 8.13.5. A persistent, stormy course with worsening fever, leukocytosis, and pain

▶ The patient is not responding to medical management, and surgery is necessary.

DISORDERS OF THE COLON

CASE 8.14. ▶ Right Lower Quadrant Pain No. 1

You see a 25-year-old woman in the emergency department for abdominal pain, which has been present for 12 hours. The pain began in the middle abdomen, and it has now migrated to the lower abdomen on the right side. She has anorexia. On physical examination, the only finding is mild pain without guarding or rebound tenderness in the right lower quadrant (RLQ). Laboratory studies and abdominal radiographs are normal, and a pregnancy test is negative.

▶ *What evaluation is appropriate?*

▶ You should be suspicious for appendicitis as well as a gynecologic problem. Part of the physical examination should include rectal and pelvic examinations. **A rectal examination can detect pain in the right pelvis due to retrocecal appendicitis (Figure 8-8).** The pelvic examination can detect ovarian pathology and pelvic inflammatory disease. If these parts of the examination are normal, management as for early appendicitis is appropriate; with hydration, NPO feeding; and observation with serial examinations, including a repeat complete blood count (CBC). Exploration with these mild symptoms is not appropriate. To avoid masking the progression of symptoms, pain medication should be avoided.

Some surgeons would also obtain an abdominal ultrasound to allow visualization of the fallopian tubes and ovaries to rule out gynecologic pathology. Some physicians would perform a CT scan of the abdomen to diagnose appendicitis. Most surgeons do not believe that this is necessary except in complicated cases.

FIGURE 8-8. Position of normally located and retrocecal appendix. **A.** Common location. **B.** Retrocecal location.

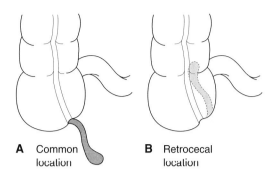

A Common location   **B** Retrocecal location

You decide to observe the patient, and she develops more pain, with localized rebound and guarding in the RLQ (Figure 8-9).

▶ *How does this alter management?*

▶ With further localization and persistence of the worsening pain, this patient fits a picture of appendicitis. Management should involve weighing the risk of appendicitis and perforation with the risk of an operation. Most surgeons would err on the side of a few unnecessary appendectomies rather than a few perforated appendices. The general guideline states that it is safe to perform 10%–15% of unnecessary appendectomies, with the hope that an appendix that ruptures while being observed will be rare.

There are two surgical options.

- Laparoscopy and visualization of the appendix, which is well tolerated and also allows removal of the appendix. However, it offers little additional benefit in terms of postoperative pain, hospital stay, or cost.
- Exploration, which is performed through a McBurney incision and the appendix visualized and removed (see Figure 8-9).

You decide to explore the patient. You find acute appendicitis and perform an appendectomy.

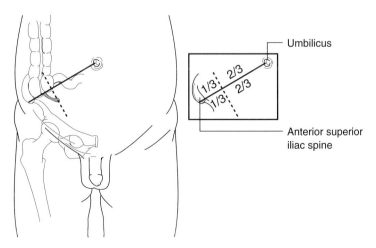

Umbilicus

1/3 · 2/3
1/3 · 2/3

Anterior superior iliac spine

FIGURE 8-9. Location of pain in acute appendicitis. The inset shows the incision that is used for an appendectomy. (From McKenney MG, Mangonon PC, Moylan JA [eds]. *Understanding surgical disease: the Miami manual of surgery.* Philadelphia: Lippincott-Raven, 1998: 318.)

▶ *What is the postoperative plan?*

▶ As soon as the patient will tolerate feeding, it should begin. Discharge is usually appropriate at that time, and follow-up may continue in the office until the patient has made a complete recovery.

CASE 8.15. ▶ **Right Lower Quadrant Pain No. 2**

You are asked to see a woman with a history and physical examination similar to that described in Case 8.14.

▶ *How might the following admission findings change the evaluation and management?*

Case Variation 8.15.1. Dysuria and a urinary WBC count of 10,000/hpf

▶ These findings are suggestive of a urinary tract infection (UTI) and could cause RLQ pain similar to appendicitis, but they could also be secondary to an appendiceal abscess in continuity with the bladder. It would be appropriate to continue to follow the patient for further signs of appendicitis, although these are less likely.

Case Variation 8.15.2. Minimal dysuria and a urinary WBC count of 8–10/hpf

▶ This finding would not be unusual in acute appendicitis, in which the local inflammatory process is in continuity with some part of the urinary tract. It would be appropriate to remain highly suspicious for appendicitis.

Case Variation 8.15.3. Urinary red blood cells (RBCs) too numerous to count

▶ This finding could be a severe UTI or a kidney stone. Most surgeons would perform an intravenous pyelogram or a CT scan without contrast (to examine for a stone).

Case Variation 8.15.4. History of pelvic inflammatory disease

▶ Pelvic inflammatory disease tends to recur. Appendicitis may still develop. A careful pelvic examination is necessary.

Case Variation 8.15.5. Tenderness of cervix on pelvic examination

▶ This finding tends to confirm pelvic inflammatory disease and should prompt gynecologic consultation.

Case Variation 8.15.6. Tenderness of adnexa on the right side

▶ This finding tends to confirm pelvic inflammatory disease, possibly with a tubo-ovarian abscess, and should also prompt gynecologic consultation.

Case Variation 8.15.7. Cervical discharge

▶ This findings tends to confirm pelvic inflammatory disease. It is necessary to stain for gonococcus and obtain gynecologic consultation.

Case Variation 8.15.8. Other family members at home with gastroenteritis

▶ It is probable that this woman has been in contact with family members who have gastroenteritis. Although she could still have appendicitis, gastroenteritis is much more likely, and she should receive treatment for this latter condition.

Case Variation 8.15.9. Voiding symptoms in a 65-year-old man

▶ This patient may have bladder outlet obstruction and a large, distended bladder. With careful physical examination, percussion of the distended bladder may be possible. Treatment involves insertion of a Foley catheter, if possible, and reexamination.

Case Variation 8.15.10. Family history of inflammatory bowel disease (IBD)

▶ The presentation of IBD, which is sometimes familial, may be similar to appendicitis. With suspected IBD, further studies may be appropriate before exploration takes place. CT may show a thickened loop of bowel or enlarged nodes in the terminal ileum. **With certain IBD, exploration is not necessary.** It is appropriate to establish the diagnosis with colonoscopy or barium enema (Figure 8-10). Initial treatment involves steroids, and maintenance therapy involves a 5-acetylsalicylic acid–containing medicine. It is prudent to remember that appendicitis may develop even in patients with established IBD. The addition of steroids to a missed appendicitis will surely create complications and delay or obscure the correct diagnosis of appendicitis.

Exploration of a patient with suspected appendicitis may reveal a normal appendix and establish the diagnosis of IBD (terminal ileitis). Gross findings such as an inflamed ileum,

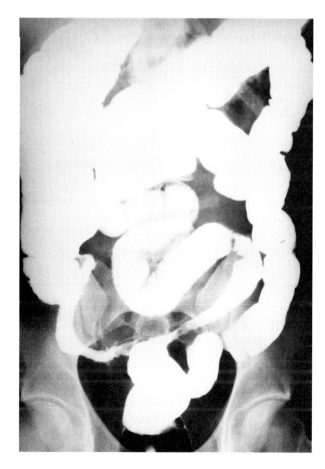

FIGURE 8-10. Barium enema showing the "string sign" typical of a distal ileal stricture due to Crohn's disease. (From McKenney MG, Mangonon PC, Moylan JA [eds]. *Understanding surgical disease: the Miami manual of surgery.* Philadelphia: Lippincott-Raven, 1998: 135.)

fat wrapping of the intestine, a thickened wall, and enlarged nodes are the basis of diagnosis of IBD. Because of the risk of anastomotic breakdown and GI fistula, most surgeons would not biopsy the bowel. It is possible to biopsy a local node, and if granulomas are present, make the diagnosis, but this is not necessary. Most surgeons remove the appendix if it is not involved with the inflammatory process; removal eliminates the possibility of a future diagnosis of appendicitis.

Case Variation 8.15.11. 2-month history of crampy pain and diarrhea

▶ It is necessary to consider a cause other than appendicitis to account for this problem. IBD, constipation, and carcinoma are all possible diagnoses. A more complete workup with imaging and colonoscopy should be considered.

Case Variation 8.15.12. Marked tenderness in the right pelvis on rectal examination

▶ When an appendix is retrocecal or deeper in the pelvis, it may not cause localized pain in the anterior abdominal wall because it is not in contact with the parietal peritoneum. Tenderness on rectal examination may be the best clue to localize this problem. If this is present, the suspected diagnosis is appendicitis, and the patient should go to the operating room.

▶ *How might the following situations change the presentation of appendicitis?*

Case Variation 8.15.13. Advanced age (75 years)

▶ Appendicitis has a bimodal distribution, with peaks in incidence around 25 years and 65 years. Older patients do not typically present with the classical history of periumbilical pain migrating to RLQ pain. Usually, they present with vague abdominal complaints, sepsis, altered consciousness, or failure to thrive.

Case Variation 8.15.14. Childhood (5 years)

▶ Children more often present with appendicitis in which the appendix has ruptured.

Case Variation 8.15.15. High doses of corticosteroids

▶ Steroids can mask most or all signs and symptoms of any inflammatory process. In addition, the body's attempt to "wall off" inflammation and abscesses is blunted with steroids. Therefore, in many cases, the warning signs are absent until perforation occurs and sepsis develops. Thus, a high index of suspicion is necessary. It is essential to be very cautious with patients who are taking steroids.

Case Variation 8.15.16. Pregnancy

▶ Appendicitis may occur during pregnancy. As the uterus enlarges, it pushes the appendix cephalad and laterally (Figure 8-11). Thus, the pain is in the upper lateral abdomen. Appendectomy can be safely performed during pregnancy with minimal risk to the mother or fetus. Early operation is appropriate. A perforated appendix carries a significant risk to both mother and child; peritonitis, not appendectomy, poses the risk.

CASE 8.16. ▶ Right Lower Quadrant Pain No. 3

You see a 28-year-old woman in the emergency department who has a typical history of appendicitis. The pain, which began in the periumbilical region and migrated to the RLQ, is now

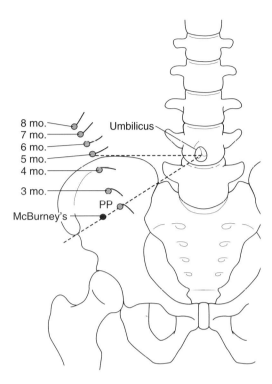

FIGURE 8-11. Location of pain of appendicitis in pregnancy. (From Yamada T, Alpers DH, Laine L, et al. [eds]. *Textbook of gastroenterology.* 3rd ed. Philadelphia: Lippincott Williams & Wilkins, 1999: 1068.)

very localized. There is marked tenderness over McBurney's point. Because her condition has worsened, you decide that exploration is appropriate.

▶ *How would you manage the following operative findings?*

Case Variation 8.16.1. A red, inflamed appendiceal tip with exudate

▶ This represents acute appendicitis, and it is necessary to ligate the appendix at its base and amputate the appendix, leaving a small stump beyond the ligature. Typically, the stump tip is cauterized, but there are many ways to handle the stump. Because the incision is a muscle-splitting incision, the muscle edges are approximated, and the skin is closed.

Case Variation 8.16.2. Acute gangrenous appendicitis with necrosis extending up to the base of the cecum

▶ When the base of the appendix is necrotic, it is still necessary to ligate and amputate the organ using sutures. Most surgeons then bury the base of the appendix into the cecum with a suture to lessen the chance of a "blowout" of the stump. If the cecum also appears involved, it is safe to invert a larger segment of the base of the cecum in most cases. If the cecum is involved in an inflammatory process or mass that seems to originate from the appendix, then a right colectomy is appropriate. This procedure is essential both to remove the necrotic appendix and cecum safely and to not miss a perforated colon cancer.

Case Variation 8.16.3. Perforated appendicitis with localized abscess

▶ It is still necessary to remove the appendix and to incise, drain, and irrigate the abscess. Many surgeons leave a closed drain in the abscess draining to the outside. They close the muscular layers but often leave the skin open because of the high likelihood of wound infection with complete closure (Figure 8-12).

Case Variation 8.16.4. Acute appendicitis with a 1-cm round, moveable mass

▶ This may be a fecalith, which is associated with appendicitis. A seed or similar-sized object was ingested. Fecaliths also are apparent on abdominal radiographs in some patients; this establishes the diagnosis of appendicitis and simplifies the decision to operate.

Case Variation 8.16.5. Normal appendix

▶ It is necessary to **examine for other causes** of the pain. These include mesenteric adenitis, inflammation of a Meckel diverticulum, terminal enteritis, ovarian and fallopian tube disorders, and diverticulitis. Except under unusual circumstances, removal of the appendix is appropriate to eliminate the diagnosis of appendicitis in the future.

CASE 8.17. ▶ Right Lower Quadrant Pain No. 4

A 34-year-old man has suspected appendicitis. On exploration, you find a mass at the tip of the appendix.

▶ *What management is appropriate for the following findings?*

Case Variation 8.17.1. A 1-cm diameter, yellow firm mass at the tip of the appendix

▶ This is most likely a **small carcinoid tumor** (Figure 8-13). Biopsy is not necessary. If the tumor is at the tip of the appendix, less than 2 cm in diameter, and there is no evidence of spread to the cecum or nearby nodes, a routine appendectomy may be performed.

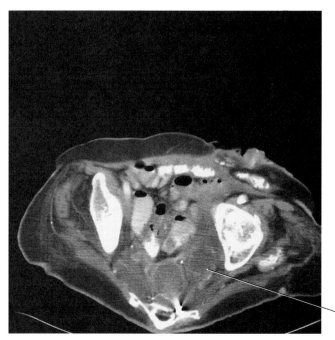

Pelvic abscess

FIGURE 8-12. Computed tomography (CT) scan showing a pelvic abscess.

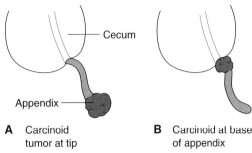

FIGURE 8-13. Location of carcinoid tumors of the appendix.

A   Carcinoid tumor at tip

B   Carcinoid at base of appendix

Case Variation 8.17.2. A 2.2-cm diameter, yellow firm mass at the base of the appendix

▶ This is most likely a larger carcinoid tumor that involves the base of the cecum. Excision, not biopsy, is appropriate.

> **QUICK CUTS**   A carcinoid tumor with a **size of 2 cm or more** or involvement of the base of the appendix or cecum **suggests malignant behavior** and is an indication to perform a **right colectomy.**

An adenocarcinoma may appear similar, although the color is different. Colectomy may require an extension of the incision cephalad for adequate exposure. Reanastomosis of the ileum and colon can usually be performed safely.

Case Variation 8.17.3. A 3-cm round pedunculated mass in the terminal ileum that appears to be obstructing the lumen (Figure 8-14)

▶ **Carcinoid tumors and adenocarcinomas** of the small intestine may manifest as **pedunculated masses** that cause intermittent small bowel obstruction that may mimic appendicitis. It is necessary to remove the involved ileum and regional lymph nodes. Examination of the remaining bowel for other lesions is also appropriate because of a **significant incidence of multiple carcinoid tumors in the bowel.**

The pathology for the appendiceal mass returns as carcinoid tumor.

▷ *What management plan is appropriate?*

▶ For each of the previously discussed carcinoid tumors (Case Variations 8.17.1 and 8.17.2), it is necessary to obtain a baseline urinary 5-hydroxyindoleacetic acid (5-HIAA) and serum serotonin level. The **principal determinants of malignancy involve the biological behavior of the tumor** rather than its histologic appearance, location, and size. Thus,

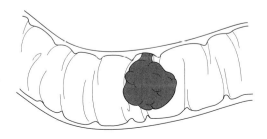

FIGURE 8-14. A pedunculated small bowel carcinoid tumor causing a small bowel obstruction.

long-term follow-up of patients with such tumors is appropriate. If there is a question of recurrence, a **CT scan of the abdomen** and **an octreotide scan,** which localizes to neuroendocrine tumors, is warranted.

CASE 8.18. ▶ Right Lower Quadrant Pain No. 5

A 60-year-old man with a ruptured appendix recovers from surgery and is discharged. One week later, he presents with fever, chills, anorexia, and malaise.

▶ *What evaluation is appropriate?*

▶ This could be a **pelvic abscess or a wound infection** if the wound has closed. If a wound infection is present, drainage is necessary. If not, then most surgeons would obtain a CT or ultrasound study of the pelvis to examine for an abscess. On palpation, a pelvic abscess feels like a tender mass on rectal examination.

You establish a diagnosis of a pelvic abscess. (Fig 8-12)

▶ *What management plan is appropriate?*

▶ Management of a pelvic abscess varies. Many surgeons would **drain the abscess** with a percutaneously placed catheter if accessible, and others would use open surgical drainage. Occasionally, transrectal or transvaginal drainage is appropriate if the abscess is intimate with either of those structures (Figure 8-15). Once drained, an abscess resolves in most cases, and an associated cecal fistula would be unusual.

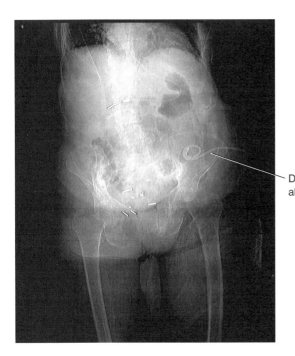

Drain in abscess

FIGURE 8-15. Computed tomography (CT) scan with guided drainage of a pelvic abscess.

MALIGNANT DISORDERS OF THE COLON, RECTUM, AND ANUS

CASE 8.19. ▶ Screening for Colorectal Cancer

A 40-year-old man is concerned about colorectal cancer. He wants to know your recommendations for screening for colorectal cancer.

▶ *What do you tell him?*

▶ Screening is aimed at **detecting cancers that are asymptomatic.** Obviously, **symptomatic patients should undergo evaluation** with an accepted routine, usually including colonoscopy. According to the 1997 recommendations of the American Gastroenterological Association, asymptomatic individuals should undergo the following screening procedure:

- Most persons who require screening for colorectal cancer have the usual or average risk for development of colorectal cancer. Average-risk individuals are defined as asymptomatic patients over 50 years of age who have no other risk factors.
- The most accepted screening test is a **yearly fecal occult blood test (FOBT)** [three samples]. If positive, further workup is warranted. The major drawback of FOBT is its false-negative rate.
- Another accepted screening test involves using yearly FOBT and combining it with **flexible sigmoidoscopy,** first at 50 years of age and then at 5-year intervals. The major disadvantage of this method is that it misses up to 50% of colorectal polyps and cancers, because these lesions occur at a higher level in the colon.
- Many physicians recommend **colonoscopy,** first at 50 years of age and then at 10-year intervals, although its benefit is less proven.

▶ *What risk factors might lead to a modification of these recommendations?*

▶ Some patients have an increased risk for colorectal cancer.

- Individuals with a first-degree relative (i.e., sibling, parent, child) with colorectal carcinoma or an adenomatous polyp should have the same options as average-risk patients, but when they are 40 years of age, not 50.
- Persons with a family history of familial adenomatous polyposis should undergo genetic counseling and yearly flexible sigmoidoscopy. The chance of developing colorectal carcinoma is nearly 100%, so colectomy is the only treatment strategy recommended once polyps are discovered on endoscopic examination.
- Individuals with a family history of hereditary nonpolyposis colorectal cancer should undergo genetic testing and colonoscopy every 1–2 years, beginning between 20 and 30 years of age and every year after 40.
- Patients with a history of a large or multiple adenomatous polyps removed by colonoscopy should have an examination of the colon 3 years after the initial examination.
- Patients with a history of resected colorectal cancer should have a colonoscopy 1 year after the initial operation, as well as screening at 3 years and then at 5-year intervals.

▶ *How might this recommendation change if the patient has previously had a colon cancer removed?*

▶ One of the most productive ways to detect cancer recurrence after primary colon cancer is by **screening with carcinoembryonic antigen (CEA) measurements.** If patients with stage II or III cancer are free of disease, CEA measurement every 2–3 months for at least

2 years is worthwhile. This method detects up to 80% of recurrences. Production of CEA does not occur in up to 30% of recurrences, especially with poorly differentiated tumors or in patients who had normal CEA measurements with their primary cancer. Physical examination, which should be performed every 3–6 months, detects up to 20% of recurrences. Screening for liver function studies is also recommended.

CASE 8.20. ▶ Heme-Positive Stool No. 1

A 45-year-old man is referred to you because he noted bright-red blood streaks on his stool intermittently for the last 3 weeks. Otherwise, he feels fine but complains of occasional constipation. His stools have been normal caliber and brown. The history (past, family, and social) and review of symptoms are negative. On physical examination, the man's vital signs are normal. He does not appear anemic. The head, neck, chest, abdomen, extremity, and neurologic examination are all normal.

▶ *What is the appropriate diagnosis or initial management of the following findings on rectal examination or sigmoidoscopy?*

Case Variation 8.20.1. Several hemorrhoids with evidence of recent injury

▶ With a negative family history of colon cancer and no history of IBD or past history of colon cancer, it is likely that the source of the bleeding is hemorrhoids (Figure 8-16). Conservative management, with sitz baths, stool softeners, and the addition of fiber to the diet, is one option. If the hemorrhoids continue to bleed despite medical management, removal in the operating room may be necessary. External hemorrhoids are surgically excised. Internal hemorrhoids can be excised or banded (Figure 8-17). **Most surgeons still recommend colonoscopy or sigmoidoscopy to absolutely rule out colon cancer.**

Case Variation 8.20.2. Thrombosed hemorrhoids

▶ Conservative management with sitz baths and stool softeners may be appropriate for thrombosed hemorrhoids. However, if individuals present with extreme pain, incision

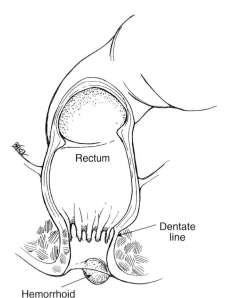

FIGURE 8-16. Location of external hemorrhoids. (From Chen H, Sonnenday CJ, Lillemoe KD [eds]. *Manual of common bedside surgical procedures.* 2nd ed. Philadelphia: Lippincott, Williams & Wilkins, 2000: 163.)

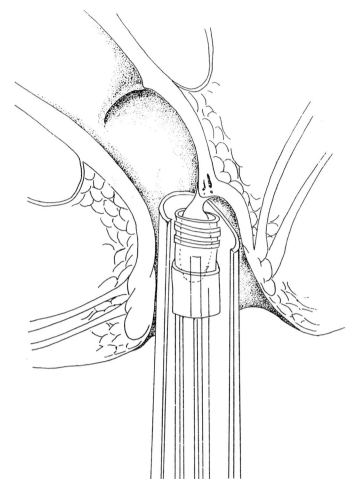

FIGURE 8-17. Banding of internal hemorrhoids. (From Lawrence PF, Bilbao M, Bell RM, et al. [eds]. *Essentials of general surgery.* Baltimore: Williams & Wilkins, 1988: 227.)

and drainage (I and D) of the hemorrhoids may be necessary. Surgeons should be certain to excise the overlying skin and subcutaneous tissue to remove the underlying vessels. It is permissible to leave the skin open. Thrombosed hemorrhoids usually heal well after I and D, with mild analgesics and sitz baths.

Case Variation 8.20.3. Bright-red blood on the glove after rectal examination

▶ Anoscopy or sigmoidoscopy is necessary to determine the cause of anorectal bleeding, which may be due to internal hemorrhoids, a fissure, a bleeding rectal or anal carcinoma, or a polyp. If the lesion is not visualized in the anus or rectum, colonoscopy is required to ensure that a polyp or cancer is not causing the bleeding.

Case Variation 8.20.4. A 5-cm perianal fungating mass

▶ It is important to obtain a biopsy of this mass, because it most likely represents an anal carcinoma. Transanal ultrasound may also be necessary to determine the depth of invasion and help guide your treatment strategy (Figure 8-18).

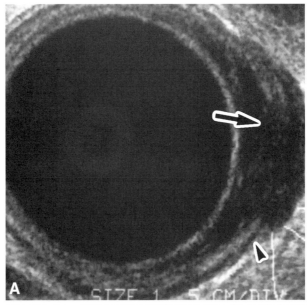

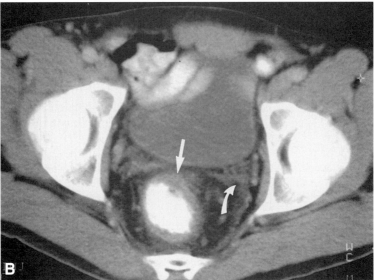

FIGURE 8-18. Rectal carcinoma. **A.** Endoscopic ultrasound (EUS) showing a T3 lesion with tumor extension beyond the bowel wall into the perirectal space. **B.** CT scan showing the same patient. (From Wanebo HJ [ed]. *Surgery for gastrointestinal cancer.* Philadelphia: Lippincott-Raven, 1997: 175–176.)

CASE 8.21. ▶ Heme-Positive Stool No. 2

A 60-year-old woman reports bright-red blood on her stool. On examination, no other abnormalities are apparent. A colonoscopy finds a **polyp in her colon.**

▶ Polyps can either be pedunculated, on a stalk, or sessile, flush with the mucosa (Figure 8-19). It is necessary to remove them because of the risk of adenocarcinoma development.

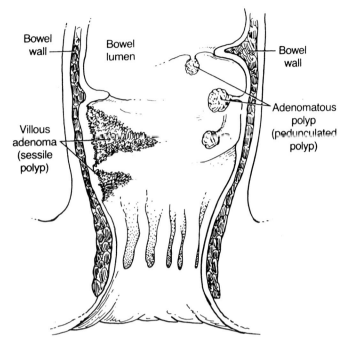

FIGURE 8-19. Types of polyps occurring in the colon: pedunculated polyps versus sessile polyps. (From Lawrence PF, Bilbao M, Bell RM, et al. [eds]. *Essentials of general surgery.* Baltimore: Williams & Wilkins, 1988: 218.)

The supposed histologic progression from formation of polyps to invasive carcinoma may take up to 10 years.

▶ *What is the management, prognosis, and recommended surveillance after treatment for each of the following findings?*

Case Variation 8.21.1. A 1-cm pedunculated polyp

▶ A **polypectomy** is appropriate, which involves placing a snare around the polyp and advancing it down the stalk. The snare is then closed as the polyp is lifted up, with the application of electrocautery to the stalk as the polyp is ensnared.

  The pathology of the lesion determines whether further resection is necessary (e.g., in the case of invasive carcinoma). Repeat colonoscopy after 3–6 months to confirm that the polyp indeed was removed is usually warranted, followed by surveillance colonoscopy every 3 years.

Case Variation 8.21.2. A 5-cm pedunculated polyp

▶ A large pedunculated polyp may require removal in a piecemeal fashion or may necessitate more than one endoscopic session for removal. These patients are at **increased risk for developing colorectal cancers** and should also have surveillance colonoscopy.

Case Variation 8.21.3. A 4-cm flat, sessile lesion

▶ Whether sessile polyps warrant **biopsy or attempted ensnaring** is controversial. One technique involves the injection of saline under the polyp and attempting to ensnare it in its entirety. Usually, sessile polyps less than 2 cm are possible to remove successfully, but those **greater than 2 cm** may require formal **surgical resection.**

Case Variation 8.21.4. Severe atypia in the removed pedunculated polyp (Figure 8-20)

▶ Polypectomy is sufficient therapy. Close follow-up with colonoscopy is warranted.

Case Variation 8.21.5. Carcinoma in situ in the head of a pedunculated polyp with no extension to the stalk

▶ **Polypectomy alone** is sufficient therapy in the case of carcinoma in situ **confined to the head** of a pedunculated polyp, because **no invasion** has occurred through the muscularis mucosa. A bowel resection is not necessary. The long-term risk of lymph node metastasis is about 1–3%. Follow-up is controversial, but the general recommendations are repeat colonoscopy in 3–6 months and then at 12-month intervals.

Case Variation 8.21.6. Carcinoma in the stalk of a pedunculated polyp

▶ The issue of carcinoma in the stalk of the polyp is controversial. Generally, if a **margin of greater than 2 mm** is present, the cancer is **not poorly differentiated** or there is **no vascular or lymphatic invasion.** In such a case, **polypectomy** is sufficient. Otherwise, marking with a tattoo and surgical resection of that segment of bowel is necessary.

Case Variation 8.21.7. Carcinoma in a sessile lesion

▶ The risk of lymph node metastasis is 15% in sessile polyps with **invasive carcinoma.** The local recurrence rate following endoscopic resection is about 20% with no further resection, so **bowel resection** is indicated in this case. Follow-up involves repeat colonoscopy after 1 year.

CASE 8.22. ▶ Heme-Positive Stool No. 3

A previously healthy 55-year-old man is referred to you for recent onset of fatigue and a 5-lb weight loss. He has no other symptoms, and history (past, family, and social) is negative. Review of symptoms is negative. On physical examination, two positive findings are evident: pale conjunctiva and black, guaiac-positive stool.

▶ *What evaluation is appropriate?*

▶ The man has suspected colon cancer, particularly of the cecum or right colon because of the anemia and black stools. Identification, localization, and histology of the lesion is necessary. **Colonoscopy** is best, and it also identifies other colonic pathology such as **second lesions** or other disease processes. Colonoscopy has largely replaced barium enema. A CXR, CEA measurement, and liver function tests are warranted to check for metastatic disease. If the liver function tests are abnormal, CT of the liver is indicated. The current spiral CT scans are highly reliable in detecting liver lesions. Further studies are unnecessary unless organ-specific symptoms are present (Table 8-2; Figure 8-21).

The patient's hematocrit is low (30%), and indices demonstrate a microcytic anemia. Serum iron is decreased. Colonoscopy reveals a 5-cm exophytic mass in the cecum. The remaining studies, including CXR and liver function tests, are normal. A biopsy reveals moderately differentiated adenocarcinoma of the cecum.

▶ *What is the next step?*

▶ **Surgery** to remove the cancer is necessary. There is no need for further evaluation for the cancer, but the patient should undergo a careful medical evaluation to assess operative risk and should also receive supplemental iron preoperatively.

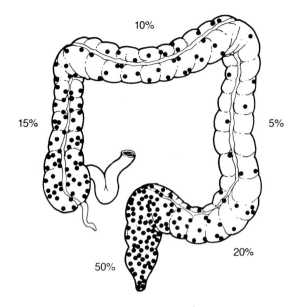

FIGURE 8-20. Common locations of colon cancers. (From Lawrence PF, Bilbao M, Bell RM, et al. [eds]. *Essentials of general surgery.* Baltimore: Williams & Wilkins, 1988: 218.)

▷ *What would you tell the patient about his operative risk and potential complications?*

▶ The operative risk for a routine colectomy is no different from that of most abdominal procedures. Postoperative complications include the usual problems.

- Wound infection, which occurs in approximately 5%–10% of cases. The risk is higher than with a clean operation.
- A small risk of an anastomotic leak.
- The need for a colostomy if an unforeseen operative problem occurs.
- Involvement by tumor or injury to the ureter. This possibility warrants discussion.
- Biopsy or removal of any suspicious lesions for metastasis, particularly in the liver.

The patient agrees to the surgery.

TABLE 8-2

Symptoms of Left-Sided and Right-Sided Lesions

	Right Colon (%)	Left Colon (%)	Sigmoid Colon (%)	Rectum (%)
Pain	80	70	50	5
Bowel complaints	30	50	70	80
Vomiting	30	15	3	0
Bleeding	10	10	30	70
Weight loss	50	15	20	30
Obstruction	10	20	30	3
Abscess/peritonitis	1	2	10	0
Tenesmus	0	0	0	15
Mass	70	50	40	0

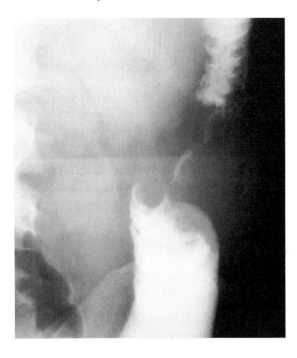

FIGURE 8-21. Barium enema showing an "apple core" lesion in the left colon. (From Wanebo HJ [ed]. *Surgery for gastrointestinal cancer*. Philadelphia: Lippincott-Raven, 1997: 174.)

▶ *What procedures are appropriate?*

> **QUICK CUTS** A **mechanical bowel "prep,"** most commonly using GoLYTELY, magnesium citrate, or another potent laxative, is necessary the day before surgery. **Oral, nonabsorbed** antibiotics are usually given to **decrease colonic bacterial levels,** along with a **single preoperative dose of a second-generation cephalosporin to diminish wound infection.**

▶ A midline incision and exploration of the abdomen is appropriate. The initial step is a **careful assessment of the primary tumor** followed by a careful assessment for **metastasis.** Surgeons should specifically seek metastasis in the small bowel mesentery, the peritoneal surface, the diaphragm, the liver, and other locations. Even if other tumor is present, resection is still appropriate to prevent obstruction and bleeding, even though the procedure is not curative.

A partial colectomy, typically a **right or hemicolectomy,** is warranted (Figure 8-22). In addition to removing the tumor-bearing colon, it is necessary to remove the mesenteric tissue, including the **regional lymph nodes.** Reanastomosis of the bowel involves connecting the terminal ileum to the transverse colon, a so-called ileotransverse colostomy. Closure of the rents in the mesentery prevents internal herniation and obstruction of the small bowel. Closure of the abdomen is the final step.

Suppose you have performed a right colectomy and excision of mesenteric lymph nodes. The remainder of the abdomen, including the liver, is normal.

▶ *What postoperative management is appropriate?*

▶ The patient should remain NPO on IV fluids until bowel function returns. Some surgeons would also use an NG tube. Once the patient can tolerate food, he can be discharged.

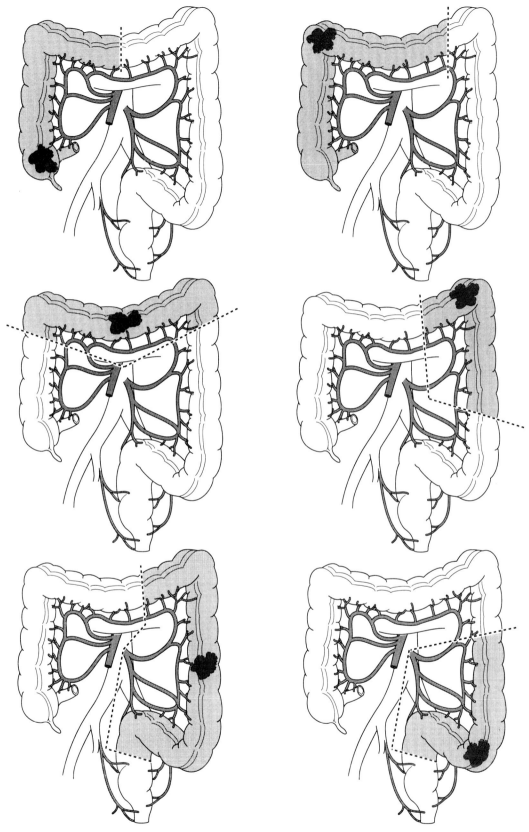

FIGURE 8-22. Types of colectomies performed based on location of the primary tumor. (From Greenfield LJ, Mulholland MW, Oldham KT, et al. [eds]. *Surgery: scientific principles and practice.* 2nd ed. Philadelphia: Lippincott Williams & Wilkins, 1997: 1139.)

On postoperative day 2, the patient's pathology result returns; it reports moderately differentiated adenocarcinoma of the cecum, with tumor penetration through serosa. Nodes are negative.

▶ *How would you stage this colon cancer?*

▶ Staging of colon cancer, which is performed after surgical resection, is based on **depth of invasion of the primary lesion, presence of regional lymph nodes, and distant metastasis.** Two methods of staging are commonly used.

1. Dukes Astler Collier classification (older)
2. Tumor–node–metastasis (TNM) system (more recent)

The TNM system is preferred. This tumor is a T3, NO, MO and represents stage II, or Dukes B classification (Table 8-3).

▶ *Is additional therapy such as radiation or chemotherapy warranted?*

▶ No studies have indicated that adjuvant chemotherapy has an advantage in stage II cancers. The therapy is termed "adjuvant" because it is given postoperatively to patients with no apparent residual disease. Research has found that radiation therapy plays no role. However, the prognosis in stage II cancers is worse for mucus-producing tumors and "signet" ring cell tumors, tumors presenting with bowel perforation, and tumors with venous or perineural invasion. Thus, some physicians would treat these patients with adjuvant chemotherapy.

Studies have shown that **adjuvant chemotherapy for stage III cancer using 5-fluorouracil (5-FU) and leucovorin or 5-FU and levamisole** is effective in reducing recurrence and improving survival by 30%–40%.

TABLE 8-3

Staging of Colorectal Cancer

Stage	Dukes Classification	TNM Stage			Description	5-Year Survival (%)
0	—	T_{is}	N_0	M_0	—	—
I	A	T_1 or T_2	N_0	M_0	Tumor limited to mucosa and submucosa (T_1) or deeper into bowel wall but not extending through muscularis propria (T_2)	>90
II	B	T_3 or T_4	N_0	M_0	Tumor extends through full thickness of bowel wall (T_3) or into adjacent structures (T_4) but does not involve regional lymph nodes	60–80
III	C	Any T	$N_1, N_2,$ or N_3	M_0	Tumor has metastasized to regional lymph nodes at various levels	20–50
IV	D	Any T	Any N	M_1	Liver or other distant metastasis	<5

The patient wants to know your plans for follow-up for recurrence of the cancer.

▶ *What do you tell him?*

▶ It is necessary to follow a patient who has undergone a curative resection for **local recurrence at the anastomosis, metastasis to the liver, distant metastasis, and occurrence of a second primary colon cancer.** Approximately 70% and 90% of recurrences become detectable by 2 and 4 years, respectively. Repeat colonoscopy at 6 months and then at 12-month intervals is necessary. More frequent monitoring of CXR, CEA, and liver function tests is essential. A rising CEA, which is 70% accurate in predicting recurrence, should prompt CT of the abdomen to examine for metastasis.

CASE 8.23. ▶ Heme-Positive Stool No. 4

You see a 62-year-old woman who has heme-positive stools. You suspect colon cancer.

▶ *How would the following additional findings change the evaluation of this patient?*

Case Variation 8.23.1. RLQ mass

▶ A **mass palpable** in the RLQ suggests a **large tumor** that may be invading local structures such as the ureter. CT would help assess involved structures.

Case Variation 8.23.2. Intermittent constipation and diarrhea

▶ This common symptom of colon cancer suggests the existence of a **higher-grade obstructive lesion,** which is perhaps more likely on the left side of the colon. Management may be more difficult, because patients may not be able to undergo a bowel "prep" preoperatively due to the urgency of the obstruction. Surgeons should attempt to perform a curative procedure, although the prognosis is worse for obstructive cancers.

Case Variation 8.23.3. Crampy abdominal pain

▶ Crampy abdominal pain also suggests intermittent obstruction. See Case Variation 8.23.2 for more information.

Case Variation 8.23.4. Family history that is positive for colon cancer

▶ A family history of colon cancer carries a higher risk of development of cancer. Genetic syndromes known to be associated with colon cancer include Lynch's syndrome and Gardner's syndrome.

Case Variation 8.23.5. Previous colonoscopy that demonstrated multiple polyps

▶ If the previous colonoscopy did not miss an additional lesion, it is unlikely that a new colon cancer has developed during the subsequent period. Epidemiologic data suggest that the **progression from polyp to invasive cancer** takes approximately 10 years. However, more recent data suggest another possibility: Cancer may arise from nonadenomatous tissue. The patient should still undergo repeat colonoscopy to establish a diagnosis.

Case Variation 8.23.6. Scleral icterus

▶ Scleral icterus could be due to a number of reasons unrelated to the tumor, but the likelihood that it is tumor-related is high. Potential tumor-related causes include **metastatic tumor replacement of the liver** and a metastasis strategically located that blocks the bile duct. An ultrasound or CT scan of the liver would help assess these possibilities.

Case Variation 8.23.7. A younger (22 years of age) instead of an older adult (55 years)

▶ In younger individuals, benign diagnoses such as inflammatory conditions are more likely. However, the scenario of colon cancer may still occur in young patients, and thus, a complete workup is necessary.

CASE 8.24. ▶ Operative Findings in Colon Cancer No. 1

You perform a colectomy for colon cancer in a 58-year-old man.

▷ *How do the following pathologic findings change the planned therapy?*

Case Variation 8.24.1. Penetration of the primary tumor into the nearby abdominal wall

▶ The portion of the abdominal wall is resected as part of a more radical procedure. Involvement of adjacent structures **makes the T classification in the TNM system a T_4 lesion and worsens the prognosis by 3%–5% over 5 years.**

Case Variation 8.24.2. Positive lymph nodes recognized at surgery

▶ The operation proceeds unchanged; however, the surgeon attempts to remove all involved nodes.

Case Variation 8.24.3. Positive lymph nodes recognized by the pathologist 2 days later

▶ The hemicolectomy remains the procedure of choice, and no further operative procedures are necessary. The patient has stage III disease and is eligible for adjuvant chemotherapy with 5-FU and levamisole.

Case Variation 8.24.4. A 1-cm lesion palpable on the surface of the liver at surgery

▶ A small lesion on the liver, particularly at the edge of the liver, usually can be wedged out as a total excision. If the lesion were contiguous with vital structures such as a hepatic vein, then a biopsy of the lesion would be appropriate, with no further therapy during that operation.

Case Variation 8.24.5. An 8-cm lesion palpable on the surface of the liver at surgery

▶ Larger lesions should not be resected when discovered at the time of surgery. A major liver resection increases both the intraoperative risk of bleeding and the overall complexity and duration of the operation. Many general surgeons also are not experienced hepatic surgeons. Postoperative complications such as infection and bile leakage are possible; none of these have usually been discussed with the patient preoperatively. Most surgeons would complete the colectomy, biopsy the liver lesion, and plan resection at a later date after further evaluation.

Case Variation 8.24.6. A poorly differentiated tumor histology obtained preoperatively from the primary tumor

▶ The operative procedure is unchanged. Factors associated with a worsened prognosis include poorly differentiated tumors, especially mucin-producing and "signet cell" tumors, tumors with venous or perineural invasion, and tumors presenting with perforation.

Case Variation 8.24.7. A 2-cm nodule apparent on CXR

▶ The nodule warrants evaluation by chest CT and biopsy by percutaneous needle biopsy if suspicious for cancer. Many surgeons would include an abdominal CT to gain further information for operative planning. A metastatic lung nodule makes a curative operation very unlikely. Therefore, the colectomy does not need to be as extensive as it might be with curable cancer. However, it is still necessary to perform a colectomy to remove the primary tumor to manage it locally and prevent further blood loss or bowel obstruction.

CASE 8.25. ▶ Complications of Postoperative Colectomy

Most patients who undergo an elective colectomy have an uneventful recovery in the postoperative period.

▷ *How would you manage the following situations?*

Case Variation 8.25.1. The patient becomes distended and vomits feculent material on the third postoperative day.

▶ This suggests that the patient's GI tract is not functional, which could be secondary to a persistent, postoperative ileus or a mechanical obstruction. Feculent vomiting results from bacterial overgrowth in the stomach and proximal small bowel due to failure to propel food and secretions distally. NPO feeding and IV fluids are appropriate, along with insertion of an NG tube. Evaluation of the abdomen with an obstructive series is necessary. The concerns are two: **(1) leakage from the anastomosis has occurred, causing a persistent ileus, or (2) a mechanical obstruction due to adhesions, an internal hernia, or an obstructed anastomosis.** These developments may require CT or a small bowel series to identify the problem, depending on the postoperative day and condition of the patient.

Case Variation 8.25.2. A reddened, fluctuant area develops at the inferior aspect of the wound.

▶ This suggests a **wound infection.** Management usually involves opening the involved portion of the wound down to the fascia, with inspection of the fascia with the finger to determine whether it is intact. Local wound care is sufficient for most uncomplicated wound infections.

Case Variation 8.25.3. Feculent material drains from the inferior aspect of the wound.

▶ This suggests a wound infection caused by an **anastomotic leak** that has spontaneously drained (necessitated) to the skin. **NPO feeding and IV fluids** are usually sufficient for most colon fistulas, the majority of which **will close with this therapy.** A CT scan of the abdomen determines whether there is **an undrained collection,** which needs draining either operatively or percutaneously, which is preferable. If any doubt about the **patency of the anastomosis** exists, a gentle Gastrografin enema or colonoscopy may be appropriate, although most surgeons would be very hesitant to do this early in the course of a fistula with a fresh anastomosis. A fistula with a distal obstruction due to a nonpatent anastomosis (i.e., obstructed) will not close. It requires operative revision and an ileostomy proximally to divert the fecal stream.

Case Variation 8.25.4. The patient returns to the hospital 10 days postoperatively with a temperature of 104°F and abdominal pain in the RLQ.

▶ This suggests an **abscess,** most likely in the right paracolic gutter or pelvis. Most commonly, diagnosis is by CT, and management is by percutaneous drainage. Concern regarding anastomotic leakage is also present, and the previously discussed management is appropriate (see Case Variation 8.25.3).

Case Variation 8.25.5. The patient returns in 6 months with crampy abdominal pain, decreased stool caliber, and constipation.

▶ These symptoms could represent **anastomotic recurrence** of the cancer, as well as a **stricture** at the anastomosis. Strictures usually result from excessive scar formation due to inadequate blood supply to the anastomosed segments. It is also possible that a second obstructing cancer, which could have been missed at initial surgery, is causing the symptoms. **Colonoscopy** usually establishes the diagnosis.

CASE 8.26. ▶ Heme-Positive Stool No. 5

A 55-year-old man presents with constipation, rectal bleeding, and a feeling of fatigue. On examination, you find a constricting hard lesion 4 cm from the anal verge. Biopsy indicates adenocarcinoma of the rectum.

▷ *What further evaluation is necessary before making a decision regarding treatment?*

▶ The following studies are necessary. **Colonoscopy** is necessary initially for visualization of the entire colon to rule out the presence of synchronous lesions. If no other lesions are found, an evaluation **determines the depth of invasion** that is warranted; this is an important prognostic sign. **Transrectal ultrasound** is useful to determine rectal wall invasion. **CT** or MRI is appropriate to determine **whether adjacent structures,** including the prostate, bladder, and ureters, **are involved.** CT scans may show **distant involvement** in the liver, as well as enlarged lymph nodes. A CXR and a CEA level are also warranted before surgery.

After studying this patient, you find that he has a circumferential lesion at 4 cm that it is not fixed to the surrounding tissues. The transrectal ultrasound indicates that the tumor is limited to the bowel wall, and no regional or local lymph nodes are evident. The CT scan shows a normal liver and no other abnormalities. The CXR is normal. The CEA is elevated, and all other laboratory studies are normal.

▷ *What is the next step?*

▶ Resection of the tumor is warranted, assuming that the patient is an acceptable operative risk. Preoperative neoadjuvant therapy is not useful in this early-stage lesion.

▷ *What procedure is appropriate?*

▶ Most surgeons would recommend an abdominoperineal resection, which involves excision of the entire rectum with the creation of a permanent colostomy (Figures 8-23 and 8-24). In addition, this procedure removes local lymph nodes.

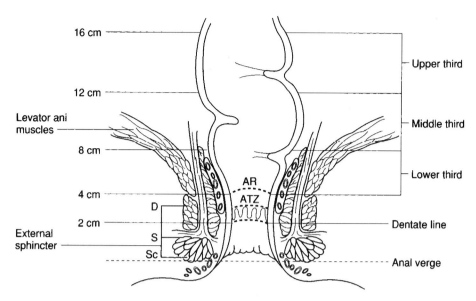

FIGURE 8-23. Local anatomy of the rectum as it relates to abdominoperineal resection. D = deep; S = superficial; Sc = subcutaneous; AR = anorectal ring; ATZ = anal transition zone. (From Greenfield LJ, Mulholland MW, Oldham KT, et al. [eds]. *Surgery: scientific principles and practice.* 2nd ed. Philadelphia: Lippincott Williams & Wilkins, 1997: 1140.)

▷ *The patient's tumor metastasizes to what nodal locations and other organs?*

▶ Rectal carcinomas spread by direct extension and lymphatics. Lymphatic spread parallels the superior hemorrhoidal vessels and includes the **internal iliac nodes, sacral nodes, and inferior mesenteric nodes.** Lesions less than 5 cm from the anal verge can **also spread** locally and to the **inguinal nodes,** and this should be determined preoperatively. Distal organ involvement most commonly includes the liver or adjacent structures.

▷ *What information should the patient receive about the perioperative risks and complications of abdominoperineal resection?*

▶ Several specific complications relate to abdominoperineal resection. Because the sympathetic plexus of nerves is located around the rectum, the chance of **impotence** following the procedure is high; it is estimated to be about 50%. It is essential that the patient be told prior to surgery about the possibility of impotence. There is also a chance that **bladder function** may be impaired following surgery. Generally, Foley catheters remain in place for 1 week after proctectomy. Other intraoperative risks include massive venous bleeding from the presacral space and injury to the ureter. Finally, a variety of colostomy complications, including retraction, prolapse, stricture, and obstruction, may occur.

Your patient decides to proceed with an abdominoperineal resection.

▷ *What are the essential elements of this procedure?*

▶ The basic principle of the abdominoperineal resection is removal of the entire rectum in continuity with its vascular and lymphatic supply. It is necessary to mark a colostomy site preoperatively, and the surgeon usually chooses the lower left quadrant. Placement of the

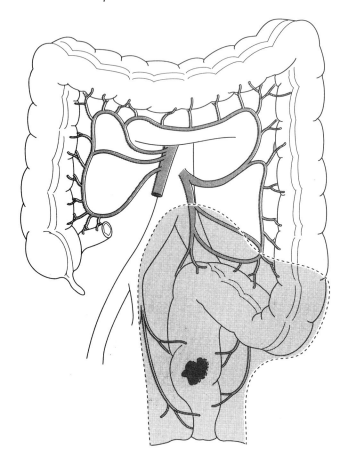

FIGURE 8-24. Bowel removal in abdominoperineal resection. (From Greenfield LJ, Mulholland MW, Oldham KT, et al. [eds]. *Surgery: scientific principles and practice.* 2nd ed. Philadelphia: Lippincott Williams & Wilkins, 1997: 1140.)

patient in the lithotomy position allows both the abdominal and pelvic dissections to be performed simultaneously.

The rectum is dissected away from the surrounding tissues, attempting to avoid injury to the nerves and urinary tract. Mesenteric lymph nodes are removed with the specimen. The colon is divided at the junction of the descending colon and the sigmoid colon, and the specimen is removed. An end colostomy is performed. The perineal wound is either closed or packed with gauze.

Pathology on the specimen returns as well-differentiated adenocarcinoma of the rectum with extension into the bowel wall to the level of the muscularis propria but not involving the serosa.

▶ *What stage is this tumor (Figure 8-25)?*

▶ This tumor is a stage I cancer.

▶ *What other factors in this primary tumor are important in the prognosis of this patient, who has no positive lymph nodes?*

▶ A poor prognosis is associated with poor histologic differentiation of the tumor, elevated CEA level, bowel perforation, and aneuploidy.

▶ *What is the appropriate management plan for this patient once he has recovered from the surgery?*

▶ Management is similar to any patient with colon cancer.

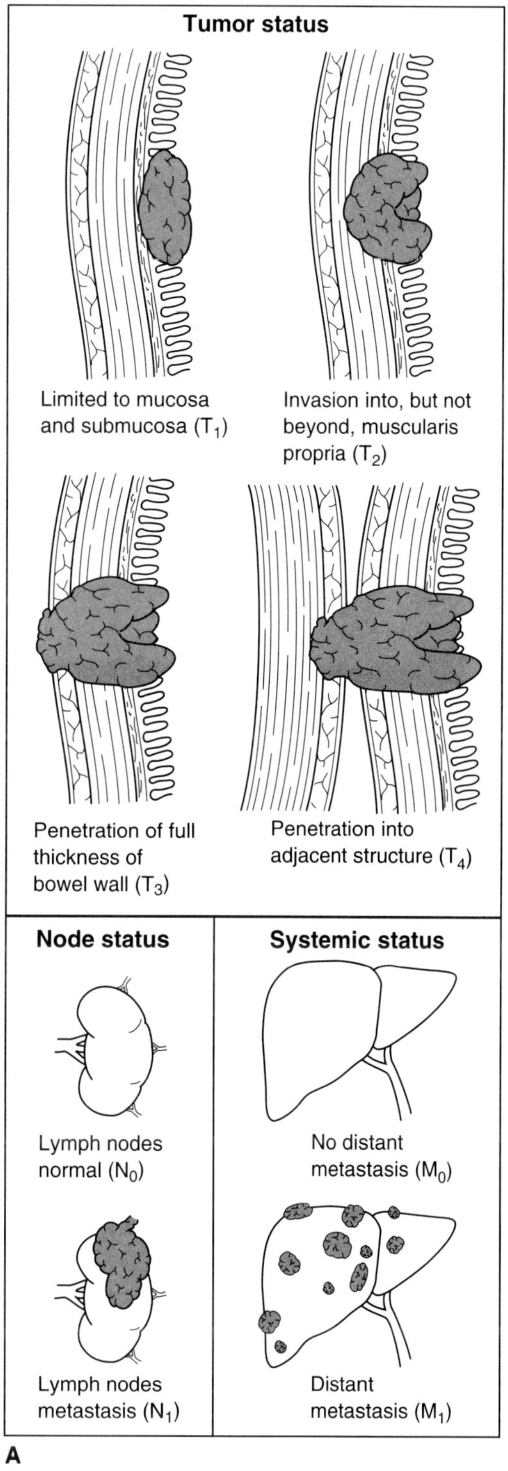

FIGURE 8-25. A. Staging of colon carcinoma. (*continued*)

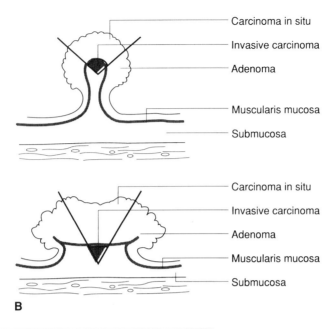

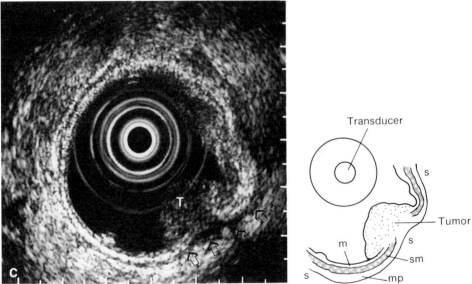

FIGURE 8-25. (*continued*) **B.** diagram showing distinction of carcinoma in situ and invasive malignancy of the colon. (From Greenfield LJ, Mulholland MW, Oldham KT, et al. [eds]. *Surgery: scientific principles and practice.* 2nd ed. Philadelphia: Lippincott Williams & Wilkins, 1997: 1132.) **C.** Stage T1 rectal carcinoma on endorectal ultrasound. (From Wanebo HJ [ed]. *Surgery for gastrointestinal cancer.* Philadelphia: Lippincott-Raven, 1997: 174.)

CASE 8.27. ▶ Heme-Positive Stool No. 6

You are asked to evaluate a 62-year-old man with rectal cancer.

▶ *How would the level of the lesion from the anal verge affect operative management?*

▶ It is possible to remove most rectal cancers that lie more than 5 cm proximal to the anal verge safely using an anterior approach. If the lesion is closer to the anal verge, abdominoperineal resection is necessary, because lesions within 5 cm of the anal verge have lateral margins of resection that include the anal sphincter mechanism. Removal or disabling of this mechanism results in incontinence, obviously not a desirable situation.

Several additional factors that influence this practice mostly relate to the type of lesion.

QUICK CUTS   **Local recurrence of rectal carcinoma is a common mode of failure. Therefore,** ample, clear margins are mandatory at the initial procedure.

For distal resection of rectal carcinomas, recommended margins are 2 cm for well- or moderately well-differentiated lesions. The recommendation is 5 cm for poorly differentiated, anaplastic, or "signet cell" carcinomas. Lesions with large lateral components also require a wider margin of resection (Figure 8-26). Thus, abdominoperineal resection is more likely for lesions larger than 5 cm. Rectal cancers that involve the regional lymph nodes (stage III) or high-risk stage II tumors also require postoperative adjuvant chemotherapy that is similar to that used with colon cancer.

▷ *When might preoperative radiation therapy be a consideration?*

▶ If lesions are large and bulky or extend outside the bowel wall into the surrounding tissue, the rate of local recurrence is higher. Thus, management usually involves **preoperative irradiation** with 45 Gy (4500 rad) over a period of several weeks to reduce local recurrence. In many cases, the radiation is so effective that the original tumor has disappeared at the time of resection.

▷ *What alternatives do patients have if they do not agree to colostomy?*

▶ The procedures previously described in this case are the standard methods for treatment of rectal cancer, but there are two additional therapeutic options.

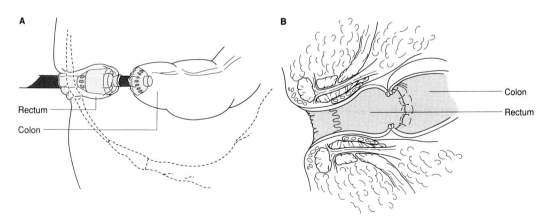

FIGURE 8-26. Low anterior bowel resection, showing (*A*) staple technique, (*B*) suture technique. (From Greenfield LJ, Mulholland MW, Oldham KT, et al. [eds]. *Surgery: scientific principles and practice.* 2nd ed. Philadelphia: Lippincott Williams & Wilkins, 1997: 1141.)

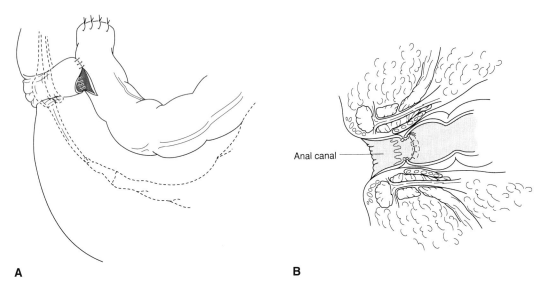

A   **B**

FIGURE 8-27. A. Sphincter-preserving proctectomy. **B.** Coloanal anastomosis. (From Greenfield LJ, Mulholland MW, Oldham KT, et al. [eds]. *Surgery: scientific principles and practice.* 2nd ed. Philadelphia: Lippincott Williams & Wilkins, 1997: 1141.)

- One approach is **sphincter-preserving proctectomy** (Figures 8-27 and 8-28). A rationale for this procedure relates to a change in thinking about the distal resection margin necessary to cure a patient with cancer. Previously, experts believed a 5-cm distal margin was necessary, but more recently, studies have found that a 2-cm margin is adequate for well-differentiated cancers. Additional improvements have occurred in the operative approach and with the preservation of anal continence. Combined with preoperative radiation to the rectum and a temporary diverting ileostomy to allow anastomotic healing to occur, these procedures have become commonplace.
- A second approach involves local resection of rectal tumors. In these cases, one method involves dilation of the anal sphincter and resection of the tumor. Another method involves using a transsacral approach to the rectum, which allows a sleeve resection of

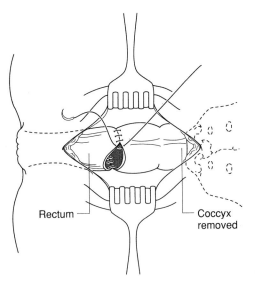

FIGURE 8-28. Transsacral resection of a rectal cancer. (From Greenfield LJ, Mulholland MW, Oldham KT, et al. [eds]. *Surgery: scientific principles and practice.* 2nd ed. Philadelphia. Lippincott Williams & Wilkins, 1997: 1141.)

the tumor-bearing bowel (see Figure 8-28). Both approaches are particularly useful for small tumors in high medical risk patients.

▶ *How does abdominoperineal resection differ in women?*

▶ In female patients with anterior rectal wall carcinoma, removal of the posterior wall of the vagina as the anterior margin of the resection is appropriate. Surgeons should be careful not to denervate the urethra. Closure of the vagina may then occur.

A patient undergoes a curative resection with an abdominoperineal resection.

▶ *What evaluation and management is appropriate for a new 0.5-cm lesion in the perineum?*

▶ **Biopsy** of the lesion is necessary. If the biopsy shows carcinoma, the patient should undergo a repeat CT scan, CEA level, and colonoscopy to determine the extent of the lesion and whether there are other lesions. Typically, a multidisciplinary approach using chemotherapy radiation and surgery is appropriate for treatment of a recurrence. In general, recurrent cancer has a poor prognosis.

▶ *What evaluation and management are appropriate for pelvic pain?*

▶ If this occurs in the early postoperative period, it may be secondary to **operative nerve injury or infection.** If it occurs later, it is necessary to rule out **local recurrence** of the tumor by physical examination and CT of the pelvis.

CASE 8.28. ▶ Metastasis in Colorectal Cancer

You perform a curative resection for colon cancer in a 49-year-old man who has stage II cancer. You decide to follow him with serial CEA measurements and yearly colonoscopy. Initial CEA values are low and stable, and repeat colonoscopy is normal at 1 and 2 years. During the next visit, the man's CEA is now significantly elevated.

▶ *What evaluation is appropriate?*

▶ A **CXR and CT of the abdomen** to look for metastasis are warranted. A repeat **colonoscopy** may be necessary, depending on when the last one was performed.

The patient's evaluation is negative except for a new 2-cm lesion in the right lobe of the liver.

▶ *What further evaluation and management is appropriate?*

▶ The patient is a candidate for **surgical resection** if he has **no extrahepatic demonstrable metastatic** cancer, **no local recurrence** of the primary cancer, an acceptable anesthetic risk from the cardiopulmonary standpoint, and a lesion that is **in a surgically resectable location.** The more current spiral CT scans and MRI studies are reliable; they demonstrate additional hepatic metastasis in more than 80% of cases. These tests are necessary if the initial CT scan is inadequate. A CXR and colonoscopy are appropriate, but further workup is unnecessary unless the patient has additional symptoms or findings.

Typically unresectable lesions are either multiple lesions in both lobes, lesions intimate with vascular structures (e.g., hepatic veins, portal vein), lesions invading local structures (e.g., the diaphragm), or lesions occurring in cirrhotic livers. Cirrhosis increases the perioperative risk as a result of limited hepatic reserve following resection, as well as technical difficulties in transecting a fibrotic liver (see Table 7-2).

▷ *What is appropriate to tell the patient about his prognosis and the variables that affect it?*

▶ Resection of liver lesions is associated with the best survival when compared to other treatment modalities, and it should be recommended if the lesion is resectable. **Patients with solitary lesions that are resected have a survival as high as 33% at 5 years.** The survival of individuals with one to four lesions is 15%, and unresectable lesions have a survival of close to 0%. Most studies have demonstrated that the following factors affect prognosis after liver resection for colon cancer metastasis.

You decide to remove the liver lesion surgically.

▷ *What procedure and follow-up do you recommend?*

▶ It is acceptable to resect a lesion with **a formal hepatic lobectomy or segmentectomy or with a nonanatomic wedge resection, as long as a greater than 1-cm margin is obtained.** The principal reasons for unresectability intraoperatively are inability to resect the lesion due to its location, multiple lesions, or evidence for metastasis outside the liver. The major surgical risk relates to uncontrollable hemorrhage related to technical problems. With most experienced hepatic surgeons, the operative mortality is approximately 1%. Recurrence may assume the form of distant metastasis or occur at the original site of resection. CXR, serial CEA measurements, and abdominal ultrasound or CT are used to check for recurrence.

▷ *What management is appropriate for unresectable liver metastasis?*

▶ There are other options for management of unresectable lesions with local methods. Most involve some form of ablation therapy with freezing–thawing techniques (cryotherapy), injection of absolute ethanol, or destruction with radio-frequency waves (**R-F ablation**). Destruction of lesions may also occur angiographically by **chemoembolization.** The hepatic artery is catheterized, and thrombotic substances such as Gelfoam are saturated with chemotherapy and injected into the region of metastasis. Most of these methods are in various stages of clinical trials.

CASE 8.29. ▶ Heme-Positive Stool No. 7

A 45-year-old man presents with rectal bleeding. On examination, you find a hard lesion that involves the anal verge. Biopsy of the lesion indicates squamous cell carcinoma of the anus.

▷ *What regional nodes are most likely to be involved with metastasis?*

▶ Squamous cell carcinomas (also called epidermoid carcinoma) are the most common tumor of the anal canal. Because the symptoms are nonspecific (e.g., bleeding, drainage, pain, pruritus), the diagnosis is often delayed while the patient is treated for a benign process. The diagnosis is made by biopsy. Squamous cell carcinomas commonly metastasize to the inguinal lymph nodes, but they also metastasize to the superior rectal lymph nodes in up to 50% of patients.

▷ *What staging system is best?*

▶ The TNM system is used for staging, and treatment differs depending on the TNM stage (see Table 8-3). CT and transrectal ultrasound are warranted to determine the depth of invasion and the presence of nodal metastasis.

▷ *How would you manage the following findings?*

Case Variation 8.29.1. A 0.5-cm diameter lesion with no local extension and negative lymph nodes

▶ **Superficial small, mobile lesions warrant treatment with local excision** alone, with close follow-up to ensure that the cancer does not recur.

Case Variation 8.29.2. A 4-cm diameter lesion with no local extension and negative lymph nodes

Surgery is not warranted. Treatment involves the Nigro protocol, which consists of **chemotherapy and radiation therapy** in order to eliminate the cancer.

▶ Abdominoperineal resection is then necessary 4–6 weeks after chemoradiation treatment is complete **only if there is biopsy-proven residual cancer.** However, even in patients with positive inguinal nodes, the Nigro protocol usually provides complete local control of the primary cancer (Table 8-4).

Case Variation 8.29.3. An 8-cm diameter lesion with clinically positive lymph nodes

▶ Chemoradiation therapy is appropriate as the initial method of treatment. Once this is complete, radical resection is probably necessary. The occurrence of positive lymph nodes worsen the prognosis.

LOWER ABDOMINAL PAIN

CASE 8.30. ▶ Left Lower Quadrant Pain No. 1

A 70-year-old woman presents to the emergency department with abdominal pain and fever that developed several hours ago. History is unremarkable, except for occasional constipation. On physical examination, she has a fever of 101°F and mild tachycardia, with a BP of 140/85 mm Hg. The abdomen is tender in the left lower quadrant (LLQ).

▷ *What is the suspected diagnosis?*

▶ **Diverticulitis** is likely in a patient with LLQ pain, tenderness, and fever. Occasionally, it is possible to palpate a mass in the LLQ.

TABLE 8-4

Treatment of Anal Cancer

NIGRO PROTOCOL
External radiation: 30 Gy to the primary tumor, pelvic, and inguinal lymph nodes from days 1–21 (2 Gy/day, 5 days/wk)
Systemic chemotherapy: 5-fluorouracil at 1000 mg/m^2/24 hr as continuous infusion for 4 days, starting on day 1 of radiotherapy and repeated on days 28–31
Mitomycin C: 15 mg/m^2 IV bolus on day 1

From Greenfield LJ, Mulholland MW, Oldham KT, et al. [eds]. *Surgery: scientific principles and practice.* 2nd ed. Philadelphia: Lippincott Williams & Wilkins, 1997: 1150.

▶ *What is the initial management?*

QUICK CUTS Generally, patients with minimal symptoms or signs of inflammation should consume a liquid diet, and they may receive **outpatient treatment with broad-spectrum antibiotics.**

▶ Because this patient is elderly and has a fever and tachycardia, more appropriate management may be **complete bowel rest, IV hydration, and parenteral antibiotics.** Morphine increases intracolonic pressure, so it is generally avoided for analgesia. Meperidine may be used instead; it lowers intraluminal pressure. If nausea or vomiting develop, NG suction may be necessary. An abdominal obstructive series is warranted to check for free air and to search for other diagnoses. A clinician may choose to perform a **CT scan to examine for inflammation, abscess, diverticula, and a thickened sigmoid bowel wall, which confirms a diagnosis of diverticulitis (Figure 8-29).** However, CT is not mandatory in uncomplicated patients.

Another concern is that the symptoms are from a **perforated colon cancer;** signs and symptoms may be similar. The management plan should include careful, **serial abdominal examinations** to check for progression of the disease.

On this management, the patient exhibits rapid improvement and becomes hungry.

▶ *What would the management plan be now?*

▶ Management may entail a high-fiber diet, which is recommended after recovery from the initial attack. If she remains afebrile, she can be discharged. Outpatient treatment with broad-spectrum antibiotics is appropriate for 7–10 days.

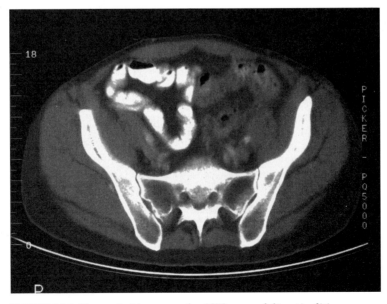

FIGURE 8-29. Computed tomography (CT) scan of diverticulitis, showing "fat stranding" and edema of the tissue near the inflamed colon.

▷ *What is the likelihood that this patient will have another episode of diverticulitis?*

▶ More than 70% of patients have no further recurrences.

▷ *What long-term follow-up is necessary?*

▶ **Colonoscopy** or barium enema may be appropriate after the patient has recovered to **confirm the presence of diverticula** and the **absence of colon cancer (Figure 8-30).**

CASE 8.31. ▶ Left Lower Quadrant Pain No. 2

The woman described in Case 8.30 returns 6 months later with a recurrence of the same problem.

▷ *How does this change the proposed management plan?*

▶ Initially, the patient should be managed in the same manner, with bowel rest, IV antibiotics, and analgesics. After the second episode of **diverticulitis, an elective resection** is usually scheduled 4–6 weeks after the inflammation has resolved. Resection is recommended because the **risk of a significant complication** such as perforation or abscess formation increases with each recurrent episode.

▷ *What procedure is appropriate?*

▶ **Removal of the diverticula-bearing colon** (colectomy) is warranted, which means that the surgeon must have a good description of the colon and the location of the diverticula. This

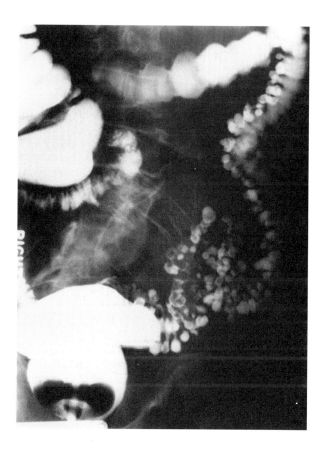

FIGURE 8-30. Barium enema showing multiple diverticula. (From McKenney MG, Mangonon PC, Moylan JA. [eds]. *Understanding surgical disease: the Miami manual of surgery.* Philadelphia: Lippincott-Raven, 1998: 154.)

necessitates either preoperative or intraoperative colonoscopy. The rectum caudad to the peritoneal reflection in the pelvis is usually free of diverticula and does not need removal. In most patients, a short segment of the sigmoid colon is involved with diverticula, with the remaining bowel free of disease. With proper planning and bowel "prep," a colonic re-anastomosis (colocolostomy) is possible without the need to perform a colostomy.

CASE 8.32. ▶ Left Lower Quadrant Pain No. 3

You admit a 75-year-old woman with LLQ pain, fever, and nausea who has a presumptive diagnosis of acute diverticulitis. An obstructive series is unremarkable, and the WBC count is 15,000 cells/mm³. Therapy with antibiotics, bowel rest, and IV fluids begins, with a plan to follow her clinically. Despite this treatment, the patient deteriorates, with continued pain, increasing fever, and rising WBC count.

▶ *What is the suspected problem?*

▶ The patient has a free perforation or an intra-abdominal abscess.

▶ *What is the appropriate evaluation?*

▶ CT may demonstrate abscess, perforation, or other complications of the acute inflammatory process. In addition, it may also reveal the presence of diverticula.

The CT scan demonstrates a loculated fluid collection in the pericolic gutter.

▶ *What management is appropriate?*

▶ A loculated fluid collection with a CT-guided needle insertion of a catheter into the collection is warranted. This method allows the fluid to be sampled and drained.

The drained fluid is purulent and contains gram-negative bacilli. With a catheter left in the collection, the patient improves.

▶ *What is the appropriate management?*

▶ It is necessary to leave the drainage catheter in place until the cavity shrinks to a small size and the drainage stops. If the patient tolerates food and remains afebrile, she can be discharged. However, many patients with a persistent ileus or functional obstruction from the edema do not tolerate food and require TPN for a period of time.

Once the inflammation is controlled and the patient has improved, usually 4–8 weeks after the bout of diverticulitis, a single-stage colectomy is appropriate. A colonoscopy is necessary prior to resection to rule out cancer, because its presentation may be similar. After bowel "prep," surgery involves a segmental colectomy performed with the proximal extent including the acute disease plus any additional diverticula-containing colon. The distal end of the resection should extend to the proximal rectum. Reanastomosis of the colon occurs during the same operation.

The colectomy is a single-stage procedure because the entire procedure is completed "in one sitting." In the past, treatment involved a two-stage or three-stage procedure. In the two-stage approach, the colon and abscess were resected and a colostomy was created, to be reconnected at a later procedure. In the three-stage approach, the first step involved drainage of the abscess, followed later by resection of the diseased bowel and creation of a colostomy, followed later by colostomy closure.

▷ *How would the proposed management change if the patient did not improve with catheter drainage?*

▶ If the patient worsens clinically, a Hartmann procedure with resection of the colon and inflammatory mass, with a colostomy, is warranted (see Figure 8-5).

CASE 8.33. ▶ Left Lower Quadrant Pain No. 4

You treat a 70-year-old woman for acute diverticulitis, who recovers without complications or need for surgery. A subsequent colonoscopy shows an area of sigmoid diverticula with scarring and a mild stricture of the involved area. Biopsies are negative for tumor. She does well at home but returns several months later with a sensation of voided air when she urinates.

▷ *What is the appropriate diagnosis and management?*

▶ **Pneumaturia** is present. Diverticulitis can form a fistula with most lower abdominal organs (Figure 8-31). In this case, it has formed a fistula with the bladder. This complicates the surgery; it is necessary to separate the diseased segment of bowel from the bladder. Otherwise, the procedure is unchanged.

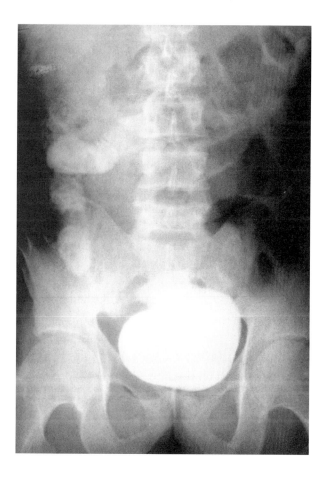

FIGURE 8-31. Contrast study of the bladder, showing a fistula between the colon and the bladder, a common occurrence. (From McKenney MG, Mangonon PC, Moylan JA. [eds]. *Understanding surgical disease: the Miami manual of surgery.* Philadelphia: Lippincott-Raven, 1998: 141.)

LOWER GASTROINTESTINAL BLEEDING

CASE 8.34. ▶ Massive Lower Gastrointestinal Bleeding

A 70-year-old woman who has been in good health presents to the emergency department with a 4-hour history of large amounts of bright-red blood per rectum. A brief history is otherwise negative. On physical examination, her heart rate is 115 beats/min with a BP of 105/70 mm Hg. She appears tired but alert. Her conjunctiva appear pale, and her mucous membranes are dry. Heart and lungs are normal except for a resting tachycardia. The abdomen is soft and non-tender, and bright-red blood per rectum is evident. She has no peripheral edema and weak but present pulses. Neurologically, she is intact.

▶ *What is the initial evaluation and management plan?*

▶ The patient's signs and symptoms, including fatigue, tachycardia, dry mucous membranes, and pale conjunctiva, are suggestive of **hypovolemia.** Like all elderly patients, this woman is particularly susceptible to volume depletion because of her higher risk of heart disease. Therefore, it is necessary to insert two large-bore IV lines and **1–2 liters of lactated Ringer's solution,** or 0.9 L normal saline, immediately to replace the isotonic fluid lost. She also requires placement on a monitor. Routine blood studies and a CXR are warranted. A coagulation evaluation is necessary to be certain that she has normal blood clotting, and blood for transfusion should be made available. Placement of a Foley catheter is indicated to help evaluate the adequacy of resuscitation.

 Placement of an NG tube for lavage is warranted to evaluate and **rule out an upper GI bleed.**

If the lavage from the NG tube is positive for blood, an upper endoscopy is necessary. **Anoscopy** should also take place in the emergency department to examine for hemorrhoids, bleeding rectal varices, or other anorectal pathology.

Once the resuscitation is under way, it is necessary to take a more careful history and perform a more detailed physical examination to evaluate for preexisting diseases, prior surgery, and other problems that might influence decision making. Constant **reevaluation of the resuscitation** should be a high priority.

▶ *What are the most likely diagnoses?*

▶ The most common causes of rapid lower GI bleeding are **bleeding diverticula and vascular ectasias.** Other causes of bright-red blood per rectum include Meckel's diverticulum, aortoenteric fistula, ischemic colitis, IBD, hemorrhoidal disease, and rectal varices. Colonic neoplasms are also a possibility, although colon cancer rarely causes massive lower GI bleeding.

After receiving IV fluids, the patient's BP and heart rate improve, and she seems more energetic. Laboratory studies reveal a hematocrit of 38% and a mildly elevated serum Na at 148 mEq/L and a blood urea nitrogen (BUN) of 30 mg/dL. Since you initially saw her, she has had no further rectal bleeding. Her NG aspirate contains bile, and anoscopy reveals no bleeding source.

▶ *What are the next management steps?*

▶ Admission for **stabilization, observation for further GI bleeding, and diagnostic workup** is warranted. Close monitoring in an intermediate or intensive care unit is necessary. Although the initial hematocrit is 38%, it takes several hours for the hematocrit to equilibrate before it is an accurate measure of blood cell volume; it should be checked every several hours. If it continues to decrease, a blood transfusion may still be required.

The patient has remained stable overnight with a heart rate of 80 beats/min, a normal BP with no orthostatic changes, and a hematocrit that has drifted down to 32%. No further episodes of rectal bleeding have occurred. She is currently hungry and feeling much better.

▷ *What is the likelihood that this patient will experience another episode of bleeding?*

▶ The likelihood that she will bleed again depends on the cause of the GI bleed. The **natural course of diverticular bleeds is to stop spontaneously.** Bleeding colonic diverticula have less than 25% likelihood of rebleeding, although 20% of affected patients continue to bleed and require operative intervention. Patients with vascular **ectasias stop bleeding spontaneously in about 90% of cases,** although the risk of rebleeding is approximately 25% and 46% after 1 year and 3 years, respectively.

▷ *What is the next step?*

▶ It is necessary to **determine the cause** of the GI bleed. In this case, in which the bleeding has stopped, the most valuable procedure is **colonoscopy.**

QUICK CUTS Whether colonoscopy is performed during this admission or as an outpatient, it is critical to not overlook this procedure. Although colon cancer is unlikely, **a missed cancer is a major oversight.**

Colonoscopy may take place during hospitalization or electively after discharge. If it occurs during admission, a bowel "prep" with 4 L of polyethylene glycol solution is appropriate.

If **vascular ectasia** is evident, treatment with **coagulation** with a monopolar current is appropriate. The most significant risk is colonic perforation from colonic coagulation. Bleeding colonic **diverticula are not amenable to endoscopic treatment,** but this approach **does permit localization** of the bleeding site on occasion. Bleeding polyps may be coagulated or, in the case of pedunculated polyps, ensnared. "Tattooing" of the bleeding site involves the submucosal injection of methylene blue or India ink, which allows precise localization if operative intervention is necessary (i.e., in the case of a colonic mass or polyp).

Colonoscopy indicates multiple diverticula in the left colon and no vascular ectasia. There is no active bleeding. The woman has a stable hematocrit and is tolerating a regular diet.

▷ *What is the next step?*

▶ Discharge with outpatient follow-up is appropriate. Most physicians would place the patient on **iron** and a high-fiber diet, which may lessen the chance of the development of additional diverticula.

▷ *Why are diverticula associated with bleeding?*

▶ Colonic diverticular bleeds result from an **underlying vasa recta artery penetrating the bowel wall** through the neck or the apex of a diverticulum and become eroded. Although most diverticula in the colon are left-sided, right-sided colonic diverticula are more apt to bleed (Figure 8-32).

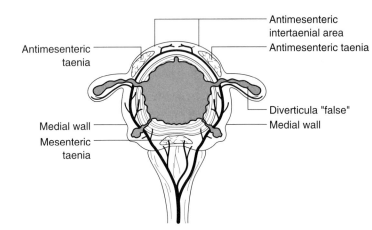

Antimesenteric intertaenial area

Antimesenteric taenia

Antimesenteric taenia

Diverticula "false"

Medial wall

Medial wall

Mesenteric taenia

FIGURE 8-32. The blood supply of the colonic wall and its association with diverticula within the wall of the colon, which explains why diverticulosis has a tendency to bleed. (From McKenney MG, Mangonon PC, Moylan JA. [eds]. *Understanding surgical disease: the Miami manual of surgery.* Philadelphia: Lippincott-Raven, 1998: 154.)

▷ *What are vascular ectasias?*

▶ Vascular ectasias, or **arteriovenous malformations,** are thought to arise from the degeneration of intestinal submucosal veins and overlying mucosal capillaries. As the disease progresses, communications between submucosal arteries and veins form. When the mucosa erodes or becomes disrupted for some reason, massive lower GI bleeding may result.

CASE 8.35. ▶ Persistent Bleeding with a Massive Lower Gastrointestinal Bleed

You admit a 68-year-old woman with bright-red bleeding per rectum. The presumptive diagnosis is bleeding from a colonic diverticulum or vascular ectasia. After resuscitation and 2 units of blood, she stabilizes. Initial evaluation reveals no evidence of an upper GI bleed, no hemorrhoids, and no evidence of a coagulopathy. You plan to further evaluate the patient the next day if she remains stable. That evening, her hematocrit is 35% after transfusion.

The next morning, she begins to bleed profusely again with bright-red blood per rectum. Her heart rate has also risen to 130 beats/min, and her BP is 100/60 mm Hg. A repeat hematocrit is 24%. You again resuscitate her and administer 2 more units of packed RBCs. Although you had planned to perform a colonoscopy, it has not yet taken place.

▷ *What is the overall management plan at this point?*

▶ The patient's **rebleeding is significant** because of her **cardiovascular instability** and a very **low hematocrit despite previous transfusion.** Medical management has failed, and surgery to stop the bleeding will most likely be necessary. Colonoscopy during active bleeding is unlikely to demonstrate the bleeding cause and is associated with a significant risk of perforation due to poor visibility of the colon.

▷ *What evaluation is appropriate at this point?*

▶ Determination of the site of bleeding is essential.

QUICK CUTS   With rebleeding, the options for diagnosing the cause of the GI bleed **include technetium-labeled RBC scan or mesenteric angiography.**

The choice between these two procedures depends on the current rate of bleeding, the instability of the patient, and the surgeon's preference.

- **Angiography** is probably better **for less stable patients,** because of better monitoring and resuscitation capability in the angiography suite, as well as **for those who are bleeding at a more rapid rate.** It can isolate a lesion bleeding at a rate of 0.5–1.0 mL/min or more.
- **Technetium-labeled RBC scanning** is better for **more stable patients** who are **bleeding more slowly.** It can detect bleeding at a rate of 0.1 mL/min or more. One limitation of RBC scanning is that it cannot precisely localize the site of the bleeding, making the results difficult to interpret. However, some physicians recommend always obtaining an RBC scan before an angiogram (Figure 8-33).

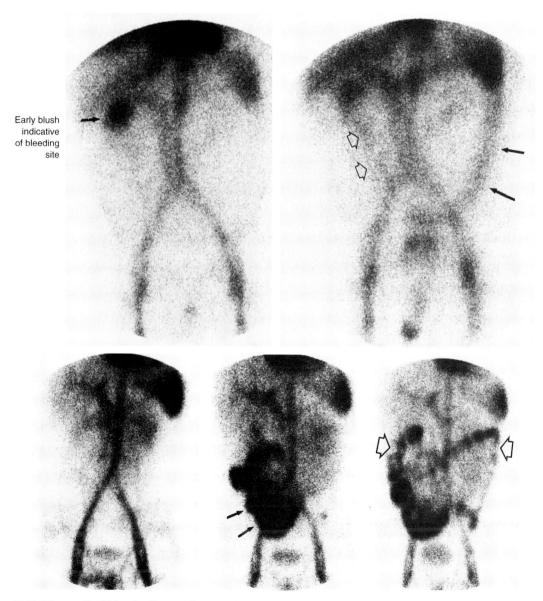

Early blush indicative of bleeding site

FIGURE 8-33. Red blood cell scan showing hemorrhage at the area of diverticulosis. (Bottom Center) Accumulation of blood in a presumed bleeding site.

An angiogram demonstrates an active bleed in the lower sigmoid area and no evidence of vascular ectasia elsewhere in the colon.

▶ *What is the management plan?*

▶ The patient has clear evidence of **continued bleeding,** has proven **cardiovascular instability,** and has now received **4 units of packed RBCs.** At no single specific point is surgery indicated, but each of these conditions is a relative indication for surgery, and the combination is certainly an indication. Many surgeons would explore most patients with lower GI bleeds once they had required **4–6 units of blood;** experience dictates that patients who have bled that much are likely to continue to bleed. A large amount of transfusion carries its own set of risks, such as transfusion reaction, coagulopathy, and infection.

Most surgeons would take this patient **urgently to the operating room.** In fact, most surgeons would say that the decision to proceed with an angiogram included a decision to perform surgery (i.e., **the angiogram is a preoperative test).** It is critical to identify the probable bleeding site prior to proceeding to the operating room. Otherwise, the surgeon does not know which portion of the colon to remove.

You have decided that operative intervention is necessary.

▶ *What operation is appropriate?*

▶ Before induction of anesthesia takes place, it is necessary to be certain that resuscitation is **adequate** and the hematocrit is acceptable. Based on the location, either a **left or right hemicolectomy** to remove the bleeding source is appropriate; this is a **preoperative decision.** It is not recommended that a surgeon try to be too precise and remove only the site of bleeding, such as a diverticulum or a particular segment of bowel; this is associated with a high rebleeding rate. It is still necessary to explore the abdomen to be certain that there is no other significant pathology. Then the planned colectomy takes place. Because of the cathartic effect of blood in the colon, most patients with massive lower GI bleeds have a sufficiently clean colon to allow performance of a **primary anastomosis.** When patients are unstable or severely malnourished, and primary anastomoses are less likely to heal, colostomy is a consideration.

▶ *Are there any situations in which it is necessary to proceed to the operating room sooner?*

▶ Certain patients should be explored *before* they require 4–6 units of blood.

- Patients who become **unstable with the bleeding** (perhaps), especially those patients with significant coronary artery disease and angina who have instability in vital signs
- Patients with **hard-to-determine blood types,** including unusual antibodies, or patients who desire no transfusion, such as **Jehovah's Witnesses.** Performing surgery at an earlier time would lessen the risk associated with hemorrhage.

▶ *If a patient is bleeding rapidly and subsequently hypotensive in the angiography suite, are there any ways to lessen the rate of bleeding?*

▶ If the bleeding site is identified, it is possible to control active hemorrhage with the direct infusion of a vasoconstrictor into the bleeding vessel. This temporary maneuver may occur during preparation for surgery. The commonly used agent is **vasopressin,** which is not given for a prolonged period of time for two reasons: (1) its coronary vasoconstrictor effect, and (2) 50% of patients have a recurrence of bleeding within 12 hours after it is discontinued. Another means of treatment during angiography is **embolization.** However, there is an increased risk of transmural intestinal necrosis in the large bowel, so this approach may be reserved for poor surgical candidates.

▶ *Why not bypass the preoperative angiogram and determine the site of bleeding in the operating room?*

▶ It is **very difficult** to attempt to determine the site of bleeding in the operating room, and the results are **unreliable.** Because they do not know the side of the bleeding, many surgeons would perform a total abdominal colectomy. In part, this is based on the experience that rebleeding after lesser procedures (i.e., blind left or right hemicolectomy) is associated with a high rebleeding rate and high mortality.

OTHER BENIGN LOWER GASTROINTESTINAL TRACT DISORDERS

CASE 8.36. ▶ Syndromes of Acute Colonic Dilation and Obstruction

An 88-year-old woman who is receiving long-term care in a nursing home is brought to the emergency department with a history of constipation and a recent deterioration in mental status. Her BP is 100/60 mm Hg, with a heart rate of 120 beats/min. She has abdominal distention and moans when you examine her abdomen. Rectal examination reveals no stool.

▶ *How would you evaluate this patient?*

▶ Hydration is necessary. Electrolytes, a CBC, and an abdominal obstructive radiographic series to rule out obstruction or other abdominal pathology are also warranted.

▶ *How would you evaluate the following radiologic findings?*

Case Variation 8.36.1. Sigmoid volvulus

▶ A sigmoid volvulus occurs most commonly in debilitated patients from nursing homes, often as a result of chronic laxative use, chronic illness, or dementia. Sigmoid volvulus develops from a clockwise twist of mobile sigmoid colon around the mesentery, leading to a closed loop obstruction. A barium enema confirms the volvulus.

 QUICK CUTS In stable patients, it is often possible to "detorse" the sigmoid colon **by rigid proctosigmoidoscopy and placement of a rectal tube.**

Definitive therapy is usually planned during the same hospital stay. The treatment is **either sigmoid colectomy** with diverting colostomy or resection with primary anastomosis, depending on the preoperative condition of the patient (Figure 8-34). If endoscopic management is unsuccessful, urgent laparotomy is required. The recurrence rate is approximately 30%.

Case Variation 8.36.2. Cecal volvulus

▶ Most patients with **cecal volvulus require urgent surgical treatment (Figure 8-35).** Attempts at detorsion with a barium enema or colonoscopy are usually not successful. Surgical options include detorsion alone, cecopexy, or right colectomy. In stable patients with viable bowel, the operation of choice is right colectomy with primary anastomosis.

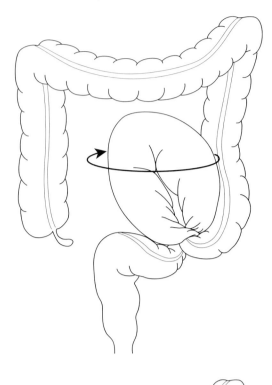

FIGURE 8-34. Detorsion of volvulus, which requires treatment with insertion of a rectal tube followed by elective sigmoid colectomy.

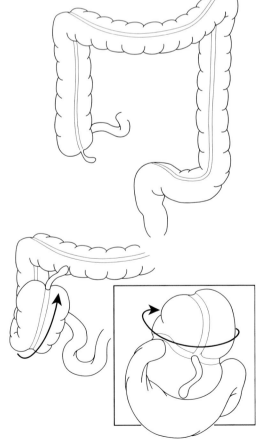

FIGURE 8-35. Types of torsion with cecal volvulus.

Case Variation 8.36.3. Massively dilated right colon to the level of the midtransverse colon with distal colonic decompression

▶ **Acute pseudoobstruction, or Ogilvie's syndrome,** is defined **as acute massive dilation of the cecum and right colon without evidence of mechanical obstruction.** This commonly occurs in hospitalized patients in the intensive care unit who are intubated and seriously ill. The cecum preferentially dilates more than the remaining colon because of Laplace's law. Conservative, nonoperative treatment is indicated when the cecal diameter is less than 9–10 cm. Serial radiographic films to follow colonic diameter are necessary.

QUICK CUTS   If the colon diameter exceeds 11–12 cm, **endoscopic decompression** is indicated. Many surgeons also attempt a brief trial of neostigmine, a parasympatholytic agent, which may increase colonic tone and counteract the dilation. If the neostigmine is unsuccessful, **surgical decompression** of the cecum or a right colectomy is necessary.

Many surgeons would perform decompression of immunosuppressed patients with Ogilvie's syndrome when the colon diameter is smaller.

Case Variation 8.36.4. Entire colon packed with stool

▶ This finding is indicative of constipation, with stool seen throughout the colon. A rectal examination to **ensure that the stool is not impacted** is necessary. Once the stool is cleared from the vault, enemas may be performed. Severe constipation causing obstruction should always be treated from below before any cathartics are administered by mouth.

CASE 8.37. ▶ Rectal Prolapse

A 65-year-old woman presents with anorectal discomfort. She says that she has trouble initiating defecation. In addition, she feels a protrusion from her rectum when she is finished moving her bowels. On examination, a patulous anus and a rectal prolapse are evident.

▷ *What management is appropriate?*

▶ Rectal prolapse, which may occur during defecation, has an unknown cause but may be related to neuromuscular deficiencies and decreased rectal sensation, particularly in the elderly (Figure 8-36). Most patients have a patulous anus and weakened external sphincters. Numerous operations are appropriate for the management of rectal prolapse. If the prolapse is entirely internal, treatment with a high-fiber diet to normalize bowel function is warranted, and it may be possible to avoid surgery. However, **if the prolapse is external and resulting in rectal bleeding** and no other causes of lower GI bleeding are discovered, surgery may be necessary.
Many operative strategies are appropriate for rectal prolapse.

- **Rectopexy,** in which the rectum is fixed to the sacrum without removing a portion of the rectum
- A low anterior resection, which removes the upper and middle portions of the rectum, along with the redundant sigmoid colon (**transabdominal rectosigmoid resection**)
- A perineal approach, which removes the prolapsed rectum and sigmoid colon with the proximal sigmoid colon anastomosed to the transitional zone 1–2 cm above the dentate line

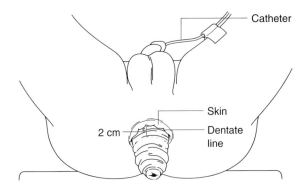

FIGURE 8-36. Rectal prolapse. (From Greenfield LJ, Mulholland MW, Oldham KT, et al. [eds]. *Surgery: scientific principles and practice.* 2nd ed. Philadelphia: Lippincott Williams & Wilkins, 1997: 1194.)

CASE 8.38. ▶ Perianal Problems

A 30-year-old man presents with rectal pain that is particularly severe during defecation. On examination, you note an ulcerated area in the anal canal that is very painful when touched.

▷ *What management is appropriate?*

▶ Anal fissures involve tears in the anoderm, which is reputedly caused by trauma from passage of hard stools, but can also result from other diseases such as IBD. They are associated with pain during bowel movements and tenderness on palpation. Blood is usually found on the toilet tissue after wiping. Anal fissures are almost always located in the posterior midline. A sentinel tag may be seen at the anal verge.

▷ *What management is appropriate?*

▶ Most anal fissures respond to **conservative treatment,** including bulk agents, stool softeners, and sitz baths. If the fissure is **deep and chronic,** lateral **sphincterotomy,** which divides a portion of the internal anal sphincter, may be necessary (Figure 8-37). The hypothesis that reflex stimulation and spasm of the internal anal sphincter is important in pathogenesis is the basis for this procedure. More than 90% of anal fissures heal after lateral sphincterotomy. **Biopsy of suspicious, chronic fissures** to rule out anal cancer is warranted.

A patient presents with a history of **persistent perianal drainage.** On examination, a sinus tract with granulation tissue is apparent.

▷ *What is the most likely diagnosis?*

▶ This patient most likely has a **fistula-in-ano,** which is the residua of a previous abscess that failed to completely heal (Figure 8-38). Instead, a chronic tract formed with an internal connection to an anal crypt and an external connection to the perianal skin.

▷ *What management is appropriate?*

▶ Treatment involves **unroofing** the tract, **draining** any undrained collection, and **allowing the tract to reepithelialize.** If the tract traverses the anal sphincter, a seton or string should be placed within the tract and allowed to traverse the sphincter without making the patient incontinent.

A patient presents with severe anal pain, a tender fluctuant perianal mass, and fever.

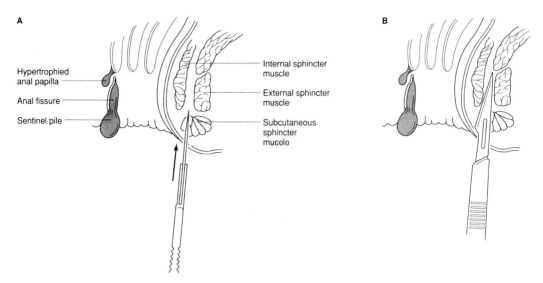

FIGURE 8-37. Location of anal fissure, which is often associated with hypertrophy of anal papilla and a sentinel pile. This may be treated by internal or external sphincterotomy, which cuts the internal sphincter but leaves the external sphincter intact. **A.** Knife is inserted. **B.** Internal sphincter is transected. (From Greenfield LJ, Mulholland MW, Oldham KT, et al. [eds]. *Surgery: scientific principles and practice.* 2nd ed. Philadelphia: Lippincott Williams & Wilkins, 1997: 1198.)

▶ *What is the likely diagnosis and appropriate management?*

▶ The most likely diagnosis is **perianal abscess,** which results from an infection that occurs in anal crypts and glands that are present at the dentate line. There are four basic types of abscess: perianal, ischioanal, intersphincteric, and supralevator. Treatment of the first two types requires drainage through a perianal incision. An intersphincteric abscess, which causes pain within the anal canal, may require drainage within the anal canal. The supralevator, a higher, more complex abscess may arise from the perianal area or higher within the abdomen; the decision regarding the site of drainage depends on its location and origin. **The primary treatment is drainage, not antibiotics.**

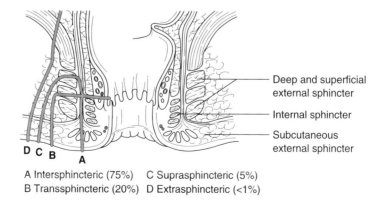

FIGURE 8-38. Typical fistula-in-ano. (From McKenney MG, Mangonon PC, Moylan JA. [eds]. *Understanding surgical disease: the Miami manual of surgery.* Philadelphia: Lippincott-Raven, 1998: 162.)

A patient complains of pain and drainage in his **sacrococcygeal area** of the lower back. You examine him and find an abscess in that location.

▶ *What management is appropriate?*

▶ This condition is a **pilonidal abscess,** which is an infection in a hair-containing sinus in the sacrococcygeal area. Treatment involves **unroofing** the abscess, removing all hair, and leaving the wound open to heal by secondary intention.

CASE 8.39. ▶ Colostomies

A 58-year-old man is having a stoma created in the operating room the next day.

▶ *What preparation is necessary?*

▶ The patient should meet with the physician and enterostomal therapist to be educated about stomas and their care. The most common complication related to a stoma is leakage around the appliance (bag) and patient dissatisfaction due to a poor location of the stoma on the abdominal wall. A stoma should be placed where it can be cared for conveniently and not in a skin fold where leakage could occur. It is best to determine this position preoperatively, with the patient in a sitting position. Other postoperative complications include parastomal herniation, bowel obstruction abscess, and fistula formation.

Your resident asks you to describe the different types of stomas.

▶ *How would you respond?*

▶ Stomas are artificially created openings between the intestine or urinary tract and the abdominal wall. Stomas may be temporary or permanent. Most temporary stomas are created to divert the fecal stream while either healing of an anastomosis occurs or an inflammatory process related to GI leakage subsides. Pairs of end stomas that act as single openings ("double barrel" stomas) or loops that are brought up onto the abdominal wall and opened are temporary stomas. Loop stomas are not totally diverting and must be separated like "double barrel" stomas for complete diversion. Distal bowel stomas are termed mucous fistulas, because their only contents are mucosal-derived mucus and no stool. If the distal bowel is closed and not brought to the abdominal wall but rather dropped back into the pelvis, it is termed a Hartmann pouch. This is commonly done for sigmoid resections for diverticulitis when the bowel cannot be safely reconnected. Loop stomas, cecostomies, and tube cecostomies can also be performed to decompress a distended segment of bowel temporarily such as in Ogilvie's syndrome (Figure 8-39).

▶ Permanent stomas are most commonly used in the following situations (presented in order of decreasing frequency):

- Following an abdominoperineal resection in which an end sigmoid colostomy is created
- An ileostomy following total proctocolectomy for ulcerative colitis. (However, many patients who previously underwent reconstruction with a continent ileostomy are now having ileoanal pull-through procedures. Typically, the surgeon creates a pouch or a reservoir and anastomoses it to the anus.)
- An ileal conduit draining the urinary system to the skin

Ileostomies and ileal conduits can be constructed in a fashion to make patients continent. After creation of a nipple valve, catheter insertion and drainage is periodically necessary.

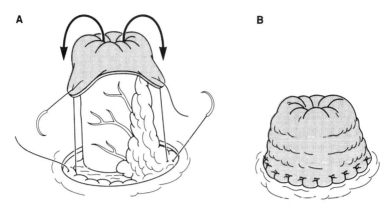

FIGURE 8-39. Performance of ileostomy. (From Greenfield LJ, Mulholland MW, Oldham KT, et al. [eds]. *Surgery: scientific principles and practice*. 2nd ed. Philadelphia: Lippincott Williams & Wilkins, 1997: 1100.)

Because the output from ileostomies is particularly irritating to the skin, ileostomies are designed to result in continence or protrude from the skin so that their output drops directly into the appliance (in the same manner as a spigot). Carefully applied appliances are critical to the success of ileostomies.

Both continent ileostomies and ileoanal pouches are susceptible to "pouchitis," an inflammatory process in the pouch hypothesized to be secondary to some form of bacterial overgrowth. Patients feel weak, have a fever, and may have abdominal or pelvic pain and malodorous stool. Symptoms usually resolve with a course of metronidazole.

Endocrine Disorders

Bruce E. Jarrell M.D., W. Bradford Carter M.D.

CASE 9.1. ▶ Thyroid Nodule Found on Examination

A 29-year-old woman presents for evaluation of a thyroid nodule that her primary care physician noted on a routine examination. She is otherwise healthy. Her only significant history is two previous normal pregnancies. On physical examination, all systems appear normal except the neck. An **isolated 1-cm firm nodule** is present in the right lobe of the thyroid gland that moves when the patient swallows.

▶ *How does a patient's **history and physical examination influence your evaluation?***

▶ Your greatest concern is that this nodule represents thyroid cancer, so it is important to obtain information regarding risk factors for thyroid cancer, including radiation history, family history, voice and airway, symptoms, and thyroid nodule pattern. A past history (10–25 years) of **low-dose ionizing radiation** (<2000 rad) to the neck carries a 40% risk of thyroid cancer; the most common cancer following radiation is papillary carcinoma. Radioactive iodine ablation has not been associated with increased incidence of thyroid cancer.

 In a patient with a history of neck radiation, it is appropriate to proceed directly to thyroidectomy. No additional evaluation is necessary.

▶ A **family history** of thyroid cancer is significant. Medullary thyroid cancer is inherited as an autosomal dominant trait, and testing for the existence of a point mutation of the *RET* gene in a family can establish a diagnosis. In a suspicious lesion, examination of serum calcitonin may be appropriate. Elevated values are highly suggestive of medullary carcinoma, and screening for the RET mutation is then warranted. Positive results suggest multiple endocrine neoplasia (MEN). Evaluation of affected patients for pheochromocytoma, adrenal medullary hyperplasia, and hyperparathyroidism is necessary before surgery.

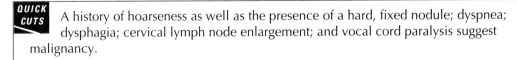 A history of hoarseness as well as the presence of a hard, fixed nodule; dyspnea; dysphagia; cervical lymph node enlargement; and vocal cord paralysis suggest malignancy.

▶ In a **solitary nodule,** the **risk of malignancy is approximately 15%.** In contrast, in a **dominant nodule in a multinodular gland,** the **risk of malignancy drops to 5% or less** except in cases involving previous neck irradiation.

You perform a complete history and physical examination and find that the woman has no risk factors for thyroid cancer. On examination, the nodule is solitary and not hard or fixed. The vocal cords move normally.

▶ *What is the **next step** in evaluation?*

▶ Most surgeons would perform a **fine needle aspiration (FNA)** of the lesion (Figure 9-1). This involves local anesthesia, aspiration of the mass using a syringe and 21–25-gauge needle, and sending the aspirate for cytology.

 QUICK CUTS   FNA poses little risk and can firmly establish a diagnosis in a majority of cases.

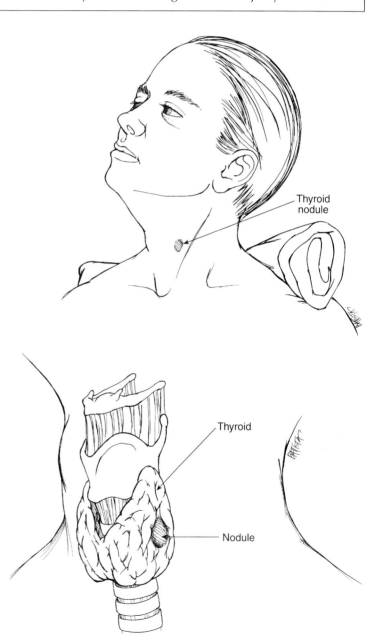

FIGURE 9-1. Technique of fine needle aspiration, shown in four steps. (From Chen H, Sonnenday CJ, Lillemoe KD [eds]. *Manual of common bedside surgical procedures.* 2nd ed. Philadelphia: Lippincott, Williams & Wilkins, 2000: 305–308.) (*continued*)

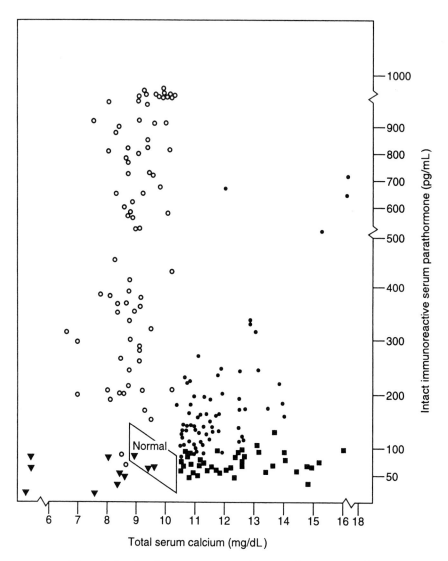

FIGURE 9-4. The relationship between serum calcium and serum parathormone levels in primary hyperparathyroidism surgically proven (●), secondary hyperparathyroidism (○), hypoparathyroidism (▲), and hypocalcemia due to metastatic bone disease (■). (From Jarrell BE, Carabasi RA III, Radomski JS. *NMS surgery.* 4th ed. Philadelphia: Lippincott Williams & Wilkins, 2000: 351.)

▶ Parathyroid **carcinoma is present in less than 2% of cases.**

You measure her PTH and plot it on Fig 9-4 and find that she has primary hyperparathyroidism.

▶ *What is your plan at this point?*

▶ Most experienced surgeons would **explore the neck** to examine the parathyroid glands. No preoperative studies to further localize or characterize the disease are necessary.

▶ *What operative strategy is commonly practiced?*

TABLE 9-1

Common Presenting Symptoms of Hyperparathyroidism

Symptom	Frequency
Muscle weakness	2/3
Myalgia	1/2
Arthralgia	1/2
Nephrolithiasis	1/3
Constipation	1/3
Polyuria	1/3
Psychiatric disorders	1/7
Peptic ulcer disease	1/8

▶ Parathyroid adenomas are resected in conjunction with the identification of all three other glands and a biopsy of a single gland to determine its normalcy. Radical resection is reserved for carcinoma.

▷ *Is there an alternative strategy?*

▶ Some surgeons practice an alternate strategy. A preoperative **sestamibi scan,** which typically demonstrates enlarged parathyroid glands, is used to determine the site of the adenoma (Figure 9-5). This localization allows the surgeon to make a small neck incision, go directly to the adenoma, and remove it without needing to explore the remaining glands. This has been termed **minimally invasive parathyroid** surgery.

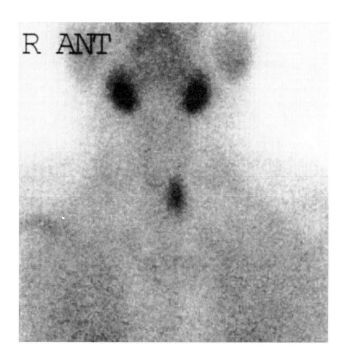

FIGURE 9-5. An example of a sestamibi scan, which demonstrates the parathyroid glands and helps visualize adenomas. The upper hot spots are the submaxillary salivary glands and the lower hot spot is a parathyroid adenoma.

You decide to proceed with a standard procedure to explore the parathyroid glands. You identify only **three glands, which are normal. No adenomas are apparent.**

▶ *What would you do at this point in the operation?*

▶ It is essential to find the single missing gland.

 The most common location for a missing inferior gland is in the thymus.

▶ It is possible to search for the missing gland through the same cervical incision used to gain access to the parathyroids. It is important to identify the location of the three identified glands and be aware of their embryologic origins. A missing lower pole parathyroid may be intrathyroidal. Additional places for the parathyroid glands are the tracheoesophageal groove and in the carotid sheath; even intravagal locations are possible (Figure 9-6).

You have failed to find the missing adenoma and stopped the operation. **Persistent calcium elevation has occurred postoperatively.**

▶ *How would you manage this situation?*

▶ This patient has **persistent hyperparathyroidism.** Management usually involves **localization studies,** including sestamibi scan, ultrasound, computed tomography (CT), magnetic resonance imaging (MRI), angiography, or venous sampling. Once the "missing"

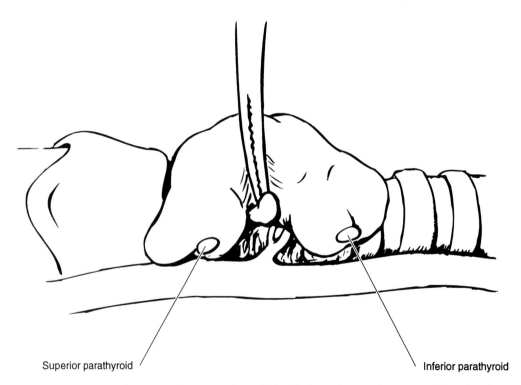

Superior parathyroid   Inferior parathyroid

FIGURE 9-6. Normal locations of the parathyroid glands, lateral view. (From Jarrell BE, Carabasi RA III, Radomski JS. *NMS surgery.* 4th ed. Philadelphia: Lippincott Williams & Wilkins, 2000: 323.)

gland has been localized, **reexploration** through a neck or a lateral direct approach is necessary. In cases where a persistent intrathymic parathyroid is found, a **thymectomy** through a cervical incision or a median sternotomy is warranted. Ectopic supernumerary glands, when present, are found most commonly in the tracheoesophageal groove.

▶ *What are the **risks** of a parathyroid exploration?*

▶ The complications are **similar to those in thyroid surgery,** including injury to the recurrent laryngeal nerve or the external branch of the superior laryngeal nerve, or hypoparathyroidism. The resection of all parathyroid tissue leads to hypocalcemia and hyperphosphatemia. In the immediate postoperative period, tetany may occur. Tapping on the facial nerve adjacent to the ear elicits a Chvostek's sign, which is spasm of the orbicularis oris muscle. If it occurs, hypocalcemia is present.

Suppose you are treating an **asymptomatic patient** who has an elevation in serum calcium found on a screening panel performed for unrelated reasons.

▶ *How would the management differ?*

▶ The treatment of the asymptomatic hypercalcemia is expectant for a minimally elevated serum calcium. Many clinicians recommend parathyroid exploration once the serum calcium exceeds 11 mEq/L to avoid the complications of hypercalcemia. The cutoff calcium level and the likelihood of development of complications is still a matter of debate.

CASE 9.3. ▶ Medical Management of Acute Hypercalcemia

A 45-year-old man presents to the emergency department with nausea, fatigue, and weight loss, as well as drowsiness, abdominal pain, and altered mental status. He has a history of bipolar disorder and kidney stones. His **serum calcium level is 16 mEq/L.**

▶ *What is the most likely cause of the man's disorder?*

▶ This patient is suffering from acute hypercalcemia.

 Parathyroid adenoma is the **most common benign cause** of hypercalcemia.

Metastatic carcinoma such as breast carcinoma is a common malignant cause of hypercalcemia; it is a common diagnosis in **women with metastatic breast cancer.** Other causes of hypercalcemia include parathyroid hyperplasia, multiple myeloma, hyperthyroidism, sarcoidosis, milk alkali syndrome, vitamin A intoxication, thiazide diuretics, renal cell carcinoma, squamous cell cancer of the lung (secretes a PTH-like substance), and familial hypocalciuric hypercalcemia.

▶ *What acute treatment should this man receive?*

▶ Hypercalcemia results in an osmotic diuresis in the earlier phases of the disease, which leads to a vicious cycle of alternating dehydration and worsening hypercalcemia. Therefore, the initial treatment must be rehydration with normal saline. After the patient is hydrated, furosemide, which leads to a brisk diuresis high in calcium, is necessary. Other agents used to control hypercalcemia on an extended basis are mithramycin, calcitonin, and glucocorticoids (Table 9-2).

TABLE 9-2

Initial Treatment of Acute Hypercalcemia with Symptoms

1. Hydration with normal saline
2. Calcium diuresis with furosemide
3. Initiation of bisphosphonates
4. Treatment of underlying cause

The man's calcium has returned to a near-normal level after several days of therapy. After you plot his PTH value on the nomogram in Figure 9-4, you note that it is inappropriately high for the corresponding serum calcium and is compatible with primary hyperparathyroidism.

▷ *What management strategy would you recommend?*

▶ With primary hyperparathyroidism, **neck exploration** and removal of abnormal parathyroid glands is recommended. Most commonly, a single adenoma is present, but **multiple adenomas occur about 5% or more** of the time and should be an object of search. Removal of an adenoma is curative in the vast majority of cases.

CASE 9.4. ▶ Secondary Hyperparathyroidism

You receive a consult from the renal service to consider parathyroidectomy in a 34-year-old man who is undergoing dialysis.

▷ *What is the most likely diagnosis?*

▶ Patients with chronic renal failure retain phosphate as their glomerular filtration rate decreases. Hyperphosphatemia causes hypocalcemia, which elevates serum PTH, and this syndrome is termed secondary hyperparathyroidism. Calcium absorption from the gut and vitamin D metabolism are also impaired.

▷ *How do you decide whether surgical management is warranted?*

▶ Medical management is usually appropriate in patients with chronic renal failure and secondary hyperparathyroidism. Surgical management is indicated when **bone pain, fractures, intractable pruritus, or ectopic calcifications in the soft tissues (calcium tachyphylaxis)** are present.

 QUICK CUTS   The common operative finding in secondary hyperparathyroidism is hyperplasia of all glands.

▶ Excision of all but 50 mg of parathyroid tissue is warranted. This remaining tissue may be left in place or transplanted to a more accessible site such as the forearm. Transplantation of the tissue is useful if the patient fails to recover from the effects of secondary hyperparathyroidism after surgery and needs removal of additional parathyroid tissue. It is much simpler to find remaining tissue in the forearm rather than in the neck, where the risks of injury to nerve and other vital structures are greater.

Occasionally, renal transplant patients develop parathyroid abnormalities.

▶ *What is the typical management?*

▶ Most patients who receive a renal transplant have a return of normal parathyroid function. Occasionally, they develop high serum calcium postoperatively; this condition is termed **tertiary hyperparathyroidism.** The parathyroid glands do not respond to the return of renal function and continue to overproduce PTH. If this condition persists for 1 year, and homeostasis does not occur, a **3 1/2-gland resection** is indicated.

CASE 9.5. ▶ Hyperparathyroidism and Severe Hypertension in the Same Patient

The same 34-year-old man undergoes **neck exploration** surgery for primary hyperparathyroidism (see Case 9.4). During the procedure, he becomes **uncontrollably hypertensive,** with a blood pressure (BP) of 210/140 mm Hg. The operative team checks routine possibilities such as improper endotracheal tube placement, inadequate oxygenation, and inadequate level of anesthesia, but this does not demonstrate a cause.

▶ *What do you advise?*

▶ This patient may be experiencing a **catecholamine release** from an undiagnosed pheochromocytoma. It is necessary to terminate the current operation and admit the patient to the intensive care unit for further evaluation. A combination of both α- and β-blockers can be used to obtain immediate control of the hypertension; it is important never to use β-blockade alone, because unopposed α-stimulation can be fatal.

You do this and the man's BP is controlled.

▶ *What is the next step?*

▶ It is necessary to test for the presence of a **pheochromocytoma.**

 QUICK CUTS Pheochromocytomas are the "10%" tumor; 10% are malignant, extra-adrenal, epinephrine producers, and bilateral.

More than 90% of pheochromocytomas result in elevated levels of **urinary catechols, metanephrine, and vanillylmandelic acid.** MRI using T2-weighted imaging may demonstrate a tumor brightness three-fold greater than the liver. This is useful in the patients with additional tumor deposits of tumor in the abdomen that are intra-abdominal but extra-adrenal. For tumors that are difficult to locate, the octreotide scan often localizes the tumor (Figure 9-7). As a last resort, a nuclear I[131] metaiodobenzylguanidine (**MIBG**) scan is used. A nuclear MIBG scan material selectively accumulates in chromaffin tissue, with a high sensitivity and even higher specificity for pheochromocytomas. After tumor localization, α-blockage should be obtained using phenoxybenzamine for 10–14 days before surgery. β-blockade is used in patients with persistent tachycardia or a previous heart history. Treatment is adrenalectomy.

You establish a diagnosis of pheochromocytoma and localize it with the imaging studies.

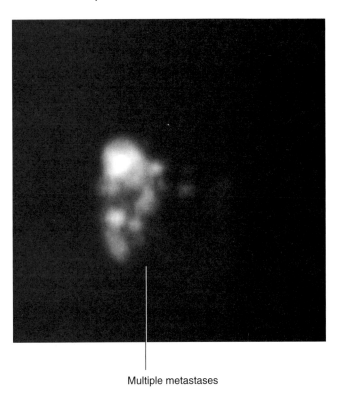

FIGURE 9-7. Octreotide scan, showing multiple metastases to the liver and duodenum.

Multiple metastases

▷ *What is the next management step?*

▶ **Transabdominal exploration** and tumor identification is necessary. A significant number of tumors are bilateral and extra-adrenal, and transabdominal exploration allows the surgeon to explore these areas more extensively. It is important to perform **resection** with minimal manipulation of the tumor to avoid a release of catecholamines. For this reason, it is necessary to ligate all venous drainage from the tumor before manipulating the tumor. Extra-adrenal pheochromocytomas occur along the abdominal aorta in a distribution similar to the sympathetic chain.

CASE 9.6. ▶ Acute Development of a Tender Neck Mass

A 38-year-old woman complains of a sudden onset of a swollen, tender thyroid gland. Her family physician has referred her for evaluation of this tender neck mass.

▷ *What is the most likely diagnosis?*

▶ This patient is presumably suffering from a case of painful thyroiditis; the acute form is **de Quervain's thyroiditis.** In the early stages of disease, patients present with hyperthyroidism due to the sudden release of thyroid hormone directly from acutely injured thyroid follicles.

The general finding associated with thyroiditis is an elevated erythrocyte sedimentation rate (ESR).

Histology is classic for giant cell granulomas around degenerating thyroid follicles.

▶ *How do you want to proceed with this patient's management?*

▶ Therapy consists of analgesics and aspirin. Steroids may be effective in more resistant cases. Surgery is not necessary. Thyroid function tests may be performed if the patient has symptoms of hyperthyroidism.

▶ *Is surgery appropriate in some cases of acute thyroid inflammation?*

▶ If it is believed that a patient has a bacterial infection, surgical drainage might be appropriate. Bacterial infection is termed **acute suppurative thyroiditis.** Pathogens usually include *Streptococcus, Staphylococcus,* and *Pseudomonas.* Other rare causes are tuberculosis, aspergillosis, actinomycoses, and syphilis. The best treatment for these infections is antibiotics or antifungal agents with the drainage of any abscesses, if present.

A patient presents with a painless thyroid mass and is hypothyroid. Biopsy indicates **Hashimoto's thyroiditis (chronic lymphocytic thyroiditis).**

▶ *How would you manage this patient?*

▶ Hashimoto's thyroiditis is an autoimmune disease that involves the replacement of immune damaged thyroid tissue with lymphocytes and plasma cells. These patients are most frequently **hypothyroid and present with enlarged painless masses** in their thyroids. Laboratory tests reveal low thyroxine and triiodothyronine levels and normal TSH levels.

 QUICK CUTS   A **higher incidence of malignancy** is associated with Hashimoto's thyroiditis, especially papillary carcinoma and thyroid lymphomas.

▶ No specific therapy for Hashimoto's thyroiditis is available, but the use of thyroid replacement is common. **Biopsy of all suspicious lesions is necessary,** and patients with **compressive symptoms of the trachea** should undergo palliative resection to relieve the obstruction.

CASE 9.7. ▶ History of Hyperparathyroidism and Intractable Duodenal Ulcers

A 40-year-old man is referred to you by his gastroenterologist for **intractable ulcers** in the stomach and the third portion of the duodenum. He has had a **parathyroidectomy for hypercalcemia** in which three glands were resected. In addition, he reports a significant history of ulcer disease and neck operations in three family members.

▶ *How would you evaluate this patient?*

▶ First-line investigation should be to rule out a chronic *Helicobacter pylori* infection, a medically treatable source of chronic ulcer disease. It is also necessary to obtain a serum gastrin level to determine if the ulcer disease is due to hypergastrinemia (Table 9-3). If the *H. pylori* test is negative and the basal serum gastrin is over 600 pg/mL (>1000 pg/mL is diagnostic), you suspect a **gastrinoma (Zollinger-Ellison syndrome).** There

TABLE 9-3

Gastrinoma

Parameter	Description
Symptoms	Peptic ulcer disease
	Diarrhea
	Esophagitis
Diagnostic tests	Serum gastrin measurement
	Gastric ulcer analysis
	Secretin stimulation test
Anatomic localization	Duodenum and head of pancreas (gastrinoma triangle)

are two forms of Zollinger-Ellison syndrome: one is sporadic, and the other is familial and associated with MEN-1. Other associated diseases are pituitary adenoma, parathyroid hyperplasia, and pancreatic endocrine tumors. Presenting features of pituitary neoplasms, which occur in 15%–50% of patients with MEN-1, include vision symptoms (local compression) or hypersecretion (lactation). Treatment involves resection of the affected side of the pituitary (partial hypophysectomy). The pancreatic endocrine tumors include gastrinoma, insulinoma, and vipomas. There has also been an association with bronchial carcinoids.

> **QUICK CUTS** The diagnosis of hypergastrinemia is established by an elevated unstimulated serum gastrin level or with a positive calcium or secretin stimulation test to augment the gastrin response.

The man's gastrin level is 1200 pg/mL.

▷ *What are the next steps in evaluation?*

▶ The presence of hypergastrinemia may result from a gastrin-secreting tumor, an incomplete previous gastric resection, or G-cell hyperplasia. Because this patient has no previous surgery, **localization** of a gastrin-secreting tumor is performed using CT and MRI. These tumors are typically located in the head of the pancreas and within the duodenal wall. Other measures used to determine localization are endoscopic ultrasound scanning, angiogram and venous sampling for gastrin (Figure 9-8).

You establish a diagnosis of a gastrin-secreting tumor, which appears to be in close proximity to the head of the pancreas.

▷ *Would you recommend surgery?*

▶ The previous philosophy in management has been to treat MEN gastrinomas nonoperatively because of their **multifocal nature.** During the past decade, there has been a **more aggressive, surgical approach to resection** in an attempt to slow the pace of disease and prevent or delay metastasis. However, malignant tumors spread to the lymph nodes and especially the liver in a majority of patients. Sporadic gastrinomas

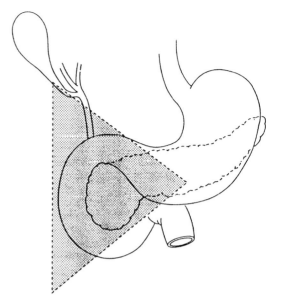

FIGURE 9-8. Location of gastrinomas. Most gastrinomas are found within the gastrinoma triangle. (From Greenfield LJ, Mulholland MW, Oldham KT, et al. [eds]. *Surgery: scientific principles and practice.* 2nd ed. Philadelphia: Lippincott Williams & Wilkins, 1997: 262.)

are usually solitary; disease is limited, and physicians generally agree that resection is appropriate.

▶ *What is the operative strategy?*

▶ **Location of the tumor and removal of as much tumor as possible** are necessary. This process includes intraoperative **endoscopy** to identify duodenal lesions, as well as intraoperative **ultrasound** to isolate the mass.

 The surgeon should use **surgical enucleation,** which preserves pancreatic mass, to remove as much tumor as possible.

▶ However, when the mass involves or abuts a large pancreatic duct, a Whipple procedure or removal of the involved pancreas, typically a distal pancreatectomy, should be performed. Treatment of malignant or metastatic gastrinomas that are not resectable involves gastric resection (traditional) or highly selective vagotomy. Streptozocin is the primary chemotherapeutic agent used for tumor control.

▶ *How might the presentation change if the gastrinoma were an insulinoma?*

▶ **Insulinomas** are the next most frequently observed lesions. Affected patients present with the Whipple triad: fasting hypoglycemia (glucose <60 mg/dL), symptomatic hypoglycemia, and relief by administration of glucose. These patients have an elevated insulin secretion (C peptide must be measured to exclude self-administration of excess insulin) (Table 9-4). Usually, insulinomas associated with MEN are small (<1 cm) and multicentric as opposed to sporadic; 80% of these are solitary. Insulinomas have only a 10% incidence of malignancy.

▶ *What would be the operative strategy for an insulinoma?*

▶ **The operative management of insulinomas is similar to that of gastrinomas.** If the tumors are unresectable insulinomas, diazoxide, an inhibitor of insulin release, is appropriate.

CHAPTER 10

Skin and Soft Tissue Disorders and Hernias

Bruce E. Jarrell M.D.

[handwritten: Amelanotic Melanoma]

MALIGNANT MELANOMA

CASE 10.1. ▶ Evaluation of a Skin Lesion

A 42-year-old man visits you for a lesion on his left forearm. The lesion, which is not painful, has been present for several months. He believes it may be enlarging.

▷ *What aspects of the history or physical examination might be important?*

▶ A **family history of malignant melanoma** increases the risk of melanoma. Other risk factors for many skin disorders are extensive exposure to sunlight and previous dysplastic nevi or atypical moles.

Physical examination can help distinguish benign from malignant lesions. Ulceration, bleeding, and recent change in size are commonly present with malignancy. Variation in pigmentation is also a significant indicator of malignancy. **Between 5% and 10% of malignant melanomas are not pigmented,** and a significant number of basal cell carcinomas and squamous cell carcinomas are pigmented. The **ABCD rule** (**a**symmetry; **b**order irregularity; **c**olor variation; diameter greater than 0.6 cm, **d**ark black color) has been established to describe the findings suggestive of melanoma in pigmented lesions. In addition, the presence of ulceration or nodularity is a concern. A search for regional lymphadenopathy is also appropriate.

▷ *Is excision of the lesion appropriate?*

▶ Excision of any lesion that has changed recently or has any of the listed attributes is necessary.

In **larger lesions (>2–3 cm) or lesions that are contiguous with important structures such as on the face, incisional biopsy** of full-thickness skin at the border of the lesion is warranted (Figure 10-1). Shave biopsies should not be performed, because they do not allow an adequate assessment of lesion thickness.

You decide to perform an excisional biopsy of the lesion.

▷ *What management is appropriate for each of the following pathologic conditions?*

Case Variation 10.1.1. Benign skin lesion

▶ No further treatment is necessary.

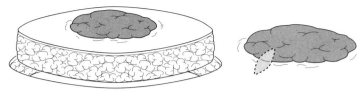

Excisional Biopsy   Incisional Biopsy

FIGURE 10-1. Excisional biopsy versus incisional biopsy. Excisional biopsy completely excises the lesion with a rim of normal tissue. It extends down to the subcutaneous tissue in order to be able to measure the depth of the lesion. Incisional biopsy excises a portion of the margin of the lesion with a segment of normal tissue.

Case Variation 10.1.2. Basal cell carcinoma

▶ These lesions rarely metastasize, but they require adequate local excision **because recurrent lesions may be locally invasive.** This patient is at risk for new lesions, especially in areas of the skin exposed to sunlight. If the histologic margins are free of tumor, then no further treatment is necessary.

QUICK CUTS   **If margins are positive, it is essential to reexcise the node to clear margins.** The margin for large or more aggressive lesions should be 2–4 mm.

Treatment for basal cell carcinoma may also involve topical 5-fluorouracil or radiation.

Case Variation 10.1.3. Squamous cell carcinoma

QUICK CUTS   Squamous cell carcinoma is more dangerous than basal cell carcinoma because of its **locally aggressive behavior and its propensity to metastasize to local lymph nodes.**

▶ Squamous cell carcinoma in situ is termed Bowen's disease. Local recurrence is more common with lesions 4 mm or greater in thickness, which necessitate excision with a 1-cm tumor-free margin. Lesions 10 mm or greater in thickness are more likely to be metastatic to regional lymph nodes. However, **lymph node excision** is generally recommended only for **clinically palpable nodes,** except where behavior of the primary lesion is very aggressive. Treatment with topical 5-fluorouracil or radiation is also appropriate.

Case Variation 10.1.4. In situ melanoma

▶ It is necessary to reexcise the lesion to a 0.5–1-cm margin of normal tissue. This approach should result in a cure.

Case Variation 10.1.5. Dysplastic nevus

▶ This benign neoplasm of melanocytes with areas of **atypia** may represent a transition between benign nevus and melanoma. Only adequate excision is necessary, with close examination for other suspicious lesions and routine surveillance.

CASE 10.2. ▶ Diagnosis of Malignant Melanoma in a Skin Lesion

After excision of the lesion from the forearm of the patient described in Case 10.1, pathologic findings indicate malignant melanoma.

▷ *How is this lesion staged?*

▶ The current methods for staging melanoma principally relate to the depth of penetration or thickness of the lesion. The two commonly used classifications are the **Clark level and Breslow thickness** (Figure 10-2; Table 10-1). The tumor–node–metastasis (TNM) stages correlate highly with patient survival (Figure 10-3; Table 10-2).

   Although there are several types of melanoma (superficial spreading, nodular, lentigo maligna, acral lentiginous), they all result in a **similar prognosis when corrected for thickness.** Nodular melanomas are another distinctive type but do not worsen prognosis when corrected for depth.

▷ *What factors in addition to histologic classification and TNM stage strongly affect survival?*

▶ The most significant finding in addition to the histologic findings and TNM stage is the presence of ulceration in the primary lesion.

QUICK CUTS Even in stage I lesions, **ulcerated lesions have about a one-third reduction in survival.**

   Individuals with lesions located on the face or trunk have a worse prognosis than those with lesions on the extremities, and women do better than men overall.

A pathologist reviews the lesion.

▷ *How would you manage the following histologic findings?*

Case Variation 10.2.1. Malignant melanoma of 0.7-mm depth

▶ This lesion is an early, superficial finding, and **with local control, the prognosis is good. Reexcising the lesion with a 1-cm margin,** which is the same treatment for Clark level II lesions, should accomplish this. It is necessary to reexcise the previous excision site down

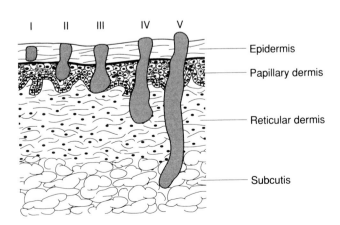

FIGURE 10-2. Clark levels in melanoma. (From Greenfield LJ, Mulholland MW, Oldham KT, et al. [eds]. *Surgery: scientific principles and practice*. 2nd ed. Philadelphia: Lippincott Williams & Wilkins, 1997: 2233.)

TABLE 10-1

Staging of Melanoma: Breslow Tumor Thickness and Clark Level

Breslow Tumor Thickness (mm)	Primary Tumor Classification	Clark Level	5-Year Survival (%)
	T_0	I	>95
≤0.75	T_1	II	89
0.76–1.49	T_2	III	75
1.50–2.49	T_3	IV	58
2.50–3.99			46
≥4.0	T_4	V	25

to the deep fascial plane, being certain that the incision goes straight down rather than beveling toward the center of the lesion. A chest x-ray (radiograph) [CXR], complete blood count (CBC), and liver function tests are appropriate; they warrant follow-up only if they are abnormal. Routine examination for additional melanomas is necessary, because additional primary melanomas occur in up to 5% of patients. Although the risk of regional adenopathy is low, it is important to check for it on physical examination.

Case Variation 10.2.2. Malignant melanoma of 1.6-mm depth

▶ This lesion, which is more advanced, has a higher rate of local recurrence. **It warrants re-excision with a larger, 2-cm margin.** The risk of regional lymph node metastasis is approximately 40%. **If palpable nodes are present, therapeutic lymphadenectomy should be performed.** Surgeons no longer perform lymphadenectomy with nonpalpable lymph nodes (so-called elective lymph node dissection, or ELND) due to the lack of a benefit in survival and a significant morbidity of lymphedema and wound complications. Studies concerning the role of lymph node mapping and selective sampling of the first, or sentinel, node in the chain to examine for tumor are ongoing.

> **QUICK CUTS** If no nodes are palpable, a sentinel lymph node biopsy is warranted. **If the biopsy is positive, elective lymph node dissection is indicated,** even in the case of nonpalpable nodes.

Case Variation 10.2.3. Malignant melanoma of 4.5-mm depth

▶ This patient, who has a poor prognosis, will **most likely die from metastatic disease.** Re-excision of the lesion with a 2–3-cm margin is appropriate. In such a case, it is more likely that lymph nodes are palpable; if so, excision of the nodes is warranted, because they have a tendency to erode the skin and become infected and painful. It is unlikely that an elective, or prophylactic, node dissection will be beneficial.

In addition, computed tomography (CT) of the abdomen and magnetic resonance imaging (MRI) of the brain to examine for metastasis is necessary. The patient should then enter a protocol for treatment with interferon, which has proven benefit for patients with T_4 primary tumors or stage III disease.

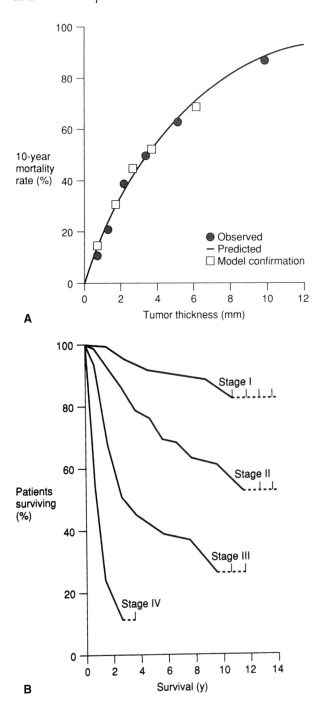

FIGURE 10-3. Survival in malignant melanoma according to thickness of lesion or cancer stage. **A.** Graphic relationship between melanoma tumor thickness and mortality. **B.** Survival according to American Joint Commission staging system (see Table 10-2) (After Balch CM, Soong SJ, Shaw HM, et al. An analysis of prognostic factors in 4000 patients with cutaneous melanoma. In: Blach CM, Milton GW [eds]. *Cutaneous melanoma: clinical management and treatment results worldwide.* Philadelphia: J.B. Lippincott, 1985: 321). (Reprinted with permission from Greenfield LJ, Mulholland MW, Oldham KT, et al. [eds]. *Surgery: scientific principles and practice,* 2nd ed. Philadelphia: Lippincott Williams & Wilkins, 1997: 2234, 2235.)

CASE 10.3. ▶ Malignant Melanoma with a Palpable Lymph Node

You remove a skin lesion from the patient in Case 10.1, and the pathologic findings indicate a Clark III malignant melanoma. After reviewing the depth of the lesion, you reexamine the patient.

TABLE 10-2

American Joint Commission on Cancer Melanoma Staging System, 1985

TUMOR–NODE–METASTASIS (TNM) DEFINITIONS

Primary Tumor (T)

T_X Unknown, cannot be assessed
T_0 Atypical melanocytic hyperplasia in situ, Clark level I
T_1 Clark level II, thickness ≤ 0.75 mm
T_2 Clark level III, thickness 0.76–1.5 mm
T_3 Clark level IV, thickness 1.51–4.0 mm
T_4 Clark level V, depth ≥ 4.0 mm or satellites within 2 cm of primary tumor

Regional lymph nodes (N)

N_X Unknown, cannot be assessed
N_0 No regional lymph node involvement
N_1 One regional node station, nodes, mobiles, 5 cm in diameter or smaller, or negative nodes and fewer than five in-transit metastases
N_2 More than one node station positive, nodes larger than 5 cm or fixed, more than five in-transit metastases, or any metastases with positive nodes

Distant Metastasis (M)

M_X Unknown, cannot be assessed
M_0 None
M_1 Involvement of skin or subcutaneous tissue beyond the regional lymph node basin
M_2 Visceral

STAGE GROUPING

Stage	T	N	M	Ulceration Present
0	T_{is}	N_0	M_0	−
IA	T_1	N_0	M_0	−
IB	T_1	N_0	M_0	+
IB	T_2	N_0	M_0	−
IIA	T_2	N_0	M_0	+
IIA	T_3	N_0	M_0	−
IIB	T_3	N_0	M_0	+
IIB	T_4	N_0	M_0	−
III	Any T	N_1	M_0	+/−
IV	Any T	N_2	M_0	+/−
	Any T	Any N	M_1	

▷ *How would the presence of a palpable axillary lymph node change the management plan?*

▶ The presence of axillary lymphadenopathy suggests metastatic disease, potentially stage III or IV disease. **Regional lymphadenectomy** to establish the diagnosis and to remove the involved nodes is warranted. With metastasis, there is a 75% chance of recurrence of melanoma in the next 5 years. Patients should undergo **complete staging** for the presence of distant metastasis. This usually includes CXR, liver function tests, CT of the abdomen, and MRI of the brain. Treatment with interferon may increase survival by as much as 40%.

Case Variation 10.6.4. A malignant melanoma of the anus

▶ Anal melanomas, along with other mucosal melanomas, are associated with a particularly **poor prognosis,** with mortality near 100% at 5 years. Thin lesions can be locally excised and most commonly occur at the dentate line. **Thicker lesions usually require abdominoperineal resection of the anorectum,** although wide local excision may also be performed. Abdominoperineal resection has a lower rate of local recurrence than local excision, but neither procedure produces a better patient survival rate. Regional lymph node excision is only indicated for positive inguinal nodes.

CASE 10.7. ▶ Small Bowel Obstruction and History of Malignant Melanoma

A patient with a stage I malignant melanoma removed 5 years ago who returns to the emergency department with abdominal distention, nausea, vomiting, and radiographic evidence of small bowel obstruction.

▷ *What management is appropriate?*

▶ Melanoma has a unique propensity to **metastasize to the peritoneal cavity** and involve the viscera; the common presentation is a small bowel obstruction. Exploration is indicated, but the prognosis is poor. Palliative treatment may be possible with solitary lesions or a resectable group of lesions, and patients may be able to leave the hospital. However, many patients succumb.

SARCOMA

CASE 10.8. ▶ Sarcoma of the Lower Extremity

A 45-year-old man presents with a painless mass on his anterior thigh. The slow-growing 5-cm lesion has been present for several months.

▷ *What facts may be important in the history and physical examination?*

▶ Soft tissue sarcomas are rare neoplasms of connective tissue; clinicians diagnose approximately 6000 new cases per year. Family history of sarcoma is uncommon, but it may increase the incidence of subsequent sarcoma. A history of therapeutic radiation (fibrosarcoma) or axillary lymphadenectomy (lymphangiosarcoma) one to two decades earlier has been associated with sarcoma development. A history of trauma with a subsequent and persistent mass can be a sarcoma misdiagnosed as a hematoma.

Physical examination is important to distinguish a sarcoma from other benign lesions such as hematoma, lipoma, fibroma, hamartoma, or hemangioma. Sarcomas occur as **firm, painless masses** that are typically larger than benign tumors. Regional adenopathy is rare (2.6%) but may be evident in several types of sarcomas (lymphangiosarcoma, epithelioid sarcoma, embryonal rhabdomyosarcoma, malignant fibrous histiocytoma, synovial cell sarcoma).

▷ *What type of biopsy or excision is appropriate?*

▶ Biopsy is directed by the size of the lesion. Excisional biopsy is indicated for masses less than 3 cm.

QUICK CUTS Incisional biopsy is the initial step for sarcomas 3 cm or more. The biopsy incision should parallel the subsequent surgical incision for a definitive resection (Figure 10-6).

Excisional biopsies performed in lesions greater than 3 cm or perpendicular to definitive resection margins are inappropriate. The larger defect makes primary closure complex or potentially contaminates additional compartments with tumor and increases the risk for local recurrence. Core biopsy may provide accurate diagnosis in select centers, but fine needle aspiration (FNA) provides nondiagnostic tissue and should be discouraged. In addition, frozen section biopsies of sarcoma do not lead to a reliable diagnosis.

The biopsy confirms a soft tissue sarcoma.

▷ *What pathologic features prompt concern?*

▶ Sarcomas can be pathologically divided into **low-grade and high-grade malignancy** based on the number of **mitotic figures and the degree of necrosis (not the cell type of**

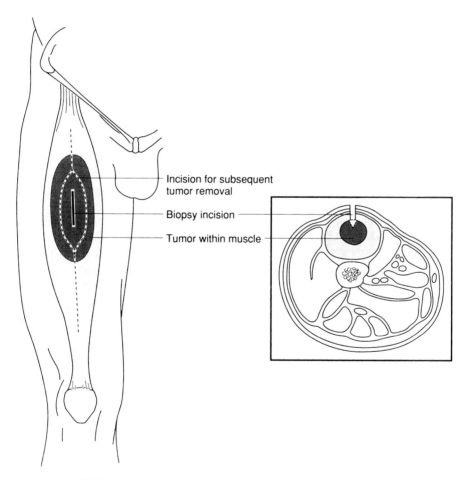

Incision for subsequent tumor removal

Biopsy incision

Tumor within muscle

FIGURE 10-6. Technique for incisional biopsy of a sarcoma. (From Greenfield LJ, Mulholland MW, Oldham KT, et al. [eds]. *Surgery: scientific principles and practice,* 2nd ed. Philadelphia: Lippincott Williams & Wilkins, 1997: 2252.)

origin). Gross **size greater than 15 cm and a symptomatic lesion** have been associated with poor outcome (Figure 10-7A).

▶ *What diagnostic tests are necessary to characterize and stage the cancer?*

▶ Sarcomas have a high rate of metastasis on presentation (22%); the most common sites for metastasis are the liver, lung, bone, and brain. Patients should have a metastatic workup prior to resection. A CT scan is very useful for detection of bony involvement, and an MRI scan detects involvement of adjacent soft tissue structures (e.g., muscle group definition, involvement of neurovascular bundles, and the interface between tumor and normal tissue).

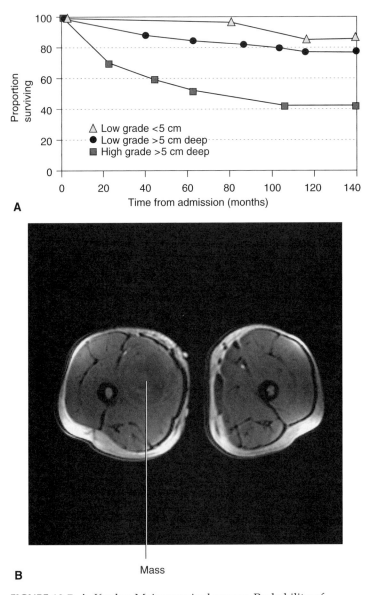

FIGURE 10-7. A. Kaplan-Meier survival curves. Probability of overall survival of sarcoma by stage. **B.** MRI of a thigh showing a large mass in the muscle compartment. **C.** Another MRI view of sarcoma of an extremity.

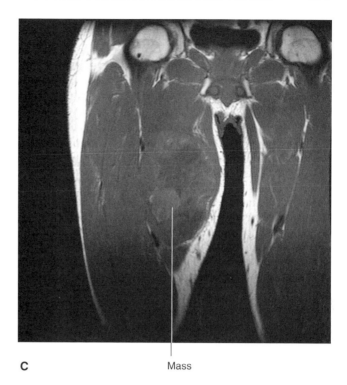

FIGURE 10-7. (CONTINUED)

C   Mass

Staging should be completed with the performance of abdominal–pelvic CT and plain CXR. A suspicious CXR should prompt a chest CT scan, and the presence of bone pain should prompt a bone scan (Figure 10-7B).

▷ *What are the staging criteria for sarcomas?*

▶ The standard TNM system is used for staging (Table 10-3.)

Pathologic findings indicate that this lesion is a low-grade sarcoma. The workup is negative for metastasis.

▷ *What type of resection is appropriate?*

▶ Surgical therapy must balance the morbidity of the resection with the risk of local recurrence.

 QUICK CUTS A basic principle in sarcoma surgery: An extensive initial resection of the primary tumor is necessary to obtain long-standing local tumor control.

Total resection of a tissue compartment or an amputation of the extremity has the highest potential for local control.

In this case, most surgeons would perform a **total compartmental resection** for two reasons: (1) it is limb-sparing and (2) it provides excellent local control (Figure 10-8). This technique removes the entire structure that involves the tumor plus all of the enclosing tissue. For example, a sarcoma of a large muscle such as the quadriceps femoris involves **removing the entire length of the muscle, its origin and insertion, and its investing fas-**

Most of the listed conditions have signs or symptoms that could be detected with a complete history and physical examination.

No additional history or physical findings indicative of other diseases are evident.

▷ *Is surgical repair of the hernia recommended?*

▶ If the physical condition of the patient is acceptable, repair of the hernia is appropriate.

> **QUICK CUTS** The **risk of intestinal strangulation** of the hernia is the most compelling reason for hernia repair.

This risk varies with the type of hernia; hernias with a narrow neck pose a higher risk. Femoral hernias are particularly prone to strangulation (Figure 10-10). Other significant reasons for repair include local pain, enlargement, inability to lift, and patient preference.

▷ *What are the surgical options for hernia repair and their advantages?*

▶ The basic surgical options for a direct or indirect hernia are open and laparoscopic repair.

Open repairs

▶ **Bassini repair** involves a reconstruction of the posterior inguinal canal, with a suturing of a superior abdominal wall layer (internal oblique muscle, transversus abdominal muscle, and **transversalis fascia**) to an inferior location on **the inguinal ligament** and iliopubic tract (Figure 10-11).

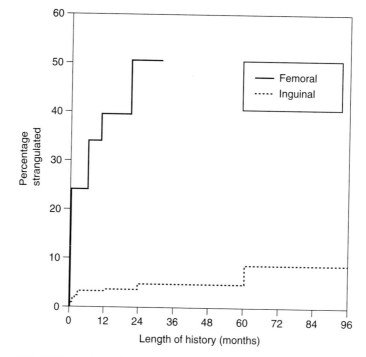

FIGURE 10-10. Cumulative incidence of strangulation with inguinal and femoral hernias.

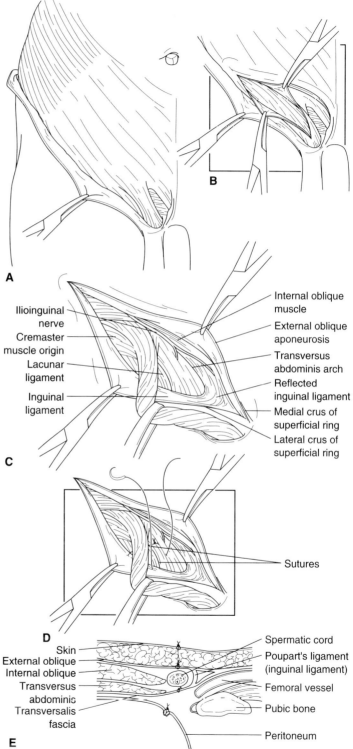

FIGURE 10-11. Bassini repair. **A.** Parasagittal section through the groin. The hernia (through a weakness in the transversalis fascia) is repaired by suturing the transversalis fascia to the shelving (reflecting) edge of the inguinal ligament. **B.** The external oblique aponeurosis and external ring are opened. **C.** The spermatic cord is elevated. **D.** The transversalis fascia and shelving (reflecting) edge of the inguinal ligament are exposed. **E.** Suturing of the two structures together follows. (Redrawn from Fitzgibbons RJ Jr, Greenburg AG [eds]. *Nyhus and Condon's hernia.* 5th ed. Philadelphia: Lippincott Williams & Wilkins, 2002: 36, 69.)

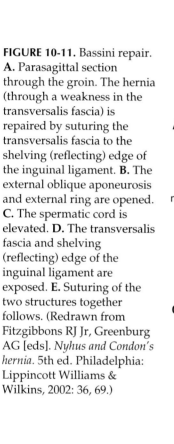

Bassini repair, a widely practiced procedure, has an acceptably low recurrence rate of several percent over multiple years. Its major weakness is the tension it places on the structure; with poor tissue, it is likely to fail.

▶ **Cooper's ligament repair** is similar to Bassini repair except that the inferior sutures are placed into Cooper's ligament, which is the **periosteum of the pubic ramus** (Figure 10-12). This approach is better for femoral hernias and attenuated inguinal ligaments.

 Most hernia repairs attach the transversalis fascia to either the inguinal ligament or the periosteum of the pubic ramus to the inguinal ligament.

▶ **Shouldice repair,** another widely practiced procedure, involves attaching a reinforced transversalis fascia to the inguinal ligament in two layers.

▶ **Lichtenstein repair** uses **prosthetic mesh** to approximate the superior abdominal wall structures to the inguinal ligament (Figure 10-13). The **use of mesh avoids creating tension on the fascial structures,** which is believed to lessen postoperative pain and recurrence. **This procedure has become popular with a high percentage of surgeons.**

Laparoscopic procedures

▶ Although laparoscopic procedures are acceptable and effective, they have not gained wide acceptance because of a **steep learning curve and unproven results** to date.

   Transabdominal preperitoneal repair involves attachment of mesh to the floor of the inguinal canal from the preperitoneal space (i.e., from within the abdominal cavity), but in a preperitoneal location (Figure 10-14). Its major complications are general anesthesia and the risk of abdominal adhesion at the laparoscopic sites.

   Totally extraperitoneal repair entails inflation of a balloon in the preperitoneal plane to expose the inguinal floor. Once exposed, the floor can be laparoscopically repaired using a prosthetic mesh to cover the defect. The anatomy and surgical procedures are more difficult to learn.

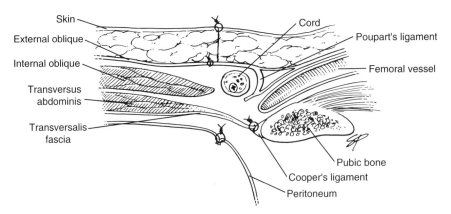

FIGURE 10-12. Cooper's ligament or McVay repair. Parasagittal section through the groin. The hernia (through a weakness in the transversalis fascia) is repaired by suturing the transversalis fascia to Cooper's ligament, which is a portion of the periosteum of the pubic bone. The exposure is similar to that shown for the Bassini repair but with deeper dissection to expose the pubic ramus with Cooper's ligament. (Redrawn from Fitzgibbons RJ Jr, Greenburg AG [eds]. *Nyhus and Condon's hernia.* 5th ed. Philadelphia: Lippincott Williams & Wilkins, 2002: 36.)

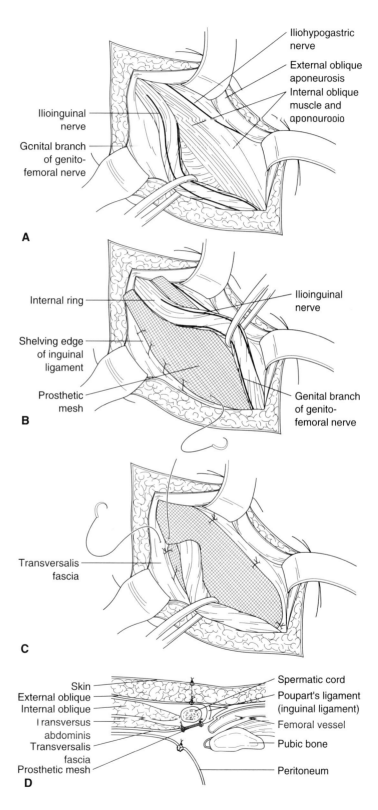

FIGURE 10-13. Lichtenstein repair. **A.** The hernia (through a weakness in the transversalis fascia) is repaired by a piece of mesh sutured to the transversalis fascia and shelving edge of the inguinal ligament. **B.** The spermatic cord together with its cremasteric covering, external spermatic vessels, and genital nerve is raised, and the cremasteric fibers are cut transversely or longitudinally at the level of the internal ring. **C.** The spermatic cord is placed between the two tails of the mesh. **D.** The lower edges of the two tails are sutured to the inguinal ligament for creation of a new internal ring made of mesh. (Redrawn from Fitzgibbons RJ Jr, Greenburg AG [eds]. *Nyhus and Condon's hernia,* 5th ed. Philadelphia: Lippincott Williams & Wilkins, 2002: 36, 151, 153.)

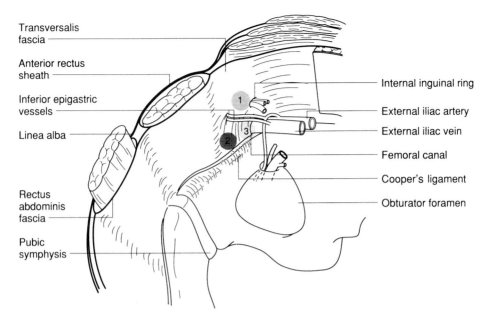

FIGURE 10-14. Laparoscopic repair of inguinal hernia. A view of the posterior aspect of the inguinal region. No. 1 is the site of an indirect inguinal hernia, which is lateral to the inferior epigastric vessels, traveling down the inguinal canal. No. 2 is the site of a direct inguinal hernia, which is medial to the inferior epigastric vessels, traveling directly though the posterior wall of the inguinal canal. No. 3 is the site of a femoral hernia, which is deep to the inguinal ligament, traveling though the femoral canal. All three types of hernia result from defects in the transversalis fascia.

There are several approaches to hernias in these locations using a laparoscope. Repairs generally involve the use of onlay mesh graphs, mesh plugs, and stapling devices. (From Greenfield LJ, Mulholland MW, Oldham KT, et al. [eds]. *Surgery: scientific principles and practice.* 2nd ed. Philadelphia: Lippincott Williams & Wilkins, 1997: 1222.)

The patient wants to know the potential complications of the procedure and his chance for cure.

▶ *How do you respond?*

▶ The principal complications of hernia repair are injuries to nerves or nearby structures. Injury to the genital branch of **genitofemoral nerve, ilioinguinal, iliohypogastric, and lateral femoral cutaneous nerves** may occur, resulting in sensory defects (Figure 10-15). The rate of recurrence, which varies according to the type of procedure and the experience of the surgeon, is 1%–10%. Other problems such as testicular atrophy, edema, and ischemia are rare. Wound infection and wound hematoma occur in less than 1% of cases.

Successful repair of the patient's hernia using the Lichtenstein method has occurred.

▶ *What instructions should the patient receive regarding short- and long-term follow-up?*

▶ The patient should **avoid lifting for the first 6 weeks** after hernia surgery. By that time, the wound should have regained 75–90% of its final strength. Gradual progression to full lifting is then possible. Most surgeons would see the patient in the office 1 week and 6 weeks postsurgery to monitor healing of the incision. Patients who have any wound complications or questions about hernia recurrence should return to the office.

CASE 10.12. ▶ Additional Hernia-Related Problems

A 32-year-old man has an inguinal hernia. You are repairing the hernia and are almost ready to make your incision. Your resident asks you to describe the surgical landmarks of the inguinal canal.

▷ *What structures would you identify?*

▶ The most important structures to identify and preserve while repairing the hernia are the ilioinguinal nerve and spermatic cord. Obviously knowledge of the internal and external rings and general anatomy are important.

Your resident asks you to briefly describe the difference between the following hernias.

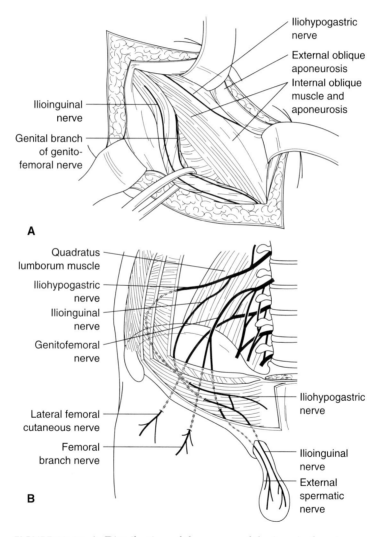

FIGURE 10-15. A. Distribution of the nerves of the inguinal region. **B.** The nerves seen from a hernia incision. The nerves exposed during repair are the most commonly injured, causing sensory defects in their distribution. (Redrawn from Fitzgibbons RJ Jr, Greenburg AG [eds]. *Nyhus and Condon's hernia.* 5th ed. Philadelphia: Lippincott Williams & Wilkins, 2002: 151, 39.)

What is your response?

Case Variation 10.12.1. An adult and a pediatric inguinal hernia

► Pediatric hernias involve no defect in the floor of the inguinal canal; thus, they are indirect inguinal hernias.

> **QUICK CUTS** Pediatric hernias differ from adult hernias in that pediatric hernias usually represent a **persistent patent processus vaginalis.**

There is a direct communication between the peritoneal cavity and inguinal canal and scrotum in hernias in children, which are usually intermittent and are detected by the child's mother. There is a **high incidence of bilaterality,** and many surgeons repair both sides simultaneously. Repair is limited to a **high ligation of the sac** with no abdominal wall repair because no abdominal wall defect is present (Figure 10-16).

Case Variation 10.12.2. An inguinal and femoral hernia

► An **inguinal hernia** is a defect in the abdominal wall allowing structures to pass down the inguinal canal, or through the floor of the inguinal canal, toward the scrotum. The **femoral hernia,** which is more common in women, **typically produces a mass below the inguinal ligament.** The hernia passes into the upper thigh through a space bounded anteriorly by the iliopubic tract (reflection of the inguinal ligament), posteriorly by Cooper's ligament (pubic ramus) periosteum, medially by the pubic tubercle and its ligamentous attachments, and laterally by the femoral vein. Repair of a femoral hernia involves closing the femoral space with either mesh or a Cooper's ligament (McVay) repair (Figure 10-17).

You are repairing an inguinal hernia.

► *In addition to nerves, what other structures can be intimate with the hernia and therefore injured in the repair?*

► Hernias, so-called sliding hernias, may involve other structures that form part of a wall of a hernia (Figure 10-18). Sliding hernias most commonly occur in indirect hernias. **The most common forms involve the bladder, cecum, or sigmoid colon.** The protrusion of a portion of the intestine wall into the hernia sac results in a Richter hernia. The protrusion of a Meckel diverticulum into the hernia sac results in a Littré hernia. Other structures such as the ovary and appendix may also occur in a hernia.

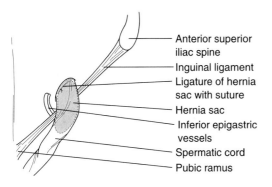

Anterior superior iliac spine
Inguinal ligament
Ligature of hernia sac with suture
Hernia sac
Inferior epigastric vessels
Spermatic cord
Pubic ramus

FIGURE 10-16. Pediatric hernias, which are characterized by a patent processus vaginalis with a communication between the peritoneal cavity and the inguinal canal, are repaired by "high" ligation of the sac at the point where it just enters the peritoneal cavity. There is no defect in the floor of the inguinal canal; no repair is necessary there. (Redrawn from Fitzgibbons RJ Jr, Greenburg AG [eds]. *Nyhus and Condon's hernia.* 5th ed. Philadelphia: Lippincott Williams & Wilkins, 2002: 78.)

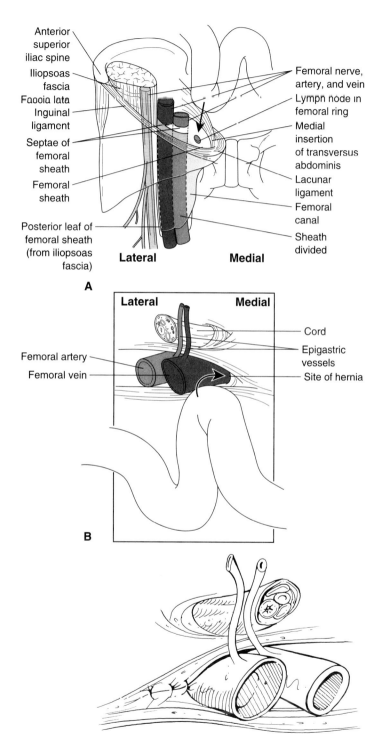

FIGURE 10-17. A. The femoral sheath and its associated structures. The anterior leaf of the sheath is continuous with the transversalis fascia of the anterior abdominal wall, and the posterior sheath is derived from the iliacus fascia (a portion of the transversalis fascia). **B.** Femoral hernias enter the femoral canal, which lies just medial to the femoral vein within its sheath.

C. A crucial, transitional suture that includes connective tissue investing the femoral vein is necessary to obliterate the defect completely. **D.** Repair of a femoral hernia involves suturing the transversalis fascia/femoral sheath to Cooper's ligament, similar to a Cooper's ligament repair. (From Fitzgibbons RJ Jr, Greenburg AG [eds]. *Nyhus and Condon's hernia.* 5th ed. Philadelphia: Lippincott Williams & Wilkins, 2002: 68, 191, 194.) (continued)

Labels in figure A:
- Anterior superior iliac spine
- Iliopsoas fascia
- Fascia lata
- Inguinal ligament
- Septae of femoral sheath
- Femoral sheath
- Posterior leaf of femoral sheath (from iliopsoas fascia)
- Femoral nerve, artery, and vein
- Lymph node in femoral ring
- Medial insertion of transversus abdominis
- Lacunar ligament
- Femoral canal
- Sheath divided
- Lateral
- Medial

A

Labels in figure B:
- Lateral
- Medial
- Femoral artery
- Femoral vein
- Cord
- Epigastric vessels
- Site of hernia

B

C

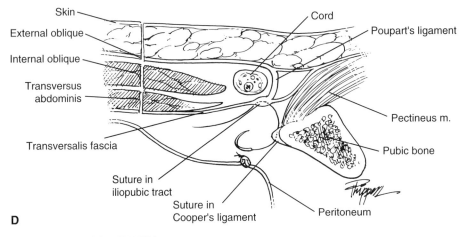

D

FIGURE 10-17. (CONTINUED)

 It is important to recognize the presence of a sliding hernia at the time of surgery so that the bowel or other contained structure is not injured.

CASE 10.13. ▶ Ventral Hernia

A 46-year-old man with a ventral hernia had a previous laparotomy for adhesions 1 year ago, and the hernia has been getting progressively larger. He has no other symptoms.

▶ *Do you recommend repair?*

▶ Hernia repair is generally recommended, because there is a risk of bowel incarceration and strangulation, which is greater for defects with a narrow neck. Progressive enlarge-

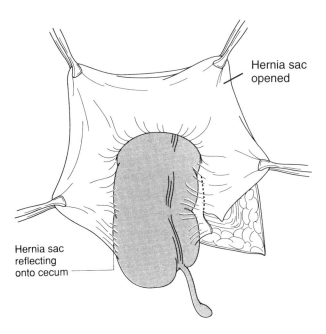

FIGURE 10-18. Sliding hernia. The visceral peritoneum covering a retroperitoneal organ is also part of the wall of the hernia sac. The organ must be dissected away from the sac and returned to the peritoneal cavity, after which the hernia is repaired using standard methods. (From Greenfield LJ, Mulholland MW, Oldham KT, et al. [eds]. *Surgery: scientific principles and practice.* 2nd ed. Philadelphia: Lippincott Williams & Wilkins, 1997: 1219.)

ment of the defect, making later repair more difficult, is also a possibility. Hernia repair might not be appropriate if the patient's medical condition is poor and the operative risk is excessive. However, repair is definitely warranted if a previous episode of bowel obstruction or other major complication related to the hernia has occurred.

▶ *How involved a procedure is repair of a ventral hernia?*

▶ Some ventral hernias are simple and easy to repair with primary closure. Larger or recurrent hernias may be very difficult to repair because of **inadequate tissue strength, insufficient tissue, infection,** or **poor nutrition.** Prosthetic mesh, which is sometimes required for closure, carries the risk of infection. In addition, most ventral hernias require entry into the peritoneal cavity and dissection of the bowel off the posterior surface of the hernia sac. This is associated with the risk of bowel injury as well as the probability of postoperative ileus, abdominal distention, and pulmonary complications such as atelectasis.

CHAPTER 11

Breast Disorders

Bruce E. Jarrell M.D., Wendy Berg M.D., Katherine Tkaczuk M.D.

CASE 11.1. ▶ Screening for Breast Cancer

A 42-year-old woman comes to you for routine evaluation. Her past history is significant for no previous visits to a physician. She asks your advice regarding prevention and early detection of breast cancer. Physical examination reveals no breast or axillary abnormalities.

▶ *What management advice should you give this woman?*

▶ It is very important that women heed the following advice; breast cancer affects 1 in 8 women at some point in their lives. Most physicians recommend **breast self-examination,** which involves monthly self-examination, as well as breast examination by a physician once yearly. In addition, all women over 40 years of age, including this patient, should have a **yearly mammogram.**

The woman asks what factors increase her risk of breast cancer.

▶ *What do you tell her?*

▶ Research has demonstrated that breast cancer has hereditary patterns.

 QUICK CUTS The most common factor that increases the risk of breast cancer is having **one or more first-degree relatives who have had breast cancer.**

▶ The majority of inherited breast cancer is associated with two genes, BRCA1 and BRCA2. BRCA1 is also associated with ovarian cancer.

Other conditions place women at a high risk for breast cancer (Table 11-1). Based on a careful history revealing a first-degree relative with breast cancer, you decide that this patient is at increased risk for breast cancer.

▶ *How might this change your advice and management?*

▶ Increased risk should prompt both a more frequent surveillance for any abnormalities and a higher degree of suspicion for any given finding. Based on degree of risk, experts have developed general guidelines for necessary screening (Table 11-2).

The woman wants to know how screening tests will improve her chances of survival if she is affected by breast cancer.

▶ *What do you tell her?*

TABLE 11-1

Risk Factors for Breast Cancer

Factor	High Risk	Low Risk
Relative Risk More Than 4×		
Age	Older	Younger
History of cancer in one breast	Yes	No
Family history of premenopausal bilateral breast cancer	Yes	No
Relative Risk 2–4×		
Any first-degree relative with breast cancer	Yes	No
History of primary cancer of ovary or endometrium	Yes	No
Age at first full-term pregnancy	Older than 30 years	Younger than 20 years
Oophorectomy	No	Yes
Body habitus, postmenopausal	Obese	Thin
Country of birth	North America, northern Europe	Asia, Africa
Socioeconomic class	Upper	Lower
History of fibrocystic disease	Yes	No
Relative risk 1–2×		
Marital status	Single	Married
Place of residence	Urban, northern U.S.	Rural, southern U.S.
Race	White	Black
Age at menarche (<12 years)	Early	Late
Age at menopause (>55 years)	Late	Early

Adapted with permission from Kelsey JL, Gannon MD. The epidermology of breast cancer. *CA Cancer J Clin* 1991;41(31):157.

TABLE 11-2

Screening Recommendations for Breast Cancer

Non-High-Risk Patients
Monthly breast self-examination starting at age 20
Breast examination by experienced professional every 2–3 years at ages 20–39, yearly after age 40
Initial mammogram at age 40
Subsequent mammograms every 1–2 years from ages 40–50 and every year after age 50

High-Risk Patients
Monthly breast self-examination starting at age 20
Breast examination by experienced professional at least twice a year starting at age 25
Initial mammogram at age 30
Subsequent mammograms every 1–2 years until age 40; yearly mammograms after age 40

Modified from the American Cancer Society and the American College of Radiology.

▶ Several studies have demonstrated that **annual mammography detects lesions when they are smaller, before they are evident on physical examination.** This benefit appears to be strongest in women between 50 and 64 years of age. The American Medical Association has more recently extended this to women between the ages of 40 and 50 years. Most screening studies for breast cancer are associated with a mortality reduction of 30% or more in women over 50 years of age.

 However, mammography does not replace the need for breast self-examination.

Mammographic screening should begin **earlier if there is a strong family history.** In women with first-degree relatives who have had breast cancer, some physicians would recommend beginning annual mammography 10 years before the age of the relative at diagnosis of the cancer. Mammograms are reliable; however, **it is never appropriate to delay biopsy of a clinically suspicious lesion just because a mammogram is negative.**

▶ *What risks do mammograms pose?*

▶ The primary risks associated with mammography are radiation exposure and false-negative results. The radiation exposure for most modern mammograms is 0.1–0.3 rads per study. For comparison, radiation exposure from chest radiography is 0.05 rads per study. Experts believe that the radiation from a mammogram is very low. The best estimates indicate that perhaps 1 death secondary to breast cancer per million women per year occurs as a result of radiation exposure. Mammograms have a false-negative rate of about 7%–20%. This rate may be higher in younger women and women with more glandular and less fatty, atrophic tissue. Mammography appears to be more accurate in older women whose glandular breast tissue has become atrophic and replaced with fat. These ambiguities in interpretation again emphasize the need for breast self-examination and the importance of clinical assessment of any palpable abnormality (Tables 11-1 and 11-2).

CASE 11.2. ▶ Evaluation of a Mammographic Abnormality

A 60-year-old woman is referred by her primary physician for an abnormality on her routine mammogram. She has a negative history for breast cancer. She is G_3P_3, and since undergoing a hysterectomy 20 years ago, she has been taking estrogen-replacement therapy. The mammogram shows a solid 1.5-cm mass in the upper outer quadrant. The surgeon to whom the patient is referred confirms that no masses are palpable in the breast. The axillary, supraclavicular, and cervical areas are negative for lymph nodes.

▶ *What are the various types of mammographic abnormalities?*

▶ Mammographic abnormalities can generally be classified as combinations of the following entities:

1. **Masses**
2. **Asymmetric densities**
3. **Microcalcifications**

▶ When an abnormality is found on screening, additional imaging is usually appropriate. The interpretation receives the Breast Imaging Reporting and Database System (BI-RADS) category O ("needs additional evaluation") designation. [For microcalcifications, spot magnification mammographic views are usually necessary (Table 11-3; Figure 11-1). For

TABLE 11-3

Mammography Categories According to the Breast Imaging Reporting and Database System (BI-RADS)

Category	Interpretation
0	Needs additional evaluation
1	Normal
2	Benign findings, recommend routine screening
3	Probably benign, recommend short initial (6-month) follow-up
4	Suspicious, biopsy should be considered
5	Highly suggestive of malignancy

From the American College of Radiology.

masses and asymmetric densities, it is often necessary to supplement additional mammographic views with ultrasound to obtain a final assessment. Asymmetric densities can result from operative procedures, previous radiation therapy, previous infections, normal variation, and other local processes.

 Comparison to old films and clinical examination is especially important.

After performance of diagnostic mammography and possibly ultrasound, it is possible to make a final assessment (Table 11-3).

▶ *How should mammographic findings be interpreted?*

▶ **"Probably benign" findings warrant follow-up. The risk of malignancy is less than 2%.** It is necessary to observe affected patients; this approach does not adversely affect the prognosis and stage of disease. Patient compliance is mandatory for follow-up. Biopsy may be essential if patients desire pregnancy, are candidates for transplantation, or have other suspicious lesions.

   "Suspicious" findings warrant biopsy. Only 15%–35% of lesions recommended for biopsy prove malignant. Initial diagnosis by core-needle biopsy is appropriate for the vast majority of lesions. A negative result may obviate the need for surgery, whereas a positive result permits directive surgical planning.

CASE 11.3. ▶ Evaluation of Mammographic Microcalcifications

A 44-year-old woman has a screening mammogram, which shows a 1-cm area of pleomorphic microcalcifications, with no associated mass. These findings are suspicious for ductal carcinoma in situ (DCIS). Breast examination is normal, with no palpable abnormalities.

▶ *What is the next step?*

▶ Because there are no palpable abnormalities, the radiologist would typically perform additional **magnification mammography.** After further evaluation, the radiologist would

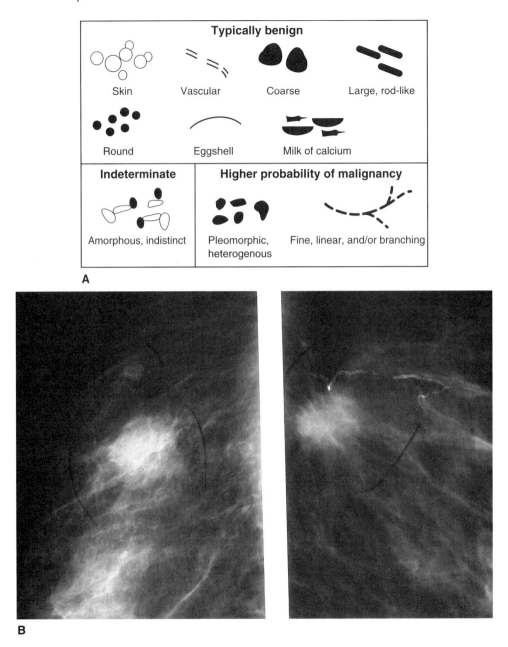

FIGURE 11-1. A. Diagram showing the morphology of typically benign calcifications and those with a higher probability of malignancy. **B.** A mammogram showing a spiculated mass in the breast that is positive for infiltrating ductal carcinoma.

recommend either a stereotactic-guided core needle biopsy or a localization and open surgical biopsy. If the **mammographic lesion is indeterminate and even less suspicious, stereotactic core-needle biopsy is preferable** because it produces a sample that allows a reliable histologic diagnosis, obviating the need for an open biopsy (Figure 11-2). Multiple cores can be taken with an 11-gauge needle. **Fine needle aspiration (FNA) is not a good technique** to use for biopsy in this case because it often produces a nondiagnostic speci-

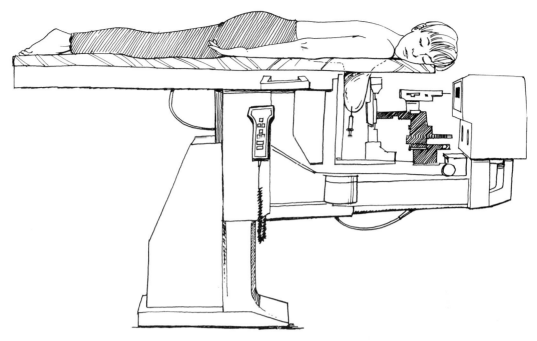

FIGURE 11-2. Stereotactic breast biopsy. The patient is positioned on a table that allows precise imaging of the breast lesion and image-guided biopsy of the lesion. (From Silen W. *Atlas of techniques in breast surgery.* Philadelphia: Lippincott-Raven, 1996: 50.)

men. **Needle localization and open surgical biopsy may be preferable if a lesion is highly suspicious for malignancy on mammography** (Figure 11-3). This approach allows complete excision of the lesion, which may be adequate therapy with one procedure.

In needle localization and open surgical biopsy, a clinician puts a needle into the mammographically demonstrated lesion under radiologic guidance and leaves it in place while the patient is transported to the operating room. Using the needle as a guide, a surgeon excises the lesion. A radiologist must then evaluate the specimen (specimen radiography) to ensure that the lesion has been removed. Ultrasound is not necessary in this case. However, ultrasound may be useful for suspicious calcifications; it can detect an occult mass often indicative of an infiltrating compound in up to one-third of patients; these patients then undergo biopsies under ultrasound guidance.

CASE 11.4. ▶ Biopsy Results in Lesions Visible on Mammography

A 40-year-old woman has her first mammogram, which reveals amorphous calcifications in one breast. She then has stereotactic core biopsy.

▶ *What evaluation and management are appropriate for the following pathologic findings?*

Case Variation 11.4.1. Ductal carcinoma in situ (DCIS) [Table 11-4]

▶ DCIS usually manifests as incidental microcalcifications on mammography, although patients may present with a breast mass. **Surgery is necessary** (Figure 11-3). Even when the

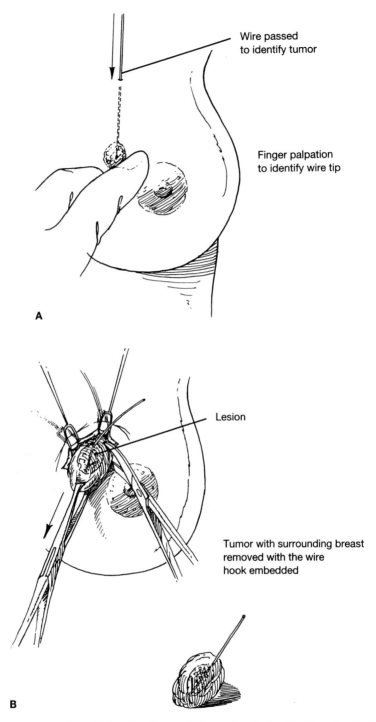

Wire passed
to identify tumor

Finger palpation
to identify wire tip

A

Lesion

Tumor with surrounding breast
removed with the wire
hook embedded

B

FIGURE 11-3. Needle localization and biopsy in a lesion that is not palpable. Under radiographic imaging, the lesion is identified and a wire with a hook is placed into the lesion to fix the wire within the lesion. The patient then goes to the operating room, where the lesion and the wire are surgically excised. A radiograph of the removed lesion and wire is then taken to be certain that the appropriate lesion has been obtained. (From Silen W. *Atlas of techniques in breast surgery*. Philadelphia: Lippincott-Raven, 1996: 52, 55.)

TABLE 11-4

Comparison of Ductal Carcinoma in Situ (DCIS) and Lobular Carcinoma in Situ (LCIS)

Feature	LCIS	DCIS
Age (years)	44–47	54–58
Incidence*	2%–5%	5%–30%
Premenopausal	2/3	1/3
Clinical signs	None	Mass, pain, nipple discharge
Mammographic signs	None	Microcalcifications
Incidence synchronous invasive carcinoma	5%	2%–46%
Multicentricity	60%–90%	40%–80%
Bilaterality	50%–70%	10%–20%
Axillary metastasis	1%	1%–2%
Subsequent carcinomas		
Incidence	25%–35%	25%–70%
Laterality	Bilateral	Ipsilateral
Interval to diagnosis	15–20 years	5–10 years
Histology	Ductal or lobular	Ductal >> lobular

*Among biopsies of mammographically detected breast lesions.
From Greenfield LJ, Mulholland MW, Oldham KT, et al. [eds]. *Surgery: scientific principles and practice.* 2nd ed. Philadelphia: Lippincott Williams & Wilkins, 1997.

best technique is used for core biopsy, **10%–20% of lesions diagnosed as DCIS have an infiltrative component at excision.** Thus, careful examination and complete excision of diseased tissue is important. If lesions are incompletely excised or untreated, the 10-year risk of invasive carcinoma is 30% or more. The risk of contralateral invasive carcinoma is 5% or less. In general, invasive carcinoma is more likely in larger lesions rather than smaller ones.

DCIS is often multifocal. DCIS has several histologic patterns, including comedo, micropapillary, and cribriform. The **comedo pattern has a higher malignant potential, with up to 30% containing invasive carcinoma.** Axillary metastasis is present in 4% of patients with the comedo variant but rare in those with other histologic patterns.

 QUICK CUTS **Simple mastectomy** with or without reconstruction is the current gold standard for diffuse and multicentric DCIS.

▶ Wide excision and radiotherapy is a preferred alternative for smaller lesions. **If wide excision is performed, it is important to document pathology-free margins in the specimen.** Most physicians would **also add radiation therapy because of the multifocal nature of the lesion** and the effect on recurrence. Local recurrence rate of DCIS falls to 22% with wide excision and radiation and 4% with simple mastectomy over a 10 year period. **Nodal dissection is not necessary,** because nodal metastases are rare except for the comedo variant. In the comedo case, axillary node sampling (by sentinel node approach) may be appropriate.

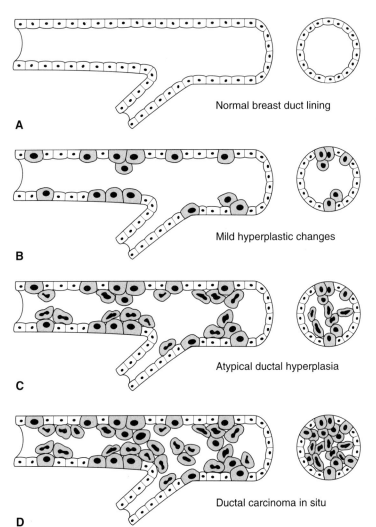

A   Normal breast duct lining

B   Mild hyperplastic changes

C   Atypical ductal hyperplasia

D   Ductal carcinoma in situ

FIGURE 11-4. Progression of breast duct lining from normal to carcinoma in situ. **A.** Normal. **B.** Mild hyperplastic changes. **C.** Atypical ductal hyperplasia. **D.** Ductal carcinoma in situ. In the normal duct, there are two layers of cells with a myoepithelial outer layer and an epithelial layer on the inside. In the usual hyperplastic lesion, there is hyperplasia of the inner lining. With atypical ductal hyperplasia, there is secondary bridging and additional hypertrophy of the epithelial layer. In carcinoma in situ, there is marked proliferation with carcinoma limited by the basal lamina.

Case Variation 11.4.2. Lobular carcinoma in situ (LCIS) [see Table 11-4]

▶ LCIS is usually an incidental finding at histopathology (Figure 11-4). Patients rarely present with a mass, and LCIS is usually not apparent on mammography. When found adjacent to a benign mass, **surveillance is appropriate.** When found on a core biopsy of a calcification, needle localization and excision of the area may be necessary, although this is controversial. LCIS is a **malignant disease marker, with a 15%–20% chance of development of invasive cancer in either breast over a 20-year period.** With LCIS, there is almost **no risk of axillary metastasis.** This disease does have a familial occurrence in some patients.

Treatment for LCIS is **close observation,** with examination and mammography every 6 months for at least the next several years. In higher-risk patients with a history of breast cancer, bilateral simple mastectomies and immediate reconstruction may be preferable.

Case Variation 11.4.3. Sclerosing adenosis

▶ Sclerosing adenosis usually manifests as clustered microcalcifications on mammography. It may appear similar to invasive tubular carcinoma histopathologically (Figure 11-4). The associated cancer risk may be slightly higher (approximately 1.5–2×). Routine follow-up is appropriate after a diagnosis of sclerosing adenosis on core biopsy, provided there is agreement with the mammographic appearance of the targeted lesion.

Case Variation 11.4.4. Atypical ductal hyperplasia

▶ Atypical hyperplasia of the ducts or lobules may be seen in breast lesions. This condition is similar in appearance to DCIS, and the two entities are often interspersed (see Figure 11-4). The **associated risk of cancer is four to five times higher.** When core biopsy results demonstrate atypical ductal hyperplasia, **needle localization and excision are appropriate.** From 15% to 50% of cases prove malignant, depending on the volume of tissue initially sampled. The relative risk for invasive carcinoma can be determined on the basis of histologic examination (Table 11-5). Treatment is similar to DCIS, involving complete excision and close observation.

CASE 11.5. ▶ Management of a Woman with a Palpable Breast Mass

A 60-year-old woman presents with a right breast mass that was palpated by her primary care physician. She denies any breast-related symptoms, and she has never had other medical problems. Her past history is significant for the following conditions:

- Menarche, age 12 years; G_2P_2, ages 23 and 25 years; menopause, age 50 years
- Family history that is negative for cancer
- Social history that is negative for alcohol and tobacco use but positive for daily caffeine use

Physical examination is normal except for the right breast, which reveals a 1.5-cm nontender mass in the upper outer quadrant that is freely movable but firm. No axillary or supraclavicular adenopathy is evident.

TABLE 11-5

Relative Risk for Invasive Breast Carcinoma Based on Histologic Examination

No increased risk (no proliferative disease)
    Apocrine change
    Ductal ectasia
    Mild epithelial hyperplasia of usual type
Slightly increased risk (1.5–2×)
    Hyperplasia of usual type, moderate or florid
    Sclerosing adenosis, papilloma
Moderately increased risk (4–5×) [atypical hyperplasia or borderline lesions]
    Atypical ductal hyperplasia and atypical lobular hyperplasia
High risk (8–10×) [carcinoma in situ]
    Lobular carcinoma in situ and ductal carcinoma in situ

Women in each category are compared with women matched for age who had no breast biopsy with regard to risk of invasive breast cancer in the ensuing 10–20 years. (Note: These risks are not lifetime risks.)
    From Greenfield LJ, Mulholland MW, Oldham KT, et al. [eds]. *Surgery: scientific principles and practice.* 2nd ed. Philadelphia: Lippincott Williams & Wilkins, 1997.

▷ *What management plan is appropriate?*

▶ The diagnosis is most likely carcinoma. The patient should undergo the following procedures:

1. A **mammogram** to better characterize the affected breast and its lesion(s) as well as to examine the contralateral breast for synchronous lesions
2. An **ultrasound of the mass if the mass feels cystic** or if there is a history of cysts. If it is a cyst, follow-up with physical examination is appropriate. If it is painful or enlarging, aspiration is warranted (Figure 11-5).
3. A **biopsy if the mass feels solid;** this procedure establishes the diagnosis in 97% of cases. Either core biopsy or an open surgical biopsy after diagnostic imaging is appropriate (see Case 11.3). Initial diagnosis by core-needle biopsy reliably establishes the specific diagnosis on which to base subsequent management. FNA for cytology, which

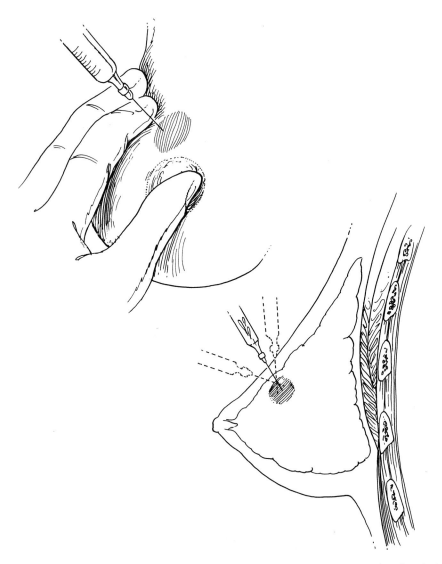

FIGURE 11-5. Method for aspiration of a breast cyst. (From Silen W: *Atlas of Techniques in Breast Surgery*. Philadelphia, Lippincott-Raven, 1996, p 38.)

is generally not sufficient to establish a diagnosis in 20% of cases, cannot distinguish in situ from infiltrating carcinomas. Open surgical biopsy should involve a wide excision with an attempt at negative margins if the mass is not too large. It is necessary to mark the biopsy and check the margins histologically, as well as to save suspicious tissue for additional studies such as estrogen receptors and flow cytologic analysis of cells.

▶ *How would the management plan change in the following women with similar physical findings?*

Case Variation 11.5.1. A 40-year-old menstruating woman

▶ **In women between 35 and 60 years of age, such breast masses are cancerous until proven otherwise.** There is no difference in the workup in the 35–60-year age group.

Case Variation 11.5.2. A 28-year-old woman

▶ **Management may differ for patients under 30 years of age, because younger women have a higher incidence of benign lesions and a higher risk of radiation from mammography.** However, a suspicion of carcinoma is always appropriate, even in young patients. Many surgeons would recommend an ultrasound study before a mammogram. If the lesion were a simple cyst, then observation or simple aspiration would be the treatment, assuming the mass completely disappeared following aspiration. If the lesion were solid and typical of a fibroadenoma, observation or elective removal without prior core biopsy would be appropriate, because 98% of solid lesions in this age group are fibroadenomas. Mammography is appropriate if clinical examination or sonography prompts a suspicion of cancer.

Observation may be indicated for selected young women in whom nodularity or breast lumps appears physiologic. A physician may observe patients for one or two menstrual cycles and then follow them if there is no change in physical findings. It is important to note that this is acceptable standard of care only in low-risk women of young age (<30 years). In older women or women at increased risk for breast cancer, definitive diagnosis is necessary. Ultrasound is warranted for evaluation of masses that develop in pregnant young women, and close follow-up is necessary. **Core-needle biopsy is appropriate if the mass persists, enlarges, or appears suspicious, because the risk of cancer is significant.**

CASE 11.6. ▶ Management of a Woman with "Lumpy" Breasts

A 35-year-old woman has tender breasts before her menstrual periods. She complains of "lumpy" breasts.

▶ *What evaluation and management are appropriate?*

▶ **Fibrocystic disease of the breast,** the most common cause of this patient's condition, is a pathologic diagnosis that includes cysts, fibrosis, sclerosing adenosis, apocrine change, and hyperplasia. This disorder is uncommon before adolescence or after menopause. Usually bilateral, it is characterized by lumpy breasts and premenstrual tenderness. Possible causes include increased sensitivity to estrogen or decreased progesterone activity.

Mammography may be warranted in fibrocystic breast disease. If a discrete, painful cyst is present, treatment involves cyst aspiration as long as the cyst completely disappears. Some physicians would also recommend elimination of caffeine from the diet and supplemental vitamin E. Follow-up in 3 months is also appropriate. If a mass is present and the diagnosis is unclear, a biopsy is necessary. **Fibrocystic breast disease is associ-**

ated with a low risk of cancer, but it increases when hyperplastic epithelium demonstrates atypia on biopsy of fibrocystic lesions.

CASE 11.7. ▶ Management of a Breast Mass in a Young Woman

A 20-year-old woman presents with a mass in her breast. The mass is 1.5 cm in diameter, and it is firm, rubbery, nontender, and freely movable. The opposite breast and axillae are normal.

▷ *What evaluation and management are appropriate?*

▶ **Fibroadenoma** is the most common breast tumor in women under 25 years of age. This benign lesion, which is more common in African Americans, is a firm, rubbery, painless, movable, well-circumscribed lesion. Excision establishes diagnosis. Biopsy or FNA may also be used. Observation may be appropriate for small lesions, but many patients desire excision. Removal of larger lesions is necessary.

▷ *The lesion is 14 cm in diameter. How would the management plan change?*

▶ A **phyllodes tumor** (cystosarcoma phyllodes, giant cell fibroadenomas), a large, bulky mass of variable malignant potential with occasional ulceration of the overlying skin, is the suspected diagnosis. Factors that determine malignancy are **(1) tumor behavior** and **(2) an increased number of mitoses** per high power field compared with benign phyllodes tumors (on histology). Treatment is local excision with generous margins that are pathologically free of disease. Fibroadenomas may also infarct and acutely enlarge, creating a similar picture.

CASE 11.8. ▶ Management of a Woman with Nipple Discharge

A 34-year-old woman sees you because of nipple discharge. She has been healthy and had two uneventful pregnancies; the rest of her history is unremarkable. On physical examination, the breasts have no masses or tenderness. A small drop of blood is noticeable on the right nipple.

▷ *What management is appropriate?*

▶ In nonlactating women, nonmilky nipple discharge is surgically significant and warrants investigation. **Important variables include whether the discharge is uni- or bilateral, contains blood, and involves single or multiple ducts. It is essential to determine whether a mass is present and whether a mammographic abnormality exists.** If a mass is palpable or a mammographic abnormality is apparent, patients should be evaluated as described in previous cases (see Cases 11.2 and 11.3).

The presence of a clear discharge from multiple ducts is usually related to fibrocystic disease (cystic mastopathy) in younger women or subareolar duct ectasia in older women. Observation is warranted. The **most common cause of bloody discharge is an intraductal papilloma** that can produce bloody or serosanguineous discharge.

 Bloody discharge from a single duct requires surgical biopsy.

After cannulating the duct to identify the lesion, the surgeon excises the duct and ductal system. These lesions may have a small increased risk for carcinoma. Bloody discharge, particularly in older women, does carry a **small risk of carcinoma (4%–13% in most stud-**

ies). Because these cancers are usually occult and often appear as early intraductal lesions, affected patients should undergo the following measures:

1. **Mammography** to examine for other breast abnormalities
2. **Close examination** of the area around the discharge to identify a single duct that is the source of the bloody discharge

A ductogram, which places radiographic dye into the duct with a small catheter, is a method for further definition of the duct. Alternatively, probing with a small (lacrimal duct) probe the duct may be useful. This allows location of the duct and defines the extent of the process within the breast. Once localized, the area should be **surgically excised** (Figure 11-6). The usual diagnosis is intraductal papilloma.

CASE 11.9. ▶ Staging and Prognosis in Infiltrating Ductal Carcinoma

A 57-year-old woman undergoes core-needle biopsy of a breast mass. The pathologic diagnosis returns infiltrating ductal carcinoma of the breast.

▶ *What is involved in staging this cancer?*

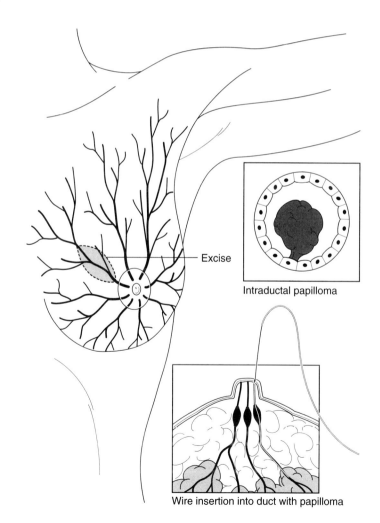

FIGURE 11-6. Intraductal papilloma. As seen in cross-section, the ductal system is radially oriented and communicates with the nipple. A fine probe is placed in the duct that has blood oozing from it, and the probe is then used as a guide for excision of that ductal system. (Redrawn from Silen W: *Atlas of techniques in breast surgery.* Philadelphia: Lippincott-Raven, 1996: 14; and Greenfield LJ, Mulholland MW, Oldham KT, et al. [eds]. *Surgery: scientific principles and practice.* 2nd ed. Philadelphia: Lippincott Williams & Wilkins, 1997: 1374.)

Excise

Intraductal papilloma

Wire insertion into duct with papilloma

▶ The first steps in staging the cancer with the system involve determination of the extent of the local tumor, involvement of regional lymph nodes, and possibility of distant spread (Table 11-6). **Mammography is necessary to assess for other lesions in the same breast and opposite breast.** Cancer staging is based on the tumor–node–metastasis (TNM) classification system (Table 11-6).

QUICK CUTS Clinical staging using the TNM system is more important than histopathology of the primary lesion in determining prognosis.

▶ Prognosis is worse in the following circumstances: when axillary lymph nodes contain metastases, when the number of nodes involved with tumor exceeds four, when the primary tumor is large, and when distant metastases are present. Local disease relates to the size of the primary tumor and direct extension to the chest wall or skin (Table 11-6).

Distant metastasis are assessed by several modalities. As a routine part of staging, all patients except those with stage 0 cancer should have a chest radiograph (CXR) to detect lung and bone metastases, as well as liver enzyme measurements to detect liver metasta-

TABLE 11-6

Staging of Breast Cancer

Primary Tumor
T_1 = Tumor 2 cm or less in greatest dimension
T_2 = Tumor greater than 2 cm but no more than 5 cm
T_3 = Tumor greater than 5 cm in greatest dimension
T_4 = Tumor of any size with direct extension to chest wall (not pectoralis major) or skin

Regional Lymph Nodes
N_0 = No palpable axillary nodes
N_1 = Metastases to movable axillary nodes
N_2 = Metastases to fixed, matted axillary nodes

Distant Metastases
M_0 = No distant metastases
M_1 = Distant metastases including ipsilateral supraclavicular nodes

Staging

Clinical Stage I	T_1	N_0	M_0
Clinical Stage IIA	T_1	N_1	M_0
	T_2	N_0	M_0
Clinical Stage IIB	T_2	N_1	M_0
	T_3	N_0	M_0
Clinical Stage IIIA	T_1	N_2	M_0
	T_2	N_2	M_0
	T_3	N_1	M_0
	T_3	N_2	M_0
Clinical Stage IIIB	T_4	Any N	M_0
Clinical Stage IV	Any T	Any N	M_1

Stage I	93% 5-year survival rate
Stage II	72% 5-year survival rate
Stage III	41% 5-year survival rate
Stage IV	18% 5-year survival rate

sis. If patients have bone pain or complain of bone-related symptoms or have neurologic signs or symptoms, it is necessary to obtain a bone scan or computed tomography (CT) scan of the head, respectively. If liver enzymes, alkaline phosphatase, or total bilirubin are abnormal, a CT scan of the abdomen is appropriate.

▷ *Are any other factors important in prognosis?*

▶ Several other factors relating to patient characteristics, lesion pathology, and molecular studies are important in prognosis. One significant variable is patient age. **Women who are younger at diagnosis tend to do worse than older women.** Certain histologic types as well as molecular factors also have prognostic implications (Table 11-7).

CASE 11.10. ▶ Some Clinical Factors That Affect Prognosis

A 49-year-old woman presents with a breast mass. You are examining the affected breast.

▷ *How would the following clinical findings affect the woman's prognosis?*

TABLE 11-7

Prognostic Indicators in Breast Cancer

Favorable Histologic Types
Tubular carcinoma
Papillary carcinoma
Mucinous (colloid) carcinoma
Paget's disease of the breast

Less Favorable Histologic Types
Infiltrating ductal carcinoma (most common type)
Infiltrating lobular carcinoma (often multicentric or bilateral)
Medullary carcinoma
  Better prognosis than in invasive ductal carcinoma but worse than in lobular carcinoma
Inflammatory carcinoma
  Very poor prognosis

Estrogen and Progesterone Receptors
Presence of receptors
  Better prognosis

DNA ploidy
Aneuploid tumors (tumors with an abnormal amount of DNA per cell)
  Worse prognosis than diploid tumors, in which metastasis may be slower and drug-resistant
    mutations may be less common

High S-phase (synthetic phase of mitosis) fraction
Ki-67, a nuclear protein associated with mitosis, correlates with S-phase fraction and mitotic index
  Worse prognosis; tumors have a higher proliferative component

Her-2-Neu oncogene (also known as *erb*-2, related to epidermal growth factor receptor)
  Worse prognosis; increased expression of gene product is associated with shorter relapse time
    and decreased survival rate in node-positive patients

Case Variation 11.10.1. An ulcerated breast lesion with an underlying mass

▶ This finding is typical of an **inflammatory carcinoma,** which has a worse prognosis than the usual infiltrating ductal carcinoma.

Case Variation 11.10.2. Edema of the skin overlying the mass

▶ This condition is also called **peau d'orange** because it appears similar to the surface of an orange. The associated tumor invasion of local dermal lymphatics worsens the prognosis.

Case Variation 11.10.3. Extensive edema of the breast

▶ This finding, which is similar to peau d'orange, implies an inflammatory carcinoma. Note that any of these findings (see Case Variations 11.10.1 and 11.10.2) could also be compatible with cellulitis or abscess of the breast, and it is necessary to interpret them in terms of the individual patient. However, they are all highly likely to represent cancer.

Case Variation 11.10.4. Retraction of the skin overlying the mass

▶ This finding suggests invasion of the breast support structures and lymphatics with tumor. It worsens the prognosis.

Case Variation 11.10.5. Retraction of the nipple

▶ This finding is similar to skin retraction (see Case Variation 11.10.4).

Case Variation 11.10.6. Two previous aspirations of fluid from the cystic mass but rapid recurrence of the mass

▶ It is necessary to excise cysts that have been aspirated but recur to rule out cancer. Prognosis depends on pathology.

Case Variation 11.10.7. A 1.5-cm mass fixed to the deeper tissues

▶ Fixation to the chest wall indicates invasion of structures outside the breast. This finding worsens the prognosis.

Case Variation 11.10.8. A lymph node palpable in the **supraclavicular** area

▶ A node in this location represents **stage IV disease** with distant metastases. It is unresectable and incurable.

Case Variation 11.10.9. A hard, fixed lymph node in the ipsilateral axilla

▶ This finding suggests the presence of a matted group of nodes with metastases, which would give the patient a node-positive N_2 status.

Case Variation 11.10.10. A soft lymph node in the ipsilateral axilla

▶ This could be an inflammatory node from some other process or a metastasis.

Case Variation 11.10.11. Small nodules on the skin of the breast

▶ These may be satellite nodules of carcinoma on the skin. Biopsy is warranted. A diagnosis of cancer worsens the prognosis.

Case Variation 11.10.12. Arm edema

▶ This finding suggests obstruction of the axillary lymphatics and worsens the prognosis.

CASE 11.11. ▶ Management of a Woman with a Nipple Lesion

A 61-year-old woman presents with a crusty lesion in the nipple of her right breast. You are examining this nipple lesion.

▶ *What evaluation and management are appropriate?*

▶ A chronic eczematoid lesion of the nipple **may be benign,** but it is necessary to rule out the possibility of **Paget's disease** of the breast. 95% of patients with Paget's disease have an underlying carcinoma, either as infiltrating ductal carcinoma or DCIS Examination for a subareolar mass and a mammogram are essential. If a mass is present, then it should be evaluated as for any mass with biopsy. **Associated masses are present in approximately 50% of cases; these patients should undergo mastectomy and staging.** If no mass is present, a biopsy of the nipple lesion is appropriate. The presence of Paget's cells prompts a high suspicion for cancer. **If the lesion is confined to the nipple (~10% of cases), treatment for cure may involve excision of the nipple areolar complex or primary radiotherapy.** Many cases are associated with extensive DCIS in the breast and treatment is controversial but is similar to Case 11.4 or adds postoperative primary radiation therapy.

▶ *How would finding a subareolar mass affect management?*

▶ Evaluation of a subareolar mass is similar to any other mass (see Case 11.3).

CASE 11.12. ▶ Surgical Management of Breast Cancer

You are making rounds with the attending surgeon, who asks what you think are the important surgical principles in the management of breast cancer.

▶ *How would you answer?*

▶ In breast cancer, it is essential to **establish a diagnosis, completely eradicate the primary tumor, and determine whether the regional nodes or distant sites are involved with metastasis.** The diagnostic procedures are discussed in other cases and will not be further described (Cases 11.2, 11.3, and 11.5). In dealing with the primary tumor, it is important to remember that the remaining breast tissue and contralateral breast also require careful evaluation. The incidence rate of multifocal and multicentric disease (as many as 60% of cases) and bilateral processes (as many as 9% of cases) is significant, and recognition of this is critical.

   Wide excision with radiation therapy may suffice for a localized, tumor if a good cosmetic result and adequate margins can be achieved. A mastectomy is usually recommended for a multicentric tumor or larger tumors. Removal of axillary nodes is necessary for accurate staging; clinical examination alone is not sufficient. Histologic status of level I and II axillary nodes and number of nodes involved are still the best markers of disease behavior and ultimate outcome. There is a linear decrease in survival with an increase in number of nodes involved, with more than 10 being a very poor prognostic indicator (10-year survival rate of 14%). Even more importantly, studies have clearly demonstrated that systemic adjuvant therapy given to patients with involved axillary nodes decreases the risk of recurrence of breast cancer by up to 30%.

Complete axillary clearance of nodes is not necessary as node dissection is used only for staging, not therapy.

The attending surgeon asks you to describe the basic anatomy of the breast.

▶ *What important structures would you identify?*

▶ Between 15 and 20 radially arranged lobes, each of which has 20–40 lobules, make up each breast. A duct, which converges on the nipple, provides the drainage for each lobe. The arterial supply is primarily from the internal mammary (60%) and lateral thoracic arteries (30%). Venous return is primarily via the axillary and internal mammary veins. Lymphatic drainage is principally to the axillary lymph node chain, which is divided into three levels, based on relationship to the pectoralis minor muscle (Figure 11-7).

The attending surgeon then asks you to describe the commonly performed surgical procedures used to remove a breast cancer.

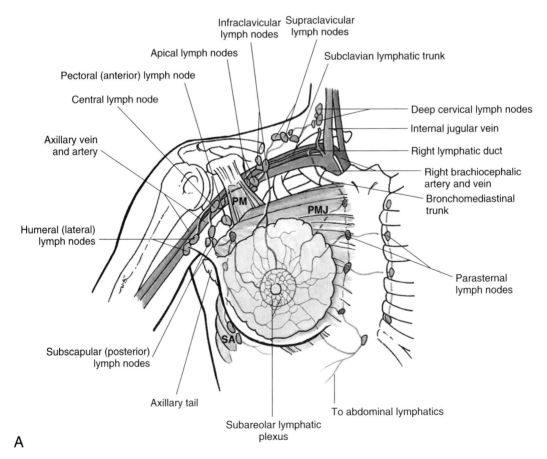

A

FIGURE 11-7. Anatomy of the breast. PM = pectoralis minor muscle; PMJ = pectoralis major muscle; SA = serratus anterior muscle. (From Moore KL, Agur AM. *Essential Clinical Anatomy.* Baltimore: Williams & Wilkins, 1995: 35, 36.)

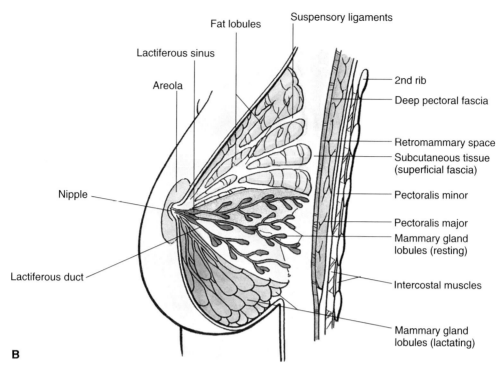

FIGURE 11-7. (CONTINUED)

▶ *How would you describe these surgical methods?*

▶ The **modified radical mastectomy** is the most commonly performed mastectomy (Figure 11-8A through E). The surgeon removes breast tissue, skin, and axillary lymph nodes, as in the radical mastectomy, but spares the pectoralis major muscle. The Auchincloss modification, which is more commonly used, spares the pectoralis minor muscle. The Patey modification involves transection of the pectoralis minor muscle and dissection of the level III nodes. Radiation therapy is not usually used with the modified procedure. However, local radiation therapy following mastectomy is indicated for patients who have tumors greater than 5 cm in diameter, that involve the margin of resection, or that invade the pectoral fascia or muscle. Axillary radiation may be indicated for patients with more than four lymph nodes involved. Radiation of internal mammary nodes may be appropriate if the nodes are apparent on sentinel node imaging. Supraclavicular node irradiation may be warranted if there is extranodal extension into the axillary fat.

The traditional procedure is the **radical mastectomy** (Halsted procedure), a very disfiguring method. The surgeon removes breast tissue, skin, pectoralis major and pectoralis minor muscles, and axillary lymph nodes. Radical mastectomies are rarely performed today; early studies found no difference in survival when patients were treated with modified radical mastectomy as compared to radical mastectomy. However, radical mastectomy is still useful for tumors that directly extend to involve pectoralis muscle.

The **simple mastectomy** involves the removal of breast tissue, nipple–areolar complex, and skin. It is often performed for LCIS or DCIS.

The **subcutaneous mastectomy** involves the removal of breast tissue only. This procedure is rarely indicated.

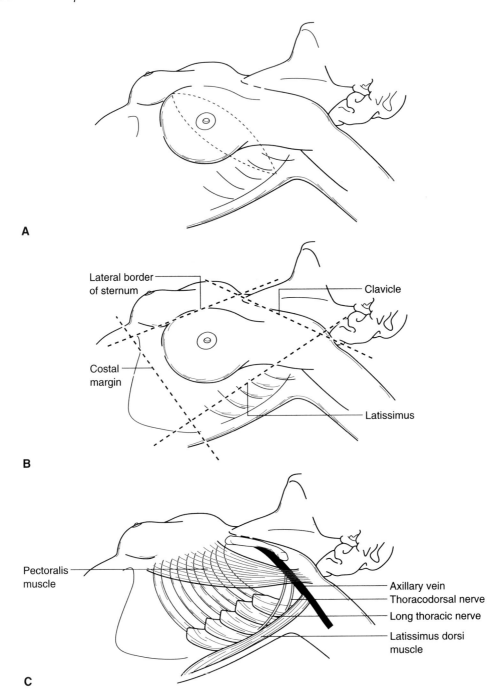

A

B

Lateral border of sternum

Clavicle

Costal margin

Latissimus

C

Pectoralis muscle

Axillary vein
Thoracodorsal nerve
Long thoracic nerve
Latissimus dorsi muscle

FIGURE 11-8. Surgical procedures for carcinoma of the breast. **A.** Mastectomy usually begins with transverse incision. **B.** Limits of dissection. **C.** Axillary dissection. **D.** Breast removed from chest wall, medially from the axillae. Pectoralis fascia is taken, and the pectoralis muscle is left. **E.** Drains are placed beneath the skin flaps, and tissue is closed over chest wall. **F.** Partial mastectomy procedures, which preserve the breast mound. Axillary nodes should be sampled. (From Lawrence PF, Bilbao M, Bell RM, et al. [eds]. *Essentials of general surgery.* Baltimore: Williams & Wilkins, 1988: 277.)

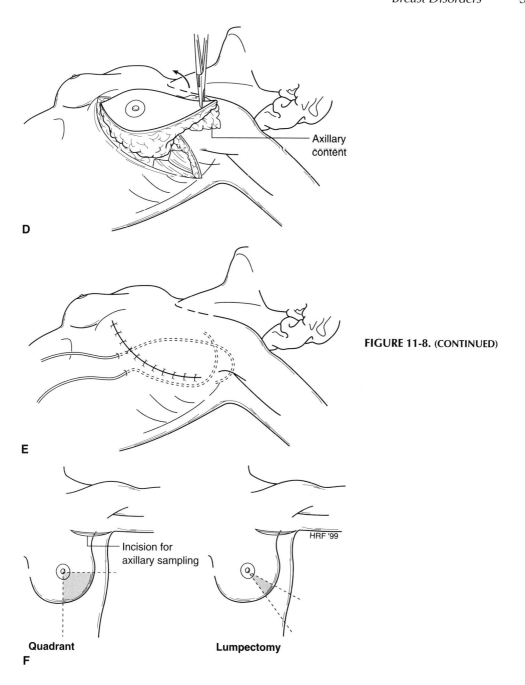

D

E

HRF '99

FIGURE 11-8. (CONTINUED)

Axillary content

Incision for axillary sampling

Quadrant

Lumpectomy

F

    The **lumpectomy/segmental mastectomy** is a breast-conserving therapy that provides a much better cosmetic result compared with modified radical mastectomy (Figure 11-8F). This procedure is appropriate for a solitary tumor less than 5 cm in size, provided the breast size is acceptable and the patient is a good candidate for postoperative radiation therapy. **Lumpectomy involves removal of the primary lesion with clear gross and histologic margins, accompanied by axillary node sampling and local radiotherapy to the entire breast.** In addition, it may involve irradiation of the axillary nodes, internal mammary nodes, and supraclavicular nodes if more than four nodes are positive or if extracapsular invasion is present.

QUICK CUTS Radiation therapy after lumpectomy greatly reduces the chance of local recurrence (Figure 11-11).

Compared to modified radical mastectomy, lumpectomy with radiation does not offer a difference in survival rates or recurrence rates.

CASE 11.13. ▶ Treatment Options for Stages I and II Breast Cancer

A 60-year-old woman has breast cancer and undergoes preliminary staging. The lesion is 1.5 cm in diameter, and no axillary nodes are palpable. A metastatic workup is negative.

▶ *What stage is this woman's cancer?*

▶ It is not possible to stage the patient correctly without knowledge of her axillary lymph node histology, which requires a biopsy of the nodes. Therefore, it is necessary to decide which surgical procedure will be used to sample the nodes and to remove the primary tumor.

▶ *What are this woman's surgical options, both for sampling the lymph nodes and treating the primary tumor?*

▶ Two methods are used for lymph node sampling. **The standard method removes the lymph nodes at levels I and II** (Figure 11-9). A more recent innovation involves a directed node biopsy performed using the **sentinel node technique,** which assumes there is a sentinel node that first receives lymphatic drainage from the primary tumor (Figure 11-10).

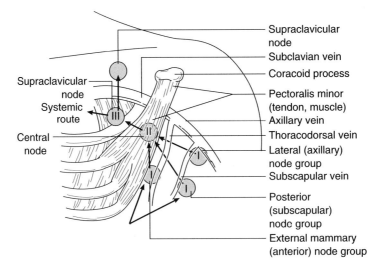

FIGURE 11-9. Lymphatic drainage of the breast, which is generally defined in three levels. Level I nodes are lateral to the pectoralis minor; level II nodes are posterior to the pectoralis minor, and level III nodes are medial to the pectoralis minor. Typically, level I nodes are sampled as a staging procedure. The *arrows* indicate the general direction of lymph flow. (From McKenney MG, Mangonon PC, Moylan JA [eds]. *Understanding surgical disease: the Miami manual of surgery.* Philadelphia: Lippincott-Raven, 1998: 79.)

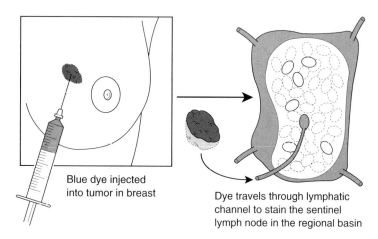

FIGURE 11-10. Sentinel node biopsy. A blue dye or a radionuclide tracer is injected around a tumor in the breast, and it moves to the axilla to the sentinel lymph node. This node, which can be identified surgically by either a radiodetector or a change in the color of the node to blue, is then removed and sampled carefully for evidence of tumor.

Blue dye injected into tumor in breast

Dye travels through lymphatic channel to stain the sentinel lymph node in the regional basin

If this node is negative for tumor, then the remaining axillary nodes are negative (>90% of cases); if this node is positive, further metastases may exist.

Sentinel node evaluation is performed by injecting a blue vital dye (isosulfan blue) or technetium-99m (^{99m}Tc)-labeled sulfur colloid (a radiotracer) around the primary tumor. The surgeon then waits for the dye or tracer to travel to the axilla. Incision and inspection of the axilla follow. The vital dye stains the lymph node blue, allowing the surgeon to identify and remove this node, the sentinel node. A handheld gamma probe identifies the node that has concentrated the radiotracer. Trials are ongoing to determine the success of this technique. It may be more sensitive for detecting micrometastasis than a standard lymph node dissection, in large part because the pathologist performs additional sections and cytokeratin stains on the sentinel node and a more careful examination. This reveals metastasis in another 10%–12% of cases that would have received a normal interpretation on routine sectioning.

Treatment of the primary tumor typically involves either modified radical mastectomy (often including immediate reconstruction) or lumpectomy with postoperative irradiation.

 QUICK CUTS Most physicians do not advocate modified radical mastectomy for tumors less than 2 cm in diameter.

▷ *How do the data relating to the efficacy of modified radical mastectomy and lumpectomy with radiation therapy compare?*

▶ Several studies compare radical mastectomy with modified radical mastectomy, a less extreme procedure with fewer problems. Although there is a difference in the chance of a local recurrence of cancer at the mastectomy site, overall survival is not significantly different.

Additional studies compare modified radical mastectomy to an even less involved procedure, lumpectomy. These studies demonstrate that survival results are similar for lumpectomy with radiation compared with modified radical mastectomy for stages I and II disease. In addition, radiation therapy after lumpectomy greatly reduces the chance of local recurrence as seen in the National Surgical Adjuvant Breast Project (NSABP) Protocol (Figure 11-11). **In conclusion, variation in the surgical treatment of local and regional disease for stage I and II patients is not important in determining their survival.**

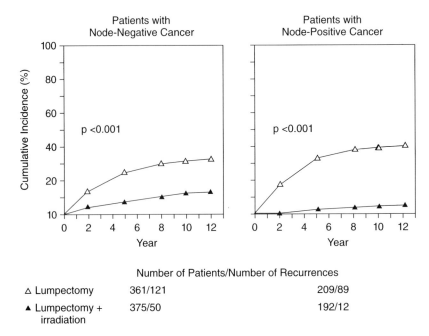

FIGURE 11-11. Life table analysis showing the incidence of recurrence of breast tumor in 1137 patients. Radiation combined with lumpectomy effectively lowers the incidence of local recurrence. **Radiation has no effect on patient survival.** (From Greenfield LJ, Mulholland MW, Oldham KT, et al. [eds]. *Surgery: scientific principles and practice,* 2nd ed. Philadelphia: Lippincott Williams & Wilkins, 1997: 576. After Fisher B, Anderson S, et al. Reanalysis and results after 12 years of follow-up in a randomized clinical trial comparing total mastectomy with lumpectomy with or without irradiation in the treatment of breast cancer. *N Engl J Med.* 1995;333:1456–1461.)

▶ *What technical considerations and patient issues are important in deciding whether modified radical mastectomy or lumpectomy with radiation should be performed?*

▶ The most important objective in treatment of the primary tumor is complete eradication of the primary tumor. This means that it is essential to obtain adequate tumor-free tissue margins. The surgeon must assess this possibility and the final cosmetic result. In patients with small breasts and large tumors, lumpectomy does not offer a good cosmetic result. In younger women, lumpectomy may be preferred by patients for cosmetic reasons. However, these patients have a higher risk for local recurrence, making modified radical mastectomy perhaps even more appropriate in this age group.

Patients with large breasts have increased complications related to radiation therapy with lumpectomy. Breast conservation may not be a viable option. Patients with connective tissue disease or prior radiation to the chest or breasts are not candidates for radiation therapy and should have mastectomies. Breast cancer support groups are effective in helping women with newly diagnosed breast cancer decide which treatment option is best for them. Patients can talk to women who have had the various procedures to learn about the pros and cons first-hand.

CASE 11.14. ▶ Breast Reconstruction

A 38-year-old woman is scheduled for a modified radical mastectomy. She is concerned about her appearance and would like to know her options for breast reconstruction.

What options should you offer?

▶ Patients undergoing a mastectomy are candidates for immediate breast reconstruction.

> **QUICK CUTS** Immediate reconstruction avoids a second operation, allows the exact defect to be duplicated and replaced, and leads to excellent cosmetic results.

▶ Depending on patient preference, the amount of skin and breast remaining, and the patient's size, reconstruction techniques involve silicone gel, saline-filled prostheses, or vascularized flaps (TRAM flaps) [Figure 11-12]. Flaps are not as successful in obese patients or smokers.

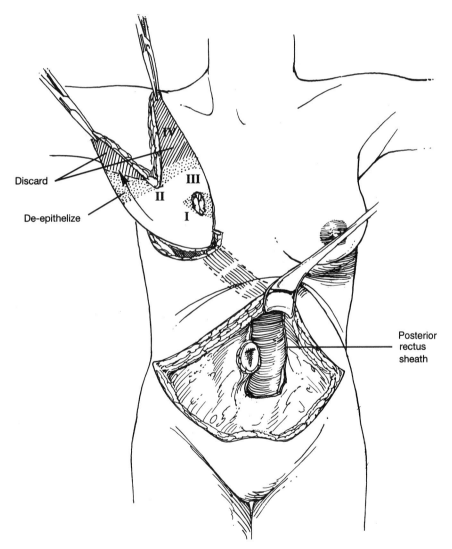

FIGURE 11-12. TRAM flap. A large segment of skin, subcutaneous tissue, and muscle is isolated and swung on its vascular pedestal to reconstruct the breast. Nipple and areolar reconstruction is done typically at a later date. (From Silen W: *Atlas of Techniques in Breast Surgery.* Philadelphia, Lippincott-Raven, 1996, p 131.)

Most mastectomies performed today are curative for in situ cancers and stage I and IIa cancers; therefore, they are amenable to reconstruction. **Typical contraindications are primary lesions involving the chest wall, extensive local or regional disease, or stage III or IV cancer.**

CASE 11.15. ▶ Medical Management of Breast Cancer

You have successfully removed the primary breast cancer from a 58-year-old woman, and you have sampled her axillary nodes. You determine the stage of her cancer. Having recovered from the procedure, she asks you about long-term medical therapy.

▷ *What are her management options?*

- For **stages 0 and I cancers with small (<1 cm) tumors** (no positive nodes), lumpectomy, axillary sampling, and radiation therapy is acceptable treatment, and no further therapy is necessary for ER Negative and hormonal therapy for ER Positive patient.
- For **stage I cancer with larger (1–2 cm) tumors** (no positive nodes), treatment is lumpectomy, axillary sampling (with either axillary dissection or sentinel node biopsy), and postoperative radiation therapy. Adjuvant therapy is beneficial in most patients. The choice of therapy is based on estrogen receptor status and menopausal status.
- For **stage II cancer** (larger primary lesions or node-positive disease), the surgical treatment is the same as for stage I, with the additional option of modified radical mastectomy for larger primary lesions or for patients with smaller breasts in which a lumpectomy could result in a poor cosmetic result. Adjuvant therapy is beneficial; it is based on estrogen receptor and menopausal status.

Generally, some combination of radiation therapy, chemotherapy, and hormonal treatment is effective (Table 11-8). Chemotherapy is appropriate for adjuvant therapy or pal-

TABLE 11-8

Nonsurgical Therapy for Node-Negative and Node-Positive Breast Disease

Node-Negative Disease	Treatment
Postmenopausal women	
ER-positive	Hormonal therapy (Aromatase inhibitor or Tamoxifen)
ER-negative	No adjuvant therapy
Premenopausal women	
ER-positive	Adjuvant chemotherapy and tamoxifen
ER-negative	Adjuvant chemotherapy and individual risk assessment

Node-Positive Disease	Treatment
Premenopausal women	
ER-negative	Chemotherapy
ER-positive	Chemotherapy followed by tamoxifen for 5 years
Postmenopausal women	
ER-negative	Chemotherapy (benefit for patients >70 years of age is not clear)
ER-positive	Tamoxifen and chemotherapy

ER = estrogen receptor.

liation for metastatic or recurrent disease. However, it is more toxic than hormonal therapy and may be poorly tolerated in elderly patients. Premenopausal patients tend to respond better to chemotherapy, whereas postmenopausal patients tend to respond better to hormonal therapy.

▶ *What follow-up surveillance is recommended?*

▶ Patients with breast cancer should see their physicians at least twice a year. An annual CXR and liver function studies are appropriate. Patients who have had lumpectomy with radiation should undergo mammography of the affected breast every 6 months for 2 years, followed by yearly mammograms. (After mastectomy, women have a 15% risk of cancer developing in the remaining breast.) The prognosis for women with early-stage breast cancer is excellent and for those with stage I disease, almost as good, with an overall 5-year survival of 93%. For stage II disease, survival is 72%.

CASE 11.16. ▶ Treatment of Stages III and IV Breast Cancer

A 63-year-old woman presents with a 6-cm breast mass that has been diagnosed as infiltrating ductal carcinoma of the breast. She has clinically positive, matted lymph nodes in the ipsilateral axilla.

▶ *What evaluation and management steps are appropriate?*

▶ **Staging** is necessary. The cancer is stage III if there is no distant metastasis or stage IV if there is distant metastasis. Many centers would dictate that the patient receive **neoadjuvant therapy, which is chemotherapy given before surgical therapy of the local disease in an attempt to reduce the tumor size.**

- For **stage III cancer** (>5-cm lesions, fixed nodes, or inflammatory lesions), it is necessary to consult an oncologist before surgery, because preoperative (neoadjuvant) chemotherapy is beneficial.
- For **stage IV cancer** (distant metastases), palliative radiation and chemotherapy is appropriate. Surgery is reserved only for local control of the primary tumor.

These management methods allow a rapid assessment of the tumor response, with the potential to change chemotherapy regimes as necessary. Two to four cycles of chemotherapy are appropriate. Pre- and posttreatment magnetic resonance imaging (MRI) of the breasts is used to assess the size and extent of the tumor accurately and plan for surgery. Patients then undergo surgery, usually a modified radical mastectomy, followed by further chemotherapy and radiation therapy. If metastatic disease is present, palliation with radiation and chemotherapy is given, and no surgical procedure is performed unless the primary tumor is painful or infected. For stage III cancer, the 5-year survival is 41%, and for stage IV, it is 18%.

CASE 11.17. ▶ Breast Mass with Cellulitis and Edema

A 38-year-old woman presents with a 3-month history of a progressively enlarging breast mass. At the time she sees you, she has a 6 × 7–cm fixed mass, with erythema and edema on the upper, outer aspect of her right breast. Clinically, her axilla is positive with enlarged, firm lymph nodes.

▶ *What is the suspected diagnosis?*

▶ This patient may have an inflammatory carcinoma of the breast.

▶ *What histologic features are typical of this condition?*

▶ The histopathology shows **cancer cells invading dermal lymphatics and vessels** with a large inflammatory component.

A surgeon confirms the physical findings and obtains a punch biopsy of the mass. Pathology reveals an inflammatory carcinoma. Estrogen and progesterone receptors are negative.

▶ *What is the recommended treatment?*

▶ **Multimodality treatment** is appropriate, and evaluation by a medical oncologist and radiation oncologist is necessary. A **staging workup,** including a complete blood count (CBC), liver enzymes, alkaline phosphatase, calcium, total bilirubin, CT scan of the chest, a bone scan, and a CT scan of the liver, is warranted. Patients would first receive chemotherapy to reduce the primary tumor size and treat any possible distant micrometastasis. **If the cancer responds to chemotherapy, four to six more cycles are appropriate. The treatment then involves modified radical mastectomy, adjuvant chemotherapy, hormonal therapy (for estrogen receptor–positive patients), and radiation therapy to the chest and regional lymph node basins.** More chemotherapy may follow. If the cancer does not shrink with chemotherapy, local treatment with surgery or radiation therapy may be required at an earlier stage to control the local disease of the breast before there is any more chemotherapy.

CASE 11.18. ▶ Events That Occur Later in Patients with Breast Cancer

A 55-year-old woman has a modified radical mastectomy for a stage II carcinoma of the breast.

▶ *What evaluation and management are appropriate for the following events that occur later in the woman's life?*

Case Variation 11.18.1. A small, 0.5-cm nodule in the suture line 5 years after surgery

▶ This is a **local recurrence** until proven otherwise.

> **QUICK CUTS** It is necessary to perform a biopsy, either a surgical biopsy or a core-needle biopsy, of any abnormality occurring in a mastectomy surgical site to rule out cancer.

▶ If the lesion is cancerous, local excision is warranted if the patient has had a previous mastectomy. After a previous lumpectomy and radiation therapy, a mastectomy is usually appropriate. Staging with a CT scan of the chest and abdomen, bone scan, CBC, liver enzymes, alkaline phosphatase, total bilirubin, and calcium is necessary to rule out metastatic disease before surgery.

Case Variation 11.18.2. A mammographic abnormality in the opposite breast

▶ This is most likely a **new primary cancer.** Evaluation of this mammographic abnormality should proceed like any other. It is important to note that patients with a history of breast cancer have a high risk for recurrence of the disease, with a threshold for conditions that require biopsy lower than that of most patients.

Case Variation 11.18.3. Elevated liver function studies

▶ Evaluation for a **metastasis to the liver** is appropriate. Most physicians would recommend a contrast-enhanced CT scan of the abdomen. MRI with gadolinium (Gd) enhancement may be necessary in patients with poor renal function.

Case Variation 11.18.4. A fracture of the femur

▶ A **pathologic fracture** secondary to a bony metastasis should be a concern. Orthopedic repair is necessary, with local cancer control with irradiation postoperatively. This controls the cancer but does not appear to inhibit fracture union.

Case Variation 11.18.5. Decreased sensation and motor function in the right leg that is new in onset

▶ This occurrence is an emergency. An **extradural metastasis to the spine** that may be impinging on the spinal cord is a concern. Localized back pain is an earlier presenting symptom. Diagnosis of cord compression necessitates an MRI scan. Steroids, cord decompression, and radiation therapy are then warranted.

Case Variation 11.18.6. New-onset seizures with focal findings

▶ This presentation should prompt concern about a possible **metastasis to the brain.** A CT scan or MRI study would determine the diagnosis. Urgent therapy with steroids is indicated to reduce the intracranial pressure followed by surgery (if indicated) or irradiation.

Case Variation 11.18.7. Presentation to the emergency department with coma or confusion and with no focal findings

▶ **Acute hypercalcemia** due to bony metastasis and parathormone-related peptide is one of the many possible diagnoses.

 The development of coma in any patient with a history of breast cancer should lead to the suspicion of hypercalcemia.

CASE 11.19. ▶ Breast Problems in Pregnancy and the Peripartum Period

A 28-year-old woman who is 3 weeks postpartum after a normal delivery presents with a painful right breast. She is currently breastfeeding and has a low-grade fever. Examination reveals a very firm, red, tender, indurated breast mass. The axilla is mildly tender; some shotty nodes are palpable. The opposite breast is normal.

▷ *What evaluation and management are appropriate?*

▶ **Mastitis** (cellulitis) of the breast related to breastfeeding is the suspected diagnosis. It most likely is secondary to skin breaks in the nipple, allowing bacteria to enter. Examination of the breast for the usual signs of infection, including abscess formation, is warranted. The usual treatment is **warm compresses** and **antibiotics** to cover staphylococcal and streptococcal organisms. Most physicians would recommend continuing breastfeeding or use of a breast pump to allow milk "let-down."

 How would management change if an area of fluctuance is present in the tender inflamed area?

▶ The presence of an **abscess** should be a concern. If definitely present, open **surgical drainage** is indicated. Needle drainage is often inadequate. If doubt exists about the diagnosis of abscess, it may be necessary to probe and aspirate the suspected area with a needle or identify under ultrasound guidance followed by drainage (Figure 11-13).

At the patient's initial visit, you decide that she has cellulitis with no abscess and decide to treat her with antibiotics. You follow her closely but she fails to improve, even after a change in antibiotics. At 3 weeks, the breast is still tender with a very firm, inflamed mass.

▶ *Would the management plan change?*

▶ Several weeks of antibiotic therapy with no resulting improvement should place the original diagnosis in question. The patient's condition may represent inflammatory carcinoma, not simple cellulitis. A **biopsy** of the lesion that includes a segment of skin to examine for carcinoma and possibly dermal lymphatic involvement is warranted.

▶ *If the woman were pregnant (first, second, or third trimester) and had a 2-cm breast lesion, how would the management plan change?*

▶ Breast cancer may occur in pregnancy.

> **QUICK CUTS** The prognosis, which is based on the stage of breast cancer at diagnosis, is similar for both pregnant and nonpregnant women.

▶ Ultrasound and biopsy are necessary for the investigation of suspicious masses. Treatment plans are identical to those of nonpregnant women but are affected by trimester. Following a diagnosis of cancer, sampling of the axillary nodes and preliminary staging are appropriate. Estrogen and progesterone receptor status is usually unreliable during pregnancy.

For **stage I and II disease,** a mastectomy or lumpectomy is safe, with an approximate 1% risk of spontaneous abortion. With lumpectomy, the remaining breast must still be irradiated after delivery. With mastectomy, irradiation is not necessary. Physicians believe that de-

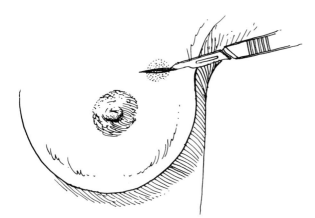

FIGURE 11-13. Drainage of a breast abscess. The area of fluctuance is palpated, and an incision is made with a scalpel to drain the abscess. Generally, needle drainage is insufficient to accomplish adequate drainage. (From Silen W. *Atlas of techniques in breast surgery*. Philadelphia: Lippincott-Raven, 1996: 43.)

laying radiation therapy until after delivery is safe for most patients in their third trimester. However, **lumpectomy is often discouraged in earlier pregnancy because of the need for radiation.** Certain chemotherapy regimens are safe in the second or third trimester.

For **stage III and IV disease,** rapid treatment with radiation and chemotherapy is essential. Thus, abortion may be necessary to allow treatment.

CASE 11.20. ▶ Breast Mass in an Elderly Woman

A 92-year-old woman with moderately advanced Alzheimer's disease presents with a breast mass. The mass is 3 cm in diameter and is hard but freely movable within the breast. The opposite breast is normal, and no axillary nodes are palpable. She lives in a nursing home.

▷ *What options should you present to the woman's family?*

▶ If the patient has moderate or greater disability, it is acceptable to do less than in a younger or more productive individual. This usually means a family meeting to discuss the options, which range from:

1. Observation with no diagnosis
2. Needle biopsy followed by diagnosis and observation
3. Needle biopsy followed by diagnosis and lumpectomy or simple mastectomy
4. Complete staging and traditional treatment (i.e., similar to a younger patient)

CASE 11.21. ▶ Breast Mass in a Man

A 42-year-old man presents with a 1-cm–diameter hard nodule beneath his right nipple. It is not painful but relatively fixed to the surrounding tissue. The left breast is normal, and no axillary adenopathy is palpable.

▷ *What evaluation and management are appropriate?*

▶ It is necessary to obtain a bilateral mammogram, which can help differentiate gynecomastia from cancer. Treatment is typically with **mastectomy and postoperative radiotherapy.**

▷ *What should you tell the man about his prognosis?*

▶ Although breast cancer in men is rare, it does develop, typically after 60 years of age. **Stage for stage, survival for men is similar to that of women.** However, men tend to present at a later stage with fixation, nipple retraction, and ulceration.

CASE 11.22. ▶ Gynecomastia

A 15-year-old boy is brought to see you by his mother about breast enlargement in the left breast. He is pubertal and his friends are making fun of him.

▷ *What is the appropriate management?*

▶ Gynecomastia, which is hypertrophy of breast tissue in men, occurs most commonly in adolescents and in adults at 40–50 years of age. The condition **usually spontaneously regresses** in adolescents.

▶ *How would the proposed management plans change in the following patients?*

Case Variation 11.22.1. A 6-year-old girl with a firm 1 cm unilateral breast mass.

▶ This condition most likely represents a **breast bud** with premature or asymmetric development. Observation with parental reassurance are necessary. Excision or biopsy are contraindicated, because this would diminish or stop development of that breast by removing the breast tissue.

Case Variation 11.22.2. A 50-year-old man

▶ Excision is indicated only if the breast enlargement fails to regress. In older men, breast hypertrophy is commonly associated with **medications,** including diuretics, estrogens, isoniazid, marijuana, digoxin, and alcohol abuse. It is rarely confused with carcinoma, which usually forms a nontender, hard, well-circumscribed mass.

CHAPTER 1 2

Trauma, Burns, and Sepsis

Bruce E. Jarrell M.D., Thomas Scalea M.D., Molly Buzdon M.D.

CASE 12.1. ▶ Primary and Secondary Assessment of Injuries

A 24-year-old man who was in an automobile crash is brought to the emergency department.

▶ *How should the evaluation proceed?*

▶ The American College of Surgeons recommends that clinicians follow an established sequence for evaluation of most trauma patients. This order of priorities is based on the relative risk of death; individuals with the most serious life-threatening problems should receive treatment before those with less severe problems (Table 12-1). These initial priorities make up the **primary survey** for trauma patients. Most clinicians reassess patients again before proceeding to the **secondary survey** (Table 12-1).

> **QUICK CUTS** **Continual reassessment** is necessary during trauma surveys, looking for cardiovascular instability and other significant changes, particularly neurologic changes.

CASE 12.2. ▶ Initial Airway Management

You are responsible for evaluating the airway of the patient in Case 12.1.

▶ *How is the initial airway evaluation performed?*

▶ Initially, it is necessary to **determine whether the airway is clear or obstructed.**

> **QUICK CUTS** **If a patient can talk, the airway is patent,** at least at that particular moment. Signs of airway obstruction include **stridor, hoarseness, and evidence of increased airway resistance** such as respiratory retractions (retraction of the soft tissues between the ribs during inspiration) and use of accessory respiratory muscles.

Visual examination of the oropharynx is appropriate in patients with altered consciousness. The presence of a gag reflex indicates that the upper airway is most likely clear. The absence of a gag reflex means that the physician should inspect the airway digitally for foreign bodies, being certain to protect the finger from being bitten. Injuries to the neck

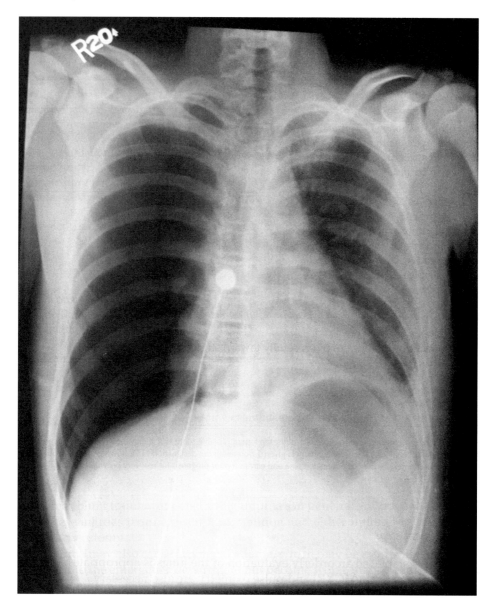

FIGURE 12-1. Simple pneumothorax

mothorax. In this situation, it is important to direct the tube toward the posterior, apical aspect of the pleural space.

▶ *What management is appropriate for a patient with a chest tube?*

▶ You would place a water seal with suction and to allow reinflation of the lung. Serial CXRs are necessary. Removal of the tube may occur **when the lung is fully inflated and no further air leak is apparent.** It is important to be certain that there are no air leaks in the tubing system and no leak at the point where the tube enters the chest wall.

▶ *How does the proposed management change in the following situations?*

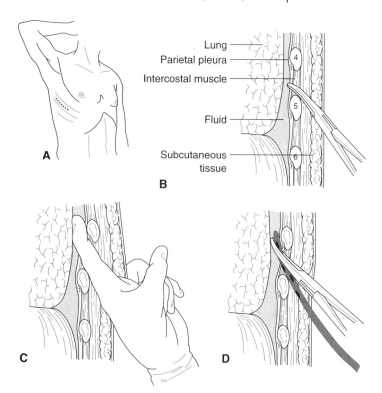

FIGURE 12-2. Treatment of a pneumothorax involves insertion of a chest tube. The tube is connected to an underwater seal drainage system to allow fluid and air to escape from the pleural space but not enter the space; thus, the lung remains expanded. **A.** Location for insertion of chest tube. **B.** Insertion of hemostat into pleural space. **C.** Palpation of pleural space to be certain no vital structures are adherent and likely to be injured. **D.** Insertion of the chest tube.

Case Variation 12.3.1. Further examination indicates a laceration on the chest wall that penetrates through to the lung and "sucks" air as it moves in and out during respiration.

▶ This is termed a **sucking chest wound.** It should be sealed with an occlusive dressing, and a chest tube should be inserted at a different location.

Case Variation 12.3.2. After insertion of the chest tube and repeating the CXR, the lung does not fully inflate.

▶ Either the chest tube is in the **wrong location or not functioning** properly. Tubes can be erroneously inserted into the subcutaneous tissues, have air leaks at their connections, or "clot off" (i.e., become occluded with debris). Management depends on the exact problem but includes repositioning or replacement of the tube or insertion of a second tube. The lung should rapidly expand with a correctly inserted chest tube.

Case Variation 12.3.3. After insertion of a chest tube, a large amount of air continues to leak into the chest tube over the next 6 hours, and the lung remains only partially inflated.

▶ This indicates that there may be a **major airway injury with disruption of a bronchus** or the trachea (Figure 12-3). This condition, which is sometimes apparent on bronchoscopy, requires a thoracotomy and partial lung resection to repair the injury.

Case Variation 12.3.4. A very small pneumothorax is apparent on CXR. Your resident asks you if simple observation and no insertion of a chest tube will be effective.

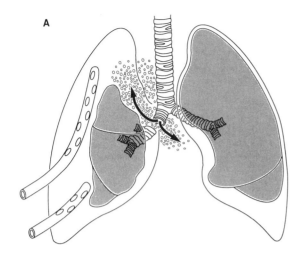

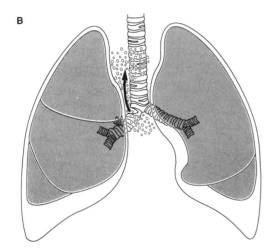

FIGURE 12-3. Ruptured bronchus demonstrating **A.** pneumothorax with intrapleural rupture and **B.** pneumomediastinum with extrapleural rupture. A ruptured bronchus, which causes persistent air leakage and pneumothorax, usually requires lung resection for repair. (From Greenfield LJ, Mulholland MW, Oldham KT, et al. [eds]. *Surgery: scientific principles and practice.* 2nd ed. Philadelphia: Lippincott Williams & Wilkins, 1997: 327.)

QUICK CUTS   Observation of a small, uncomplicated pneumothorax is appropriate if it is not enlarging, if there is no free fluid in the pleural space (i.e., a hemothorax) and if the patient is asymptomatic and has no other significant injuries, especially chest injuries.

▶ Insertion of a chest tube is necessary regardless of the size of the pneumothorax or symptoms if the patient has an injury such as a fractured femur that necessitates surgery in the operating room. General anesthesia, endotracheal intubation, and **assisted ventilation place the tracheobronchial tree at a positive pressure** of 20–40 mm Hg, which increases the risk of converting a small pneumothorax into a larger or even tension pneumothorax.

CASE 12.4. ▶ Initial Management of Pneumothorax in a patient with Hypotension

You clear the airway of the patient in Case 12.1. Absent breath sounds in the right chest are notable. The patient has a BP of 80/60 mm Hg. Distended neck veins are present.

▶ *What management is appropriate?*

 QUICK CUTS   With **hypotension** and absent breath sounds, the suspected problem is a **tension pneumothorax.**

▶ The usual etiology of this entity is a lung laceration that acts like a one-way valve, allowing air to enter the pleural space but preventing it from escaping, thus creating a progressively inreasing positive pressure in the pleural space. As this pressure reaches venous pressure, venous return and cardiac output fall, and hypotension results and neck vein distention occurs. If immediate insertion of a chest tube is not possible, **needle aspiration** of the left chest is necessary. With a diagnosis of tension pneumothorax, the patient should experience **immediate improvement in BP.** Tube thoracostomy should immediately follow needle aspiration.

Tension pneumothorax is a clinical diagnosis (Figure 12-4). It is necessary to perform the needle aspiration and thoracostomy prior to the CXR, because the CXR takes time to complete. **Time is of the essence** in patients with hypotension.

CASE 12.5. ▶ Initial Management of Hypotension and Neck Vein Distention with Normal Breath Sounds

A 42-year-old man who was in a motor vehicle crash comes to the emergency department, where you clear his airway. He has intact, normal breath sounds bilaterally and appears to be ventilating and oxygenating well. Initial assessment of the cardiovascular system reveals hypotension with a BP of 80/60 mm Hg, a heart rate of 110 beats/min, and distended neck veins.

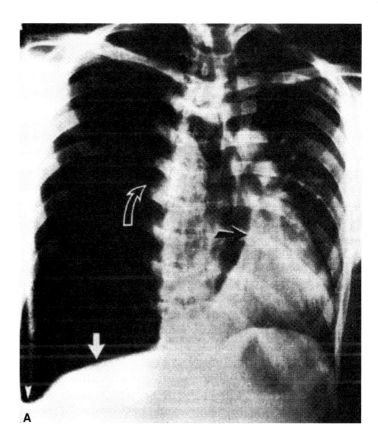

FIGURE 12-4. A. When air progressively accumulates in the pleural space of a patient with a pneumothorax, a tension pneumothorax develops. As the pressure increases in the pleural space, the mediastinum and trachea shift away from the pneumothorax and venous return is impaired with resultant jugular venous distention and decreased cardiac output. (From Schulman HS, Samuels TH. The radiology of blunt chest trauma. *J Can Assoc Radiol.* 1983;34:204.) (*continued*)

▶ *What is the next step?*

► Blood on the urethral meatus indicates possible **urethral injury.** Other reasons to suspect urethral injury on secondary survey include a high-riding prostate gland on rectal examination or a penile or scrotal hematoma. Before placing a catheter in any male trauma patient, it is necessary to perform a rectal examination to search for a prostatic injury. Attempts to place a urinary bladder catheter are contraindicated, because the catheter may complete a partially transected urethra and worsen the trauma. A **retrograde cystourethrogram** is used to determine whether an injury is present. Insertion of a suprapubic catheter is appropriate if an injury has occurred.

CASE 12.7. ▶ Initial Cervical Spine Management

An 18-year-old man who was in a motor vehicle crash is brought to the emergency department. You are responsible for evaluating the patient's cervical spine.

▷ *What management is appropriate in the following situations?*

Case Variation 12.7.1. The patient is awake and alert.

► **Cervical spine precautions** include neck immobilization with a collar or a board, as used by paramedics. If no stabilization is in place, it is necessary to maintain **in-line cervical stabilization** until the neck has been stabilized by one of these methods.

QUICK CUTS   The next step is **palpation of the neck** along the posterior aspect to detect **tenderness,** deformity, or other abnormalities. In addition, a rapid assessment of the basic **motor and sensory function** of the arms and legs is necessary.

A simple way to perform this assessment involves asking the patient to move his fingers and toes and to tell you if he can feel you touch them. In addition, a **lateral cervical spine** radiograph to examine for obvious bony abnormalities is necessary (Figure 12-6). If the initial evaluation is negative, a radiologist should view the cervical spine series, including anterior and oblique views, and be convinced that no abnormalities exist. The cervical spine precautions may be discontinued at that time.

Case Variation 12.7.2. The patient is comatose.

► An examiner **cannot clear the cervical spine** in a patient who is comatose, disoriented, or combative. Therefore, the precautions must continue until the patient's condition improves. Some surgeons obtain a magnetic resonance imaging (MRI) scan of the cervical spine in the comatose patient, and if no abnormalities exist, clear the patient.

Case Variation 12.7.3. The patient has loss of neurologic function below the neck.

► Negative radiographs do not rule out an injury, particularly if neurologic symptoms or neck tenderness is present.

QUICK CUTS   If neurologic deficits, radiologic abnormalities, or cervical spine tenderness are present, then a cervical spine injury should be suspected.

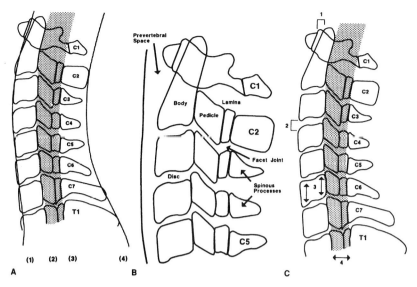

FIGURE 12-6. A. On lateral radiography, the seven cervical vertebrae plus the top of the body of T1 should be visible. **B.** Injuries are suspected if a bony structure is fractured or crushed. Other indications of injury include misalignment of the vertebrae, fluid in the prevertebral space, "step-offs" from one vertebra to another, fracture of the odontoid, and misalignment of the facet joints. **C.** #1 shows the proper alignment of C1 and C2, #2 shows normal disk space and vertebral alignment, #3 shows normal vertebral body structure and firces in a shearing fracture, and #4 shows normal canal for spinal cord. (From Wilson RF [ed]. *Handbook of trauma: pitfalls and pearls.* Philadelphia: Lippincott Williams & Wilkins, 1999: 8.)

Treatment includes continued cervical spine precautions, a neurosurgical consultation, complete evaluation with imaging, and immediate administration of steroids to maximize recovery of the neurologic loss due to damage caused by edema to the adjacent areas of the spinal cord. **Intubation requires extreme caution.** If tracheal intubation is necessary, the head cannot be tilted; oropharyngeal intubation with in-line traction to maintain spinal column alignment or nasotracheal intubation is required (Figure 12-7).

Case Variation 12.7.4. The patient has priapism.

▶ Priapism is a finding in patients with a **fresh spinal cord injury.** Other findings include loss of anal sphincter tone, loss of vasomotor tone, and bradycardia due to loss of peripheral sympathetic activity and intestinal ileus.

CASE 12.8. ▶ Initial Assessment of Thoracic Injury

A 25-year-old man presents with a stab wound to the left chest lateral to the nipple. He is verbally complaining of pain. His vital signs are BP, 120/60 mm Hg; heart rate, 90 beats/min; and respiratory rate, 20 breaths/min.

▶ *Is any immediate action necessary?*

▶ It is very likely that the pleural space has been violated and that a hemopneumothorax exists. Chest tube insertion or tube thoracostomy (≥38F) should occur in the left side, fifth intercostal space.

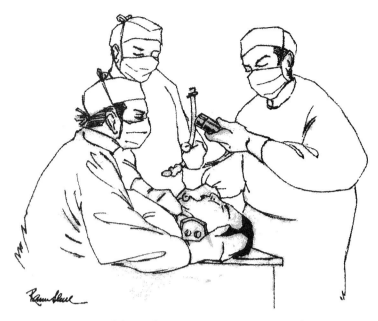

FIGURE 12-7. To safely intubate a trauma patient, an assistant must maintain stability and inline traction to prevent injury to the potentially unstable cervical spine. (From Peitzman AB, Rhodes M, Schwab CW, et al. [eds]. *The trauma manual.* 2nd ed. Philadelphia: Lippincott Williams & Wilkins, 2002: 90.)

You perform the tube thoracostomy.

▶ *What management is appropriate in the following situations?*

Case Variation 12.8.1. Immediately, 1700 mL of blood is evacuated.

▶ The decision to perform an **emergent thoracotomy** is usually based on where the stab wound is located (e.g., close to a vital structure such as the heart or great vessels) and the initial volume of blood evacuated. Generally, if a tube thoracostomy is placed with 1500 mL evacuated in a brief amount of time, a thoracotomy should be performed to evaluate for lung hilar injury or an injury to the heart.

Case Variation 12.8.2. The initial volume output from the chest tube is 1000 mL, but the patient continues to have blood loss from the chest tube.

 In thoracic injuries, the rate of blood loss is as important as the initial blood loss.

Usually, a blood loss of greater than 200 mL/hr for 3 hours also requires thoracotomy to evaluate the injury.

Case Variation 12.8.3. The patient initially presents with hypotension with a BP of 80/50 mm Hg.

▶ Hypotension in this setting is most likely **secondary to blood loss in the left chest** (Figure 12-8). Although a tension pneumothorax is a possibility, it is a less likely cause, and

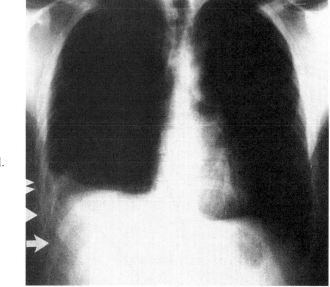

FIGURE 12-8. Chest radiograph demonstrating a right hemothorax with multiple rib fractures. (From Greenfield LJ, Mulholland MW, Oldham KT, et al. [eds]. *Surgery: scientific principles and practice.* 2nd ed. Philadelphia: Lippincott Williams & Wilkins, 1997: 321.)

the rapid placement of a chest tube in the left thorax is necessary. If the hypotension does not respond quickly to insertion of a chest tube, the bleeding is extremely rapid, and urgent thoracotomy is indicated.

Case Variation 12.8.4. The injury is immediately inferior to the clavicle.

▶ A **subclavian arterial or venous injury** with a stab wound below the clavicle is a concern. If the patient is stable, it is necessary to perform an angiogram to inspect the vessels, because operative evaluation of structures in this location is difficult and requires planning the approach. If the patient is not stable, urgent exploration is necessary (Figure 12-9).

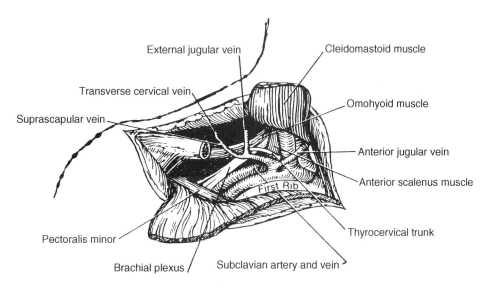

FIGURE 12-9. Penetrating injuries immediately below the clavicle can injure many vascular structures. (From Peitzman AB, Rhodes M, Schwab CW, et al. [eds]. *The trauma manual.* 2nd ed. Philadelphia: Lippincott Williams & Wilkins, 2002: 195.)

Case Variation 12.8.5. The injury is below the nipple on the left side (Figure 12-10).

▶ Suspected injury to the diaphragm and organs inferior to the diaphragm occurs as a result of gunshot entrance wounds and stab wounds below the nipple. **Diaphragmatic injuries** may be missed on initial survey, because herniation of intra-abdominal contents into the thorax may not occur in the initial period. For this reason, if suspicion of a diaphragmatic injury is high, **exploration throughout the abdomen** for related injuries, including the stomach, small bowel, colon, pancreas, and other visceral organs, is necessary. Thoracoscopy and laparoscopy are sometimes useful in this setting if the patient is stable.

Suppose the patient has a gunshot wound to the chest rather than a stab wound (see Figure 12-10).

▶ *How does the proposed management change?*

 The difference in management between gunshot wounds and stab wounds relates to the **unpredictable path of bullets.**

Because the path of a bullet is not predictable, abdominal exploration is essential if the wound is near the abdomen. It is necessary to mark the entrance and exit wounds with a metallic marker and perform radiography to determine the current location of the bullet.

Suppose the patient has blunt trauma to the chest. You place a chest tube and find a hemopneumothorax and significant blood output.

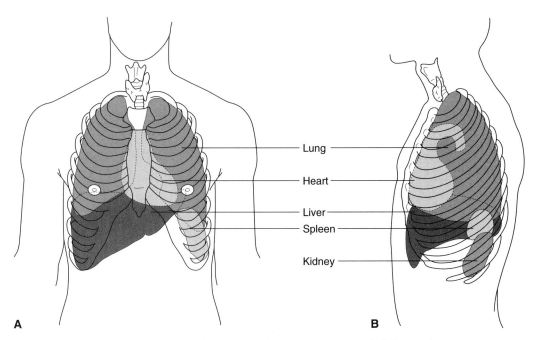

A   **B**

FIGURE 12-10. Penetrating injuries below the nipple may injure several abdominal organs. (Redrawn from Peitzman AB, Rhodes M, Schwab CW, et al. [eds]. *The trauma manual.* 2nd ed. Philadelphia: Lippincott Williams & Wilkins, 2002: 195.)

▷ *How does the proposed management change?*

▶ The management is similar to that described for the patient with the stab wound (see Case Variation 12.8.2).

CASE 12.9. ▶ Management of an Indistinct or Widened Mediastinum

A 46-year-old man who was in an automobile crash is brought to the emergency department, where he undergoes initial survey and resuscitation. On CXR, the mediastinum is wide on a portable anteroposterior film.

▷ *How should this finding be interpreted?*

▶ The possibility of a partial or complete **thoracic aortic transection is a concern.** A **portable anteroposterior CXR is unreliable** for diagnosing this condition because it tends to magnify the mediastinum. A slightly rotated CXR can also distort the mediastinal structures.

The patient is stable and has no other significant injuries.

▷ *What is the next step?*

▶ If the patient is stable and normotensive, a **posteroanterior CXR** is warranted.

▷ *What findings are associated with an aortic disruption?*

▶ A widened mediastinum has been traditionally associated with a thoracic aortic injury (Figure 12-11). However the most reliable findings are an indistinct aortic knob or descending aorta; they are associated with a high incidence of aortic injury. In addition, a variety of findings may also be present (Table 12-4).

The posteroanterior CXR shows a widened mediastinum.

▷ *What is the next step?*

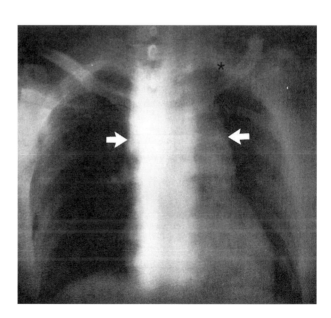

FIGURE 12-11. Chest radiograph in a patient with an aortic disruption showing loss of the aortic knob and a left apical pleural cap. Other findings include left pleural effusion and a widened mediastinum. (From Greenfield LJ, Mulholland MW, Oldham KT, et al. [eds]. *Surgery: scientific principles and practice.* 2nd ed. Philadelphia: Lippincott Williams & Wilkins, 1997: 327.)

TABLE 12-4

Radiographic Findings in Aortic Transection*

Obliteration of aortic knob
Deviation of trachea to right
Pleural cap, which is pleural fluid at top of lung cupola, suggestive of hematoma
Obliteration of aortic–pulmonary window
Deviation of esophagus to right
Depression of left mainstem bronchus or elevation of right mainstem bronchus

*An aortic transection may also be present with a normal chest radiograph or any one of these findings.

▶ The accepted methods of establishing this diagnosis are aortic angiography (the "gold standard") and dynamic computed tomography (CT) scanning of the chest (Figure 12-12).

A partially transected aorta is apparent on aortogram.

▶ *What is the next step?*

▶ The patient should **proceed to the operating room** for repair of his aorta.

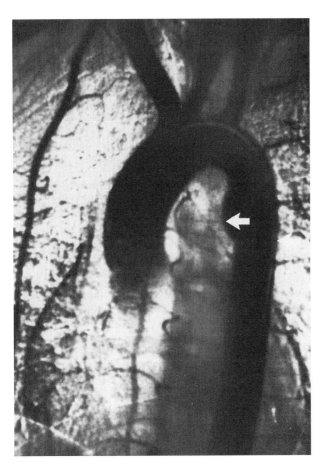

FIGURE 12-12. Thoracic aortogram showing a traumatic aortic aneurysm. (From Greenfield LJ, Mulholland MW, Oldham KT, et al. [eds]. *Surgery: scientific principles and practice.* 2nd ed. Philadelphia: Lippincott Williams & Wilkins, 1997: 369.)

CASE 12.10. ▶ Initial Abdominal Assessment Based on Mechanism of Injury

While a pedestrian, a 40-year-old man who was struck by an automobile sustained blunt trauma. When he is brought to the emergency department, he is awake and alert, with a patent airway. Initial assessment reveals adequate ventilation and a BP of 120/80 mm Hg. You are responsible for evaluating his abdomen and making management decisions.

▷ *How does the mechanism of injury influence the approach to the patient?*

▶ Trauma patients require careful abdominal evaluation when obvious injury to the abdomen is present, the mechanism of injury is associated with a **high risk of injury or a limited reserve to tolerate injury** (Table 12-5). Injury by a mechanism described in Table 12-5 warrants further abdominal imaging.

On questioning, you discover that the patient was struck by an automobile traveling at a speed of 25 miles/hour. Physical examination reveals no abdominal distention and minimal pain on palpation. Vital signs are stable and unchanged from admission.

▷ *Is additional abdominal evaluation necessary, or is simple observation sufficient?*

▶ Based on the previously described mechanism of injury, most trauma surgeons would further evaluate this patient despite the fact that no other findings are present.

Suppose the patient has a gunshot wound instead of blunt trauma.

TABLE 12-5

Injuries That Require Further Evaluation Based Solely on the Mechanism of Injury

Unprotected trauma
Pedestrians hit by motorized vehicles
Motorcycle crashes
Bicycle crashes
Assaults with objects

High-energy trauma
Motor vehicle crashes with the following:
   No restraints
   Substantial deformities
   Known high speeds
   Death at the scene
   Substantial vehicular damage
Falls >15 feet

Minor trauma in patients with limited reserve to tolerate injury
Elderly patients
Patients with chronic debilitating diseases
Immunosuppressed patients

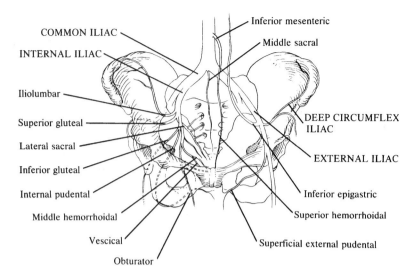

FIGURE 12-16. Arterial supply to the pelvis. These pelvic arteries and associated veins bleed profusely with certain pelvic fractures that disrupt the continuity. The treatment of choice is embolization. (From Peitzman AB, Rhodes M, Schwab CW, et al. [eds]. *The trauma manual.* 2nd ed. Philadelphia: Lippincott Williams & Wilkins, 2002: 311.)

CASE 12.12. ▶ Management of Abdominal Injuries Visible on CT Scan

A 52-year-old woman who was in an automobile crash is brought to the emergency department. After the initial survey and resuscitation, the patient is stable. No abdominal injury is obvious, but you decide to perform a CT scan of the abdomen based on the mechanism of injury.

▶ *What is the appropriate management of the following CT findings?*

Case Variation 12.12.1. Splenic laceration with fluid adjacent to the injury (Figure 12-17)

▶ This patient has a ruptured spleen with a localized hematoma. Unstable patients should go to the operating room. Different approaches may be useful in stable patients such as this one. All approaches have the following principle in common: **Preserve the spleen if possible** to avoid postsplenectomy sepsis. Most surgeons also agree with the following statement: **Avoid blood transfusions if patients can be safely managed without them.** The management of splenic injury represents a balance between these two principles.

A splenic injury in an unstable patient should be explored. In stable patients splenic injuries are graded with CT by the extent of injury (Table 12-6). For most grade III and lesser injuries, observation is safe and appropriate. Different management is necessary for grade IV and V injuries. Grade IV or V injuries most likely require exploration, even in stable patients. Some surgeons routinely explore patients and perform either splenectomy or splenorrhaphy, or a splenic repair. Other surgeons perform splenic angiography and embolize bleeding splenic vessels. Infarction is rarely a problem when embolizing a portion of the spleen because of the rich collateral blood supply from the short gastric vessels. Any patient who has had a splenectomy should receive immunization with vaccines for diplococcus, *Meningococcus*, and *Haemophilus*.

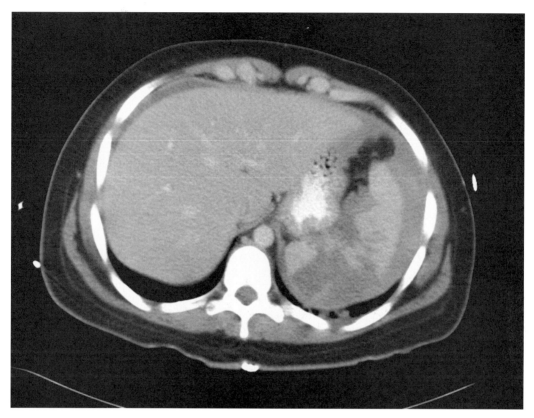

FIGURE 12-17. CT scan of splenic laceration

Case Variation 12.12.2. Liver laceration

▶ This patient has a liver injury (Figure 12-18). CT is used to grade liver injuries (Table 12-7). **Abdominal exploration is necessary regardless of grade in unstable patients, particularly in those with grade IV, V, and VI injuries.** In stable patients, attempted observation is standard practice. The risk of serious bleeding is related to the grade (Table 12-7).

Case Variation 12.12.3. Injury to the mesentery

▶ Injuries at the root of the mesentery require injury forces that are significantly large. These forces **may also tear or rupture the bowel.** Leaking bowel is obviously a serious injury that requires operative intervention. It is **particularly difficult to detect these injuries on CT.** Therefore, they must be suspected based on either mechanism or associated injuries seen on CT scan.

Case Variation 12.12.4. Rupture of the left kidney and an associated retroperitoneal hematoma around the kidney

▶ **In unstable patients, kidney ruptures require operative intervention,** although most patients are stable with isolated kidney fractures. In the setting of urgent operative inter-

TABLE 12-6

Grades of Splenic Injury

	Grade	Description of Injury
I	Hematoma	Subcapsular, nonexpanding, <10% surface area
	Laceration	Capsular tear, nonbleeding, <1 cm parenchymal depth
II	Hematoma	Subcapsular, nonexpanding, 10%–50% surface area
		Intraparenchymal, nonexpanding, <2 cm in diameter
	Laceration	Capsular tear, active bleeding; 1–3 cm parenchymal depth, which does not involve trabecular vessel
III	Hematoma	Subcapsular, >50% surface area or expanding; ruptured subcapsular hematoma >2 cm or expanding; intraparenchymal hematoma >2 cm or expanding
	Laceration	> 3 cm parenchymal depth or involving trabecular vessels
IV	Hematoma	Ruptured intraparenchymal hematoma with active bleeding
	Laceration	Laceration involving segmental or hilar vessels producing major devascularization (>25% of spleen)
V	Laceration	Completely shattered spleen
	Vascular	Hilar vascular injury, which devascularizes spleen; hematoma >2 cm and expanding

From Wilson RF [ed]. *Handbook of trauma: pitfalls and pearls.* Philadelphia: Lippincott Williams & Wilkins, 1999: 361.

vention, it is important to **document the presence of two kidneys** before removing the injured kidney. A single intravenous pyelogram obtained in the resuscitation area or operating room can determine this. **In stable patients,** the injury can be assigned a grade. **Angiography** is useful for the study of high-grade disruptions or intimal tears to examine for major vascular injuries. Some vascular injuries warrant planned operative repair.

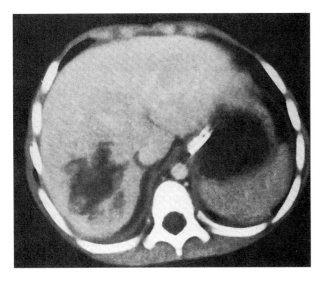

FIGURE 12-18. Computed tomography (CT) scan demonstrating a hepatic hematoma secondary to blunt trauma. (From Greenfield LJ, Mulholland MW, Oldham KT, et al. [eds]. *Surgery: scientific principles and practice.* 2nd ed. Philadelphia: Lippincott Williams & Wilkins, 1997: 383.)

TABLE 12-7

Grades of Liver Injury

	Grade	Description of Injury
I	Hematoma	Subcapsular, nonexpanding, <10% surface area
	Laceration	Capsular tear, nonbleeding, <1 cm parenchymal depth
II	Hematoma	Subcapsular, nonexpanding, 10%–50% surface area
		Intraparenchymal, nonexpanding, <2 cm in diameter
	Laceration	Capsular tear, active bleeding; 1–3 cm parenchymal depth, <10 cm
III	Hematoma	Subcapsular, >50% surface area or expanding
		Ruptured subcapsular hematoma with active bleeding
		Intraparenchymal hematoma >2 cm or expanding
	Laceration	>3 cm parenchymal depth
IV	Hematoma	Ruptured intraparenchymal hematoma with active bleeding
	Laceration	Parenchymal disruption involving 25%–50% of hepatic lobe
V	Laceration	Parenchymal disruption involving >58% of hepatic lobe
	Vascular	Juxtahepatic venous injuries (i.e., retrohepatic vena cava/major hepatic veins)
VI	Vascular	Hepatic avulsion

From Wilson RF [ed]: *Handbook of trauma: pitfalls and pearls.* Philadelphia: Lippincott Williams & Wilkins, 1999: 342.

Case Variation 12.12.5. Hematoma located centrally in the area of the superior mesenteric artery

▶ Centrally located hematomas suggest major injuries to either the **upper abdominal aorta or major aortic branches or direct injury to the pancreas and duodenum** (Figure 12-19). In unstable patients, urgent exploration is necessary. In stable patients, angiography and further assessment prior to exploration are appropriate.

Case Variation 12.12.6. Partial transection of the pancreas (Figure 12-20)

▶ This serious injury requires exploration and evaluation of the pancreas and duodenum. With relatively minor injuries, the area is debrided and drained. With more complex injuries, resection of devitalized pancreatic tissue and repair of duodenal injuries is necessary. In severe cases, the intestinal fluids can be diverted from the injury to allow time for healing to occur. This procedure has been termed a duodenal diverticularization or diversion.

Case Variation 12.12.7. Hematoma of the duodenum, with no other injuries in the abdomen (Figure 12-21)

▶ A duodenal hematoma is a common injury in children who hit their abdomen on bicycle handlebars. Typically, it is an intramural hematoma that obstructs the duodenal lumen and can be diagnosed on upper gastrointestinal (GI) series. If it is an isolated injury, management involves observation and no oral intake until the obstruction resolves, commonly in 5–7 days. If the hematoma persists, exploration is appropriate after several weeks.

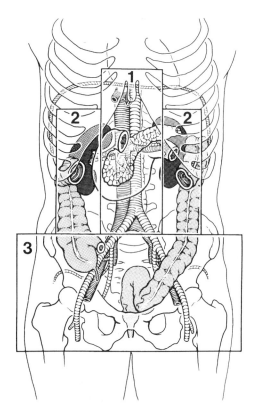

FIGURE 12-19. A zone 1, or central hematoma, is a retroperitoneal hematoma that may involve injury to a major vascular structure, and it is usually surgically explored. A zone 2, or flank hematoma, frequently is secondary to a renal parenchymal injury, and it can be observed in stable patients. A zone 3, or pelvic hematoma, is observed in stable patients; if bleeding is present, the bleeding site is located angiographically and embolized. (From Peitzman AB, Rhodes M, Schwab CW, et al. [eds]. *The trauma manual.* 2nd ed. Philadelphia: Lippincott Williams & Wilkins, 2002: 265.)

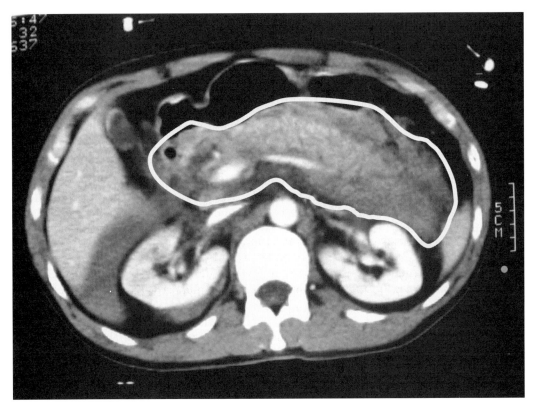

FIGURE 12-20. Pancreatic injury

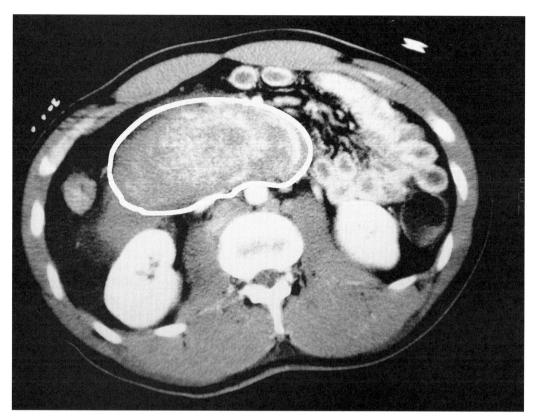

FIGURE 12-21. Duodenal hematoma

Case Variation 12.12.8. Large pelvic hematoma (see Figure 12-19)

▶ Pelvic fractures are associated with significant vascular injuries and pelvic hematomas.

 QUICK CUTS **Angiography and embolization** is appropriate in patients with continued bleeding or instability.

Surgical exploration of these patients is not likely to control bleeding because the bleeding is somewhat tamponaded by the intact peritoneum covering the pelvis. When the surgeon opens the peritoneum, the tamponade is released, making the bleeding worse. In addition, it is extremely difficult to locate a bleeding pelvic vessel for two reasons: (1) the interior of the pelvis is difficult to visualize surgically and (2) the large mass of hematoma obscures the structures.

Case Variation 12.12.9. Ruptured diaphragm (Figure 12-22)

▶ A ruptured diaphragm requires **surgical repair.** The abdominal organs are returned to the abdomen, and the diaphragm is either primarily repaired or repaired with a prosthetic mesh.

Case Variation 12.12.10. Free fluid in the peritoneal cavity and no evidence of solid organ injury

▶ Free fluid in this setting could be **blood or intestinal contents.** One should be suspicious for bowel injury and confirm it either by surgical exploration or by serial examinations and imaging.

CASE 12.13. ▶ Management of Operative Findings with Abdominal Trauma

You are caring for a 47-year-old man who was in an automobile crash. The CT scan shows a small liver laceration and a grade 3 splenic laceration. The patient's vital signs continue to be stable, and no other major injuries are present. You chose treatment with close observation. Thirty minutes later the patient deteriorates, becoming hypotensive and combative.

▶ *What is the next step?*

▶ Management of trauma patients is based on **continual assessment** of the clinical condition. Most patients with significant injuries have a dynamic course, with sometimes rapid and unexpected changes. Nonoperative management has failed in this case, and urgent surgical abdominal exploration is warranted.

On entering the peritoneum, there is a moderate amount of blood.

▶ *What should the basic steps in the operative plan be?*

QUICK CUTS The initial step is to **stop the bleeding** as quickly as possible by **packing all four quadrants of the abdomen** with gauze packs.

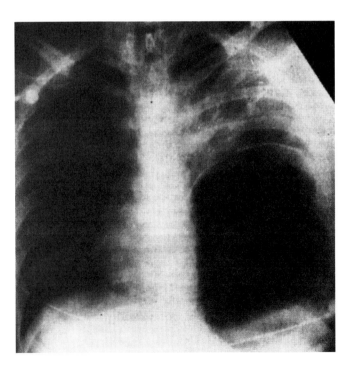

FIGURE 12-22. Plain chest radiograph showing the stomach herniated into the left chest in traumatic rupture of the diaphragm. (From Wilson RF [ed]. *Handbook of trauma: pitfalls and pearls.* Philadelphia: Lippincott Williams & Wilkins, 1999: 333.)

▶ Injuries are "attacked" in the order of their severity, with more severe injuries receiving priority. After removing one pack, the surgeon quickly assesses the area and attempts hemostasis. This is repeated in all four quadrants. Liver injuries are commonly treated by packing the laceration to achieve control rather than attempting to suture vessels.

It is possible to control the bleeding by packing the liver laceration and repairing the splenic injury.

▶ *What is the next step?*

▶ After the bleeding has been controlled, it is necessary to **inspect the remainder of the abdominal contents and repair the injuries.** Primary repair is appropriate for simple injuries, such as small bowel and stomach injuries. However, many injuries are complex and require involved procedures, including duodenal and pancreatic injuries. Primary repair of low-risk colonic injuries without a colostomy is safe. Patients with multiple injuries, hypotension, major bleeding, or significant treatment delay with peritoneal contamination are considered to be at high-risk for complications, so management with resection and colostomy is usually necessary. Careful inspection of the duodenal and pancreatic areas is essential for detection of injuries.

None of the previously listed injuries are present, but a retroperitoneal hematoma is found.

▶ *What is the appropriate management?*

▶ Retroperitoneal hematomas are classified into three groups (Table 12-8; Figure 12-19). Management depends on the location of the hematoma and the stability of the patient.

CASE 12.14. ▶ **Initial Neurologic Injury Assessment and Management**

An 18-year-old man appears to have sustained an isolated major closed head injury in a motorcycle accident.

▶ *What is involved in the initial evaluation?*

▶ Evaluation of head trauma must always begin with a **primary survey: a**irway, **b**reathing, **c**irculation (ABCs). Once an adequate airway is established and the patient is adequately ventilated, vital signs can be obtained. If vital signs are stable and initial assessment reveals no other injuries requiring immediate attention, evaluation of the patient's neurologic status should take place.

The patient has stable vital signs and a head injury but evidence of no other injury.

▶ *What is involved in the assessment of the severity of the neurologic injury?*

> **QUICK CUTS** A **rapid neurologic examination** and assessment of pupillary responses and other cranial nerve functions, peripheral motor and sensory function, and any deficits or focal findings, along with level of consciousness, is appropriate.

▶ It is also necessary to examine the head for evidence of direct trauma, such as a depressed skull fracture or scalp laceration. If available, the patient's state of consciousness at the scene of the accident is useful.

TABLE 12-8

Classification of Retroperitoneal Hematomas (see Fig 12-19 on pg 376 for description)

Type	Management
Zone 1 (central hematomas)	**Usually abdominal exploration,** because major injuries to the great vessels, pancreas, and duodenum might otherwise be overlooked (patients with blunt abdominal trauma). With hemodynamic instability, preoperative angiogram is useful.
Zone 2 (usually involve kidney)	**No exploration is warranted, unless hematoma is expanding. Exploration is typically appropriate** in unstable patients or in those with **penetrating trauma** to exclude major vascular injuries. With exploration, proximal arterial control of the kidney as the first step is desirable, if possible. Knowledge of presence of contralateral functional kidney is also necessary.
Zone 3 (pelvic hematomas)	**No exploration is warranted in blunt trauma. Exploration is typically appropriate** in patients with **penetrating trauma** to exclude major vascular injuries. **Angiographic embolization** and **pelvic fracture reduction** are appropriate, especially in unstable patients after other sources of hemorrhage have been evaluated.

Patients with **penetrating trauma** typically have zones 1, 2 and 3 hematomas **explored** to exclude major vascular injuries.

▷ *What signs might be present with a basal skull fracture?*

▶ A basal skull fracture is a fracture at the base of the skull where it connects to the spine. Fractures at this location may cause loss of consciousness, sinus fractures, and local hemorrhage. Blood in this location can migrate to sites visible to the surgeon, such as the ear, mastoid bone, and orbits.

▷ *How is level of consciousness assessed?*

▶ The Glasgow Coma Scale provides a quantitative measure of a patient's level of consciousness (Table 12-2).

On examination, the patient responds to verbal stimuli, moves all extremities normally, and has intact sensation and no focal findings.

▷ *What is his Glasgow Coma Score?*

▶ In this example, the patient opens his eyes spontaneously (4 points), responds to verbal stimuli (5 points), and moves all extremities spontaneously (6 points). The Glasgow Coma Score is 15 (Table 12-2).

▷ *What is the next step?*

▶ It is necessary to take a more complete history and perform a neurologic assessment to confirm that there are no other findings. Some physicians would observe a patient who has suffered a brief loss of consciousness (under 5 minutes) for a period of time (several hours). Other surgeons would perform a CT scan because of the loss of consciousness. Neurologic change warrants a CT scan of the head. Otherwise, the patient can be sent home if someone is there to continue the observation.

A normal CT scan virtually eliminates the possibility of a serious head injury and makes discharge from the hospital very safe. The decision to admit a patient should be based on the length of unconsciousness, the reliability of the individual, and the existence of symptoms such as nausea and vomiting. Generally, a patient who has been unconscious for more than 5 minutes should be observed in the hospital for 24 hours. However, if a patient is neurologically intact, has no symptoms, has a normal head CT scan, and a reliable home situation, the risk of a subsequent neurologic event is very low.

CASE 12.15. ▶ Other Neurologic Problems

You are evaluating a 38-year-old man in the emergency department. He has an isolated head injury and loss of consciousness.

▶ *What therapeutic measures warrant consideration during the evaluation?*

▶ The possibility that a **severe head injury will cause edema of the brain, increasing the intracranial pressure and decreasing the cerebral perfusion pressure,** should be a concern. Decreasing perfusion leads to further ischemia, edema, and eventual brain herniation and death if left untreated.

 Initial management should include neurosurgical consultation and **maintenance of good pulmonary ventilation and tissue perfusion.**

Maneuvers that may lessen the amount of brain edema when the patient is first seen include elevation of the head to 30° and hyperventilation to a level of P_{CO_2} at 26 to 28 mm Hg. Mannitol is also useful because it dehydrates the brain within 15–20 minutes, leading to decreased intracranial pressure. Mannitol administration should be slow, because rapid infusion can cause asystole. Phenytoin (Dilantin) loading with continuation for at least 1 week to prevent seizures may be useful. Medications that depress central nervous system (CNS) function should be avoided during this phase of the evaluation.

Once a CT scan and a neurologic evaluation have been performed, many neurosurgeons recommend maintaining the patient in a normocarbic state (stopping the hyperventilation). Routine hyperventilation is no longer practiced and may worsen the neurologic outcome. **In general hyperventilation is currently reserved for the patient has apparent signs of impending brain herniation such as the development of a blown pupil or lateralizing signs.**

▶ How should the following different situations be managed?

Case Variation 12.15.1. Glasgow Coma Score of 3

▶ The patient is considered comatose (Glasgow Coma Score < 8) [see Table 12-2]. Endotracheal intubation is necessary, and a neurosurgery consult is warranted. To minimize the risk of cerebral edema, it is necessary to elevate the head of the bed 30° and limit fluid volume. Hyposmolar fluids should not be used, because they lead to increased cerebral edema in this severe injury. Hyperventilation to keep the Pco_2 at 26–28 mm Hg is recommended to reduce intracranial blood volume and intracranial pressure by cerebral vasoconstriction.

 QUICK CUTS   **Unequal pupils or a lateralizing motor deficit suggest a large focal lesion.**

An immediate head CT is necessary, and the patient may require emergent operation to evacuate the lesion. This patient may have a focal injury that needs surgery, but he could also have diffuse axonal injury, which occurs in 45% of coma-producing head injuries. Diffuse axonal injury is caused by microscopic injury that is distributed throughout the brain. An affected patient may remain deeply comatose with decorticate or decerebrate posturing. This condition is associated with a high mortality that is not improved by surgery.

Case Variation 12.15.2. Glasgow Coma Score of 10 and a dilated right pupil that sluggishly reacts to light

▶ This is a sign of development of a **space-occupying CNS lesion.** A immediate CT scan is necessary, and a neurosurgical consult is warranted. The typical signs and symptoms of epidural hematoma include a loss of consciousness followed by a lucid interval, a second loss of consciousness, and a dilated and fixed pupil on the same side as the lesion. Temporal lobe intracerebral hematoma can also exhibit the same signs and symptoms, because it also arises from tentorial herniation. Emergent evacuation of the hematoma is required in either case.

Case Variation 12.15.3. Blood behind the tympanic membrane

▶ Blood behind the tympanic membrane indicates a **basal skull fracture,** as do ecchymosis in the mastoid region (Battle's sign) or around the eyes (raccoon eyes). The patient may also have cerebrospinal fluid (CSF) leaking from the ear (otorrhea) or the nose (rhinorrhea. A skull fracture may be evidence of an underlying intracranial hematoma.

　　Patients with skull fractures may require admission for observation. A neurosurgical consult is warranted. Most surgeons do not place these patients on prophylactic antibiotics, but when a CSF leak is present, some do. If the patient requires a nasogastric (NG) tube or a nasotracheal tube for ventilation, physicians should take extreme caution to ensure that the tube does not perforate fractured skull bones, particularly the cribriform plate, and enter the brain. Safer alternatives are an orogastric tube and an endotracheal tube.

Case Variation 12.15.4. Sodium level of 125 mEq/L

▶ Brain injury can lead to secretion of inappropriate antidiuretic hormone (SIADH), which is thought to be in direct response to stimulation of hypothalamic osmoreceptors. This produces a syndrome characterized by hyponatremia, concentrated urine, elevated urine sodium concentration, and a normal or mildly expanded volume of extracellular fluid. The extracellular hypotonicity leads to intracellular edema, which may cause severe cerebral edema. When hyponatremia is acute in onset, it leads to restlessness, irritability, confusion, and eventually convulsions or coma. Treatment is **water restriction.** If symptoms are severe, 3% sodium chloride solution, 200–300 mL, given over 3–4 hours, is appropriate.

> **QUICK CUTS** It is important not to correct the hyponatremia too rapidly, because this may lead to **central pontine myelinosis.** The general recommendation is to correct half the sodium deficit over 24 hours.

Case Variation 12.15.5. Sodium level of 160 mEq/L

▶ Just as head trauma can lead to SIADH, severe head trauma has also been associated with diabetes insipidus. This is caused by failure of release of antidiuretic hormone, resulting in polyuria, polydipsia, and excessive thirst (if the patient is conscious). If the thirst mechanisms are restricted either by unconsciousness or inadequate access to water, dehydration may develop, leading to symptoms of weakness, fever, psychic disturbances, and death. Clinically, rising serum osmolality and serum sodium concentration, which can exceed 175 mmol/L, occurs. Diabetes insipidus can be diagnosed by measuring urine osmolality after dehydration and after administration of antidiuretic hormone. Treatment is either subcutaneous **vasopressin** or desmopressin (synthetic vasopressin, also called ddAVP) and administration of **free water.**

CASE 12.16. ▶ Management of Continuing Hemorrhage

A 23-year-old man has sustained a liver injury in a motor vehicle accident. The injury is a large stellate fracture in the dome of the right lobe, which can be controlled only by packing the injury and closing the abdomen. You plan to reexplore the patient the next day.

 What is the appropriate management for the following postoperative conditions?

Case Variation 12.16.1. Temperature of 95°F

▶ Studies have shown that hypothermia is a predictor of poor outcome in trauma patients.

> **QUICK CUTS** **Hypothermia leads to coagulopathy from platelet dysfunction and prolongation of the prothrombin time (PT) and partial thromboplastin time (PTT).**

It is important to rewarm the patient with blankets, heating pads, or heating lamps. In this case, it is difficult to determine whether coagulopathy is secondary to liver dysfunction, massive transfusion, or hypothermia. Once the patient is rewarmed, it is possible to discover the existence of other causes. If the coagulopathy is not corrected by normalization of the temperature, the treatment is administration of fresh frozen plasma to restore coagulation factors.

Case Variation 12.16.2. Platelet count of 30,000/mm^3

▶ A decline in platelet number to 30,000/mm^3 may result from inadequate replacement of circulating platelets, and it worsens the overall coagulopathy. Decreased platelets can also result from disseminated intravascular coagulation (DIC) from a transfusion reaction or sepsis, which may result from lysis of blood products. Due to the severity of injury and the risk of ongoing bleeding, platelet transfusions to keep the platelet count above 60,000/mm^3 are necessary.

Case Variation 12.16.3. Metabolic acidosis

▶ Metabolic acidosis may result from **hypothermia or hypovolemia and subsequent tissue hypoperfusion.** Both conditions require correction.

Case Variation 12.16.4. Development of abdominal distention and oliguria

▶ Abdominal distension and oliguria may indicate **continued hemorrhage** from the liver and accumulation of intra-abdominal fluid and blood. The oliguria may be caused by decreased renal blood flow resulting from a tense abdominal compartment, so-called abdominal compartment syndrome. Affected patients may also have difficulty with ventilation due to increased inspiratory pressures required because of elevated diaphragms. In either case, a hematocrit can confirm continued hemorrhage, in which case emergent exploration in the operating room is necessary.

CASE 12.17. ▶ Management of Postoperative Problems in Trauma Patients

A 25-year-old man ruptures his spleen in a motorcycle accident. The injury requires splenectomy, with an estimated blood loss (EBL) of 500 mL in the operating room. He is now in the recovery room.

▶ *What is the appropriate evaluation and management in terms of fluids and electrolytes?*

▶ It is appropriate to both review the patient's operative blood loss and fluid replacement in the operating room and assess whether he has received adequate replacement. Any deficits should be corrected. Blood losses should be replaced with packed RBCs ml. for ml. or with 0.9 normal saline (3 ml saline per ml blood loss). At that point, if his urine output is adequate (0.5–1 mL/kg/hr), his vital signs are stable, and he does not appear to be hemorrhaging, maintenance fluid replacement is appropriate.

Suppose the patient has multiple additional injuries such as a lung contusion and a fractured femur in addition to the spleen injury.

▶ *How should the management plan be modified?*

▶ Because of the multiple injuries, the body has sustained greater stress and will mount a greater inflammatory response. Additional fluid loss into the third space will necessitate greater fluid replacement. However, physicians should avoid overaggressive volume administration in the setting of a pulmonary contusion in which the damaged lung is more susceptible to edema.

You replace his fluid losses to an appropriate level, and since then, he has been stable during your frequent visits. You see him 48 hours postoperatively and there is a change. His BP is 105/60 mm Hg, and his urine output has been 10 mL/hr over the past 4 hours.

▶ *What is the next step in his evaluation and management?*

▶ This patient most likely has large third-space losses due to the multiple injuries, and he is most likely again hypovolemic. A fluid challenge with 1–2 L of normal saline or lactated Ringer's solution is necessary.

You give him a fluid bolus of 2 L and see no response in urine output or BP.

▶ *What is the next step?*

▶ If the patient does not respond to a 2-L bolus, measurement of his **CVP** is necessary to determine if hydration is adequate. CVP provides an index of the preload of the right ventricle. If the CVP is decreased, this indicates hypovolemia, and additional volume replacement is appropriate.

The patient's CVP is 10 cm H_2O, and he remains oliguric and hypotensive.

▶ *What is the next step?*

▶ The patient appears to be adequately hydrated as measured by the CVP and yet is still not responding to the fluid challenge. One explanation is a low cardiac output from an abnormally functioning heart. A second, more likely, explanation is that the CVP is not a correct reflection of the left heart filling pressures; the patient is still volume-depleted with decreased preload, resulting in a low cardiac output.

There are limitations to the use of CVP alone. One is the assumption that right ventricular function parallels left ventricular function, which is usually true in normal individuals but not necessarily true in sick patients. Decreased preload to the left ventricle and decreased cardiac output may be present despite a normal CVP. A **pulmonary artery catheter** permits measurement of the cardiac output, right atrial, pulmonary artery and pulmonary capillary wedge pressure (PCWP), and systemic vascular resistance (SVR). These measurements allow you to assess ventricular function and guide the administration of fluids or cardiac medications designed to enhance pump function. At this point, placement of a pulmonary artery catheter to determine filling pressures to both sides of the heart is appropriate.

Your resident asks you to describe a Swan-Ganz catheter and the method for its insertion.

▶ *How do you respond?*

▶ The Swan-Ganz catheter allows measurement of CVP and pulmonary artery pressure (Figure 12-23). When the balloon near the tip is inflated, the catheter tip measures a pulmonary artery occlusion pressure, or **PCWP,** which correlates closely with left atrial pressure. The PCWP can be interpreted in the left atrium similarly to the CVP in the right atrium. If the **PCWP is low, hypovolemia** and decreased left heart preload are present. If the PCWP is high (in the range of 20–25 mm Hg), pulmonary edema and fluid overload, caused by either left heart failure or overhydration, are present.

The Swan-Ganz catheter also has a highly sensitive temperature probe near its top, which allows for the performance of cardiac output measurements. More sophisticated catheters that can measure the venous blood oxygen saturation in the pulmonary artery are available.

FIGURE 12-23. Pressure tracing seen while inserting a Swan-Ganz catheter. (From Sabiston DC [ed]. *Davis-Christopher textbook of surgery.* 13th ed. Philadelphia: WB Saunders, 1986: 71.)

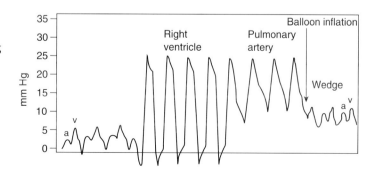

The catheter is inserted through a central venous access line, and the balloon is inflated, which tends to drag the catheter in the direction of blood flow through the heart. During passage through the line, the location of the catheter can be determined by monitoring the pressure readings at the catheter tip. When the catheter is in the right ventricle, arrhythmias are common and should be managed by either advancing or withdrawing the catheter.

▶ *What is the normal SVR, and what conditions change this value?*

▶ The normal SVR should be 800–1400 dynes-sec/cm^5. SVR elevation may occur in cardiogenic shock, hypovolemic shock, hypertension, or with administration of vasoconstrictors. SVR reduction may occur in septic shock, neurogenic shock, or with administration of vasodilators. (Table 12-10)

You measure the patient's PCWP and cardiac output (Table 12-9).

▶ *What is the correct interpretation of the results and the proper management of the patient in Example 1 (Table 12-9)?*

▶ In Example 1, the PCWP is low, indicating hypovolemia, which results in decreased venous return, eventually lowering cardiac output. The low cardiac output stimulates increased SVR by vasoconstriction. The value of 2.5 is low enough to suggest that the tissues are not being adequately perfused, and more volume is needed. Treatment involves restoration of circulatory volume.

The patient has the hemodynamic findings presented in Example 1 (Table 12-9). On the basis of these data, he is hypovolemic, and the administration of IV fluids until his PCWP reaches 15 mm Hg appears to be appropriate. He initially responds with an improvement in BP. However, over the next 24 hours, he again becomes oliguric and hypotensive. Measurement of hemodynamic parameters yields the values presented in Example 3 (Table 12-9).

▶ *What is the correct interpretation of the findings in Example 3 (Table 12-9)?*

▶ In Example 3, the patient is in a **hyperdynamic state** because the cardiac output is high; this finding is characteristic of high output septic shock. SVR falls and cardiac output increases for two reasons: (1) the left ventricle has little resistance against which to pump and (2) an adequate preload is restored.

TABLE 12-9

Calculation of Systemic Vascular Resistance (SVR)

$SVR = (MAP - CVP)/CO \times 80$

Example (see text)	PCWP (mm Hg)	CO (L/min)	SVR (dynes-sec/cm^5)
1	3	2.5	2000
2	20	2.0	2400
3	15	9.5	300
4	20	15.0	300

CO = cardiac output (L/min); CVP = central venous pressure; MAP = mean arterial pressure; PCWP = pulmonary capillary wedge pressure; SVR = systemic vascular resistance.

The sequence described here is not atypical of sepsis. Early sepsis causes fluid sequestration (third-space losses) and venodilation that results in hypovolemia and decreased cardiac preload, leading to an early decrease in cardiac output. Once the fluid deficit is replaced, the low-SVR, high cardiac output picture appears.

▶ *What management is appropriate?*

▶ Treatment includes **antibiotics and elimination of the infectious source.** In the surgical patient, elimination of the septic site often means careful examination of the patient and abdominal imaging to locate a septic site. If an abscess is present, it should be drained surgically or percutaneously. Many patients improve as a result of this treatment if it is implemented expeditiously. If this is not performed, the patient may progress to late sepsis and a septic shock characterized by decreased cardiac output and continued decreased SVR. Mortality is greatly increased in patients who progress to hypodynamic septic shock.

Suppose your patient had the findings in Example 2

▶ *What is the correct interpretation of the results and management of the patient in Example 2 (Table 12-9)?*

▶ In Example 2, the patient may be suffering from cardiogenic shock, in which the CVP or PCWP is increased and the cardiac output is severely decreased. The SVR is increased due to an outpouring of sympathetic impulses. In this situation, the CXR would most likely reveal pulmonary edema. This type of shock does not respond to IV fluids. The etiology of heart failure may be due to a traumatic injury to the myocardium or due to preexisting myocardial disease. To care for the patient appropriately, it is necessary to determine the exact cause of the problem.

Suppose your patient has a spinal cord injury at the C5 level.

▶ *What are the expected hemodynamic parameters?*

▶ Hypotension secondary to spinal cord injury is termed **neurogenic shock,** the type of shock seen most commonly in trauma victims. Impairment of the sympathetic nervous system leads to systemic vasodilation and decreased contractile force of the heart. The diagnosis is usually made in a hypotensive trauma patient with a normal or slow pulse and evidence for a spinal cord injury. Pulmonary artery catheter measurements typically demonstrate a low SVR, a low PCWP, and a low cardiac output due to decreased cardiac preload and contractility. Treatment is adequate replacement of intravascular volume. The addition of vasoconstrictors such as dopamine, phenylephrine, or norepinephrine to increase the SVR and cardiac drugs to increase the heart rate is usually not necessary.

CASE 12.18. ▶ Traumatic Arteriovenous Fistula

A 25-year-old man presents to the emergency department with acute shortness of breath, which has progressed over the past several months. His past history is significant for a stab wound to the left groin area 5 years ago, which was treated with observation. He has no other illnesses. On physical examination, he has a BP of 120/80 mm Hg, a heart rate of 125 beats/min, bilateral rales, and jugular venous distention. Cardiac examination reveals a systolic ejection murmur and an S_3 gallop.

TABLE 12-10

Normal Cardiovascular Pressures

Location	Pressure (mm Hg systolic/mm Hg diastolic)
Right atrium	0–6
Right ventricle	20–30/0–6
Pulmonary artery	20–30/6–12
Pulmonary artery mean	12–18
PCWP	6–12
Left atrium	4–12
Left ventricle	100–140/5–14
Arteries	100–140/60–80

Mean arterial pressure = 75–100 mm Hg

Cardiac output = 4–8 L/min

SVR = 800–1400 dynes-sec/cm^5

PCWP = pulmonary capillary wedge pressure; SVR = systemic vascular resistance.

▶ *Could the patient's stab wound from 5 years ago possibly cause his current problem?*

▶ The patient could have an undiagnosed traumatic arteriovenous fistula from the injury. At the time of injury, the fistula was small, but over time, it has enlarged and become hemodynamically significant. **High-output cardiac failure** is now present.

▶ *How is confirmation of this diagnosis obtained?*

▶ On physical examination, the patient would most likely have a **palpable thrill and audible bruit over the fistula.** Occlusion of the fistula with direct pressure leads to an expected significant drop in heart rate as a result of the rise in peripheral resistance. A drop of 10 beats/min or more is thought to be significant and is termed **Branham's sign.** A duplex study or angiogram could also confirm the diagnosis.

The patient has a significant arteriovenous fistula causing cardiac failure.

▶ *What is the next step?*

▶ Surgical repair of the fistula is necessary, but until the patient's cardiac status improves, repair should not be undertaken. A cardiologist should be consulted, and the patient's cardiac status optimized. The best intraoperative management probably is a pulmonary artery catheter.

A pulmonary artery catheter is inserted.

▶ *What values would you expect to find?*

▶ The expected values are presented in Example 4 (Table 12-9).

The patient undergoes repair of the fistula.

▶ *How do you repair the fistula?*

▶ It is necessary to control the artery and vein proximal and distal to the fistula, disconnect the connection, and repair the vessels. Typically, the artery is very dilated, thin-walled, and difficult to handle. Clamping the artery should result in a rapid improvement in hemodynamics.

▶ *Do hemodynamically significant fistulae in surgical patients occur in any other situations?*

▶ This condition commonly occurs in two other situations. The first situation involves patients with chronic renal failure who are on hemodialysis with one or more **arteriovenous fistulas for dialysis access.** Significantly high blood flow rates (3–6 L/min) may occur and be hemodynamically significant, especially in the presence of the anemia of renal failure. The second situation involves patients with **an abdominal aortic aneurysm that ruptures into the inferior vena cava.** This creates a large fistula over a very brief period of time that results in rapid decompensation of the patient and pulmonary edema. Hemorrhage into the surrounding tissues usually does not occur.

CASE 12.19. ▶ Management of Continuing Pulmonary Problems

A 30-year-old woman is hit by an automobile while she is a pedestrian. She sustains multiple bilateral rib fractures, a right pneumothorax, and multiple severe soft-tissue contusions. Her airway is patent, and she is ventilating adequately. You perform a right tube thoracostomy (insert a chest tube).

▶ *What is the correct interpretation and management of the following situations?*

Case Variation 12.19.1. Severe rib pain

▶ The patient's rib pain is most likely secondary to **rib fractures** and the presence of a thoracostomy tube. It is important to administer adequate analgesics to prevent excessive splinting, which leads to atelectasis, hypoxia, and increased risk of pneumonia.

Case Variation 12.19.2. Pulse oximetry of 90% and a respiratory rate of 28 breaths/min

▶ At this time, the patient is exhibiting **moderate respiratory distress,** and reassessment of airway patency is essential. Examination of the patient's chest and breathing, looking for symmetry of respiratory movement, is necessary, along with auscultation of the chest. It is important to send an arterial blood gas (ABG) to determine the patient's ventilatory status as well as oxygenation. Placement on oxygen to increase the arterial oxygen saturation to more than 95% is also appropriate. The patient should have a CXR to confirm the position of the chest tube and complete expansion of the lung.

One possible source of the patient's hypoxemia is a persistent pneumothorax related to a problem (leak or kink) in the tube thoracostomy system. It is necessary to assess if the Pleurovac chamber is bubbling correctly and is connected to wall suction. Other causes of hypoxia are chest splinting from pain, atelectasis, and pulmonary contusion.

After giving the patient a dose of morphine, her arterial oxygen saturation drops from 92% to 85% and her respiratory rate drops from 32 breaths/min to 10 breaths/min with shallow breaths. An ABG indicates that the P_{CO_2} is 55 mm Hg. Inspection and palpation of the chest wall indicates a large, painful anterior area that does not move and expand with inspiration in the normal expansion direction but instead depresses.

▷ *What is the diagnosis and management?*

▶ The patient has two problems, **hypoventilation related to oversedation** and most likely a **flail chest,** which occurs when multiple rib fractures leave a segment of chest wall unstable (Figure 12-24). This causes paradoxical movement of the chest wall. The examiner may also feel crepitus overlying the ribs, and there is often severe injury to the underlying lung, which contributes to the hypoxia.

Treatment includes adequate ventilation, administration of oxygen, and careful fluid balance to avoid pulmonary edema. The patient is not ventilating adequately with narcotic treatment, and several management options are appropriate. One possibility is **intubation.** A second option is regional anesthesia with a **thoracic epidural catheter** for relief of rib pain. Typically, bupivacaine, a local anesthetic, and morphine are infused into the epidural space to relieve pain and improve respiratory dynamics. If it is effective, the narcotic can be eliminated; it can cause sedation and other undesirable neurologic effects in older patients and patients who have the catheter at a high thoracic level. Epidural anesthesia can be especially helpful in the elderly because it may avoid mechanical ventilation, which leads to a high likelihood of pneumonia and other complications. A third option is **patient-controlled analgesia,** which lowers the peak narcotic levels and perhaps improves the risk–benefit ratio.

This patient's current ventilatory state requires urgent intubation and mechanical ventilation. More careful observation might have avoided intubation.

Case Variation 12.19.3. Chest injury requiring a chest tube

You are managing a patient similar to the one described in Case Variation 12.19.2 who has a chest injury requiring a chest tube. Pulse oximetry is 86% on 4 L of nasal oxygen, and the respiratory rate is 40 breaths/min.

▷ *What management is appropriate?*

▶ This patient has severe respiratory distress and requires immediate treatment with **emergent intubation** to avoid respiratory arrest. She cannot maintain a respiratory rate of 40/min for very long.

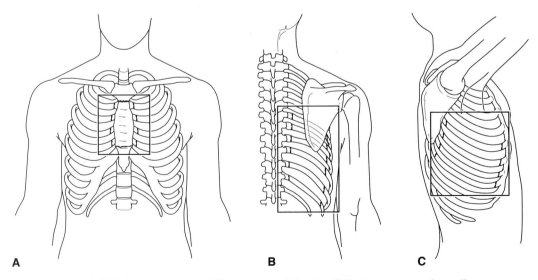

A   **B**   **C**

FIGURE 12-24. A flail chest causes a mobile segment of chest wall that moves paradoxically with respiration. **A.** Anterior view. **B.** Posterior view. **C.** Lateral view. (Campbell DR. Trauma to the chest wall, lung and major airways. *Curr Probl Surg.* 1998:726.)

CASE 12.20. ▶ Management of Respiratory Distress

The woman described in Case 12.19 develops further respiratory distress and requires intubation and mechanical ventilation. On CXR, bilateral hilar infiltrates and an infiltrate over the area of the flail chest are apparent. The fractional concentration of oxygen in inspired gas (FIO_2) is 40%, arterial oxygen saturation is 85%, and ABGs reveal a PO_2 of 54 mm Hg.

▶ *How should the following conditions be interpreted and managed?*

Case Variation 12.20.1. PCO_2 of 55 mm Hg

▶ The patient is **underventilated.** It is necessary to correct this condition by increasing the ventilatory rate or volume. This may also improve her hypoxia. Her CXR indicates a lung contusion and the probability of acute respiratory distress syndrome (ARDS) suggested by the hilar infiltrates.

Case Variation 12.20.2. PCO_2 of 25 mm Hg

▶ The **ventilatory rate is excessive.** By bringing the PCO_2 closer to 40 mm Hg, it is possible to decrease the rate. You will still have to reassess her oxygenation.

Case Variation 12.20.3. You increase her FIO_2 to 60%, which fails to increase the patient's oxygenation above 56 mm Hg

▶ This could signify **worsening ARDS, a mucous plug, or possible malposition of the endotracheal tube.** It is necessary to repeat the CXR to determine placement of the endotracheal tube. If the CXR shows massive atelectasis on one side, it could mean significant underventilation of that lung due to tube misplacement or occlusion of the tube by a mucous plug. Treatment entails repositioning or suctioning the tube. If suctioning does not resolve the problem, bronchoscopy should be performed to remove mucous plugs, obtain sputum samples, and open occluded airways. Bronchoscopy should always be performed cautiously in hypoxic patients because of the risk of worsening the hypoxia and causing cardiac arrest. It is appropriate to continue to increase the FIO_2 to bring the PO_2 above 60 mm Hg. To accomplish this, the addition of positive end-expiratory pressure (PEEP) to the ventilator may be necessary. PEEP maintains a constant baseline pressure on the airway, which recruits more alveoli to remain patent and available for gas exchange.

Case Variation 12.20.4. You increase her FIO_2 to 80%, which still does not improve oxygenation

▶ At this point, it is necessary to bring the FIO_2 up to 100% until the cause of the hypoxia is determined. PEEP should be added to the ventilator and started at 10 cm H_2O. An arterial line should be placed both to monitor BP and to allow frequent blood gas measurements. A CXR should be obtained to help determine the cause of the hypoxia.

The addition of PEEP for adequate ventilation is necessary.

▶ *She is now on PEEP. How would you manage the following situations?*

Case Variation 12.20.5. When you add 10 cm H_2O PEEP, it results in a decline in BP from 120/80 mm Hg to 90/60 mm Hg

QUICK CUTS **The addition of 10 cm H_2O of PEEP causes the cardiac output to drop by impairing venous return to the heart.**

▶ A pulmonary artery catheter may be necessary to monitor the patient's cardiac output and preload. This allows the physician to counterbalance the negative cardiovascular effects of PEEP by altering preload and cardiac function.

Case Variation 12.20.6. When you add 10 cm H_2O PEEP, it results in a decline in the patient's urine output, which remains at 10 mL/hr

▶ Likewise, the high level of PEEP is causing the cardiac output to drop, decreasing perfusion to the renal parenchyma and resulting in oliguria. The treatment is the same as in Case Variation 12.20.5.

The patient's oxygenation and hemodynamics stabilize with 10 cm H_2O PEEP. During evening rounds, the intensive care unit (ICU) nurse urgently calls you because the patient has suddenly become extremely hypoxic and hypotensive and cannot be ventilated.

▶ *What intervention is appropriate?*

▶ With hypoxia, hypotension, and difficulty ventilating, it is necessary to determine if the patient has a **tension pneumothorax.** This is an *emergent* diagnosis. First, place the patient on 100% oxygen and attempt to bag the patient by hand. Listen to the lungs on both sides to determine whether breath sounds are present. If you cannot hear breath sounds on one side, it is necessary to perform a needle thoracostomy with an angiocatheter in the second intercostal space in the midclavicular line. If you hear a rush of air and note improvement in the patient's vital signs, your action has most likely solved the problem. In either event, you should place a thoracostomy tube in the fifth intercostal space in the midaxillary line and then obtain an upright CXR.

CASE 12.21. ▶ Stab Wound to the Neck

A 25-year-old man is brought to the emergency department with a stab wound to the neck. He has no other apparent injuries.

▶ *What are the initial management steps?*

▶ The initial step is evaluation of the airway. With neck injuries, the chance of airway problems, including direct injury such as a transection of the trachea in the neck, is significant. Injuries to other structures can also cause airway compromise by compression and distortion of the airway such as might occur with an expanding hematoma, placing pressure on the pliable trachea. If airway injury is indicated, early elective intubation is preferable to emergent intubation or tracheostomy. If there is active hemorrhage from the wound, a quick assessment of the injury and application of direct digital pressure to control the bleeding is also appropriate.

The patient is able to talk normally. Assessment of the airway indicates that it is patent and that ventilation is good. There are no other injuries apparent elsewhere on his body. His vital signs are stable, with a normal BP and a heart rate of 80 beats/min.

▶ *What is the next step in the evaluation of the patient's neck?*

▶ It is necessary to perform a careful examination of the neck to determine what structures are injured as identified by palpation (Table 12-11). In addition, you should ascertain whether a hematoma is present and, if so, whether it is expanding and threatening the airway.

Examination indicates that the injury, which is in the anterior triangle of the neck at the level of the thyroid cartilage, penetrates the platysma. There is a 4-cm–diameter hematoma that appears to be enlarging in size. A small amount of blood is leaking from the wound. The patient's vital signs remain stable.

▶ *What is the next step?*

▶ Exploration of the neck is necessary because the patient has evidence of a vascular injury in zone II, (Figure 12-25). During intubation, examination of the vocal cords is warranted to determine whether an injury has occurred.

Exploration indicates an injury to the internal jugular vein, which is repaired.

▶ *What other features of the neck should be examined?*

▶ The surgeon should follow the path of the knife and examine all nearby structures. It is necessary to explore the carotid artery and vagus nerve. In addition, the trachea and esophagus may also warrant exploration if the stab path is in proximity with these structures.

You complete the exploration and close the wound. The patient returns to the floor. That evening, the nurse calls you to see the patient because there is some blood on the dressing. On examination, you note a 3-cm–diameter hematoma beneath the incision that was not present

---

TABLE 12-11

Important Structures to Examine in a Stab Wound to the Neck

Airway structures: tenderness, mobility, distortion or displacement, air in soft tissues, bubbling from wound, voice quality (e.g., hoarseness)

Vascular structures: evidence of active or recent bleeding, stable or expanding hematoma

Salivary glands: proximity of injury to major or minor salivary glands

Esophagus: pain or difficulty on swallowing, saliva in wound

Nervous system: neurologic deficits

Lungs: breath sounds in the cupola of lung, chest radiograph

Muscular structures: degree of platysma penetration, position in relation to sternocleidomastoid muscle (anterior or posterior)

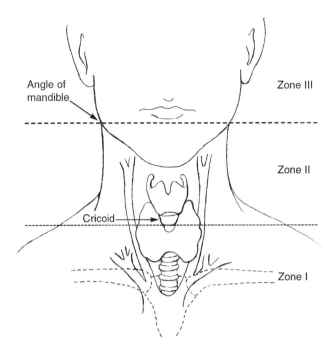

Angle of mandible

Zone III

Zone II

Cricoid

Zone I

FIGURE 12-25. The neck can be divided into three zones. In stable patients, injuries to zones I and III are often managed by assessment, with preoperative angiography to ascertain vascular injury due to exposure of certain areas. (From Peitzman AB, Rhodes M, Schwab CW, et al. [eds]. *The trauma manual.* 2nd ed. Philadelphia: Lippincott Williams & Wilkins, 2002: 192.)

at the end of the procedure. The patient tells you that he feels fine, but says that he feels a tightness in his neck and is having some trouble taking deep breaths.

▶ *What is the next step?*

▶ Airway compromise from a postoperative neck hematoma should be a concern. This situation requires urgent intervention. The removal of several sutures from the neck incision and release of the hematoma should relieve the pressure on the trachea and improve the patient's breathing. If not, then urgent intubation is necessary. Either way, he should return to the operating room for evacuation of the hematoma and hemostasis.

CASE 12.22. ▶ Other Injuries to the Neck

You are caring for a 51-year-old woman with a traumatic injury to the neck.

▶ *How do the following findings influence decision making?*

Case Variation 12.22.1. Gunshot wound to the neck, with a BP of 80/60 mm Hg

▶ A patient who is hypotensive should go directly to the operating room for resuscitation and simultaneous exploration of the neck wound. In addition, gunshot wounds are more likely to have significant associated injuries due to the blast effect of the projectile.

Case Variation 12.22.2. Stab wound to zone I (Figure 12-25)

▶ Injuries to zone 1 may involve structures such as the subclavian vessels that are technically difficult to expose and repair surgically. If patients are hemodynamically stable, a preoperative angiogram to define the location of an injury and to allow planning of the surgical approach is very useful. If patients are unstable, they should directly proceed to the operating room. It is necessary to remember that the thoracic outlet is part of zone I. Thus, injuries to the lung and brachial plexus can also occur.

Case Variation 12.22.3. Stab wound to zone III

▶ The management of this injury is similar to that of an injury in zone I; a preoperative angiogram is very useful in stable patients. Injuries to the carotid artery are possible, and surgical control and repair is very difficult in that location.

Case Variation 12.22.4. Subcutaneous emphysema in the neck

▶ This finding suggests that there is an airway injury, and exploration of the neck is indicated. Other findings associated with airway injury include air bubbling from the wound and an obvious tracheal deformity. If an airway injury is suspected, but there is no firm evidence and no other indication to explore the patient, bronchoscopy and laryngoscopy to rule out injury may be appropriate.

Case Variation 12.22.5. Difficulty swallowing

▶ This suggests an injury to the esophagus. This would be managed similarly to the injury in Case Variation 12.22.4, with use of esophagoscopy or a barium swallow to rule out injury if there is no other clear indication for surgery.

Case Variation 12.22.6. Hoarseness

▶ Hoarseness could represent an airway injury similar to other airway injuries but could also indicate direct laryngeal trauma, laryngeal dislocation, or injury to the recurrent laryngeal nerve. Exploration or direct laryngoscopy is necessary.

Case Variation 12.22.7. Hemiparesis

▶ A carotid artery injury or thrombosis should be a concern. The patient should have an angiogram. It is necessary to define the injury and base the treatment on the specific findings in consultation with a vascular surgeon or neurosurgeon.

Case Variation 12.22.8. Blunt trauma to the neck

▶ Marked extension of the neck or direct blunt trauma may result in intimal disruptions and dissection of the carotid artery, which can produce carotid thrombosis and neurologic deficits. Management of asymptomatic carotid injuries and thromboses usually involves anticoagulation. The management of symptomatic carotid occlusions is controversial. Some surgeons would attempt thrombectomy if a thrombosis is less than several hours old and is associated with significant neurologic deficits. Other surgeons would recommend anticoagulation alone.

Whether to repair a carotid injury or thrombosis is a decision that should be made in consultation with an experienced surgeon; these injuries often involve the carotid artery where it enters the base of the skull. This makes the surgical exposure very difficult and increases the complexity of the procedure.

Case Variation 12.22.9. Zone II stab wound with no symptoms, no other physical findings, and stable vital signs

▶ Management varies. Some surgeons would routinely explore the patient's neck, while others would take a nonoperative approach, either with observation or further diagnostic evaluations. Nonoperative methods include bronchoscopy, esophagoscopy, and CT imaging of the neck.

CASE 12.23. ▶ Burn

A 22-year-old man who is brought to the emergency department with extensive burns is conscious and breathing. History reveals that he was trapped in his house trailer when it caught fire. He has no other known medical problems.

▶ *What are the first steps in evaluation and management?*

▶ Initially, the basic principles of trauma management as assessment of **a**irway, **b**reathing, and **c**irculation (ABCs). Most burn patients do not die as a result of the burn but from later complications. It is necessary to remove the clothes and stop any further burn injury. Cooling injured areas is appropriate, but prolonged cooling can cause core hypothermia. The patient should be placed on clean sheets.

> **QUICK CUTS** In the initial assessment of the airway, determine whether an **airway burn** is likely. Suggestive factors are **carbonaceous sputum, facial burn, facial or nasal hair burns, hoarseness, low oxygen saturation, or dyspnea.**

Burns that occur in closed spaces are more likely to be associated with airway burns.

▶ *What is involved in assessment of the patient's burns?*

▶ This assessment is most easily performed in three steps.
   1. Determine the **depth of burn** (Table 12-12).
   2. Identify the **type of burn.** Common types include flame burns, contact burns with a hot object, scald burns with a hot liquid, and steam burns.
   3. Determine the **percentage body surface area (BSA) burned** (Table 12-13). The area of a burn wound is expressed as a percent of the total BSA.

   The "**rule of 9s**" is the most common way of estimating the BSA burn. Using this rule, different body parts account for certain percentages, and the sum of these values represents the total area burned. Note that this rule is not used in children because their heads take up a larger percentage of their BSA. Separate burn charts are available for children to determine percentage BSA burn. It is possible to obtain another good estimate of the BSA by measuring the size of the burn using the size of the patient's hand as representative of 1% of the BSA.

▶ *Under what conditions would it be necessary to transfer the patient to a burn center?*

▶ Several reasons for transfer are generally accepted (Table 12-14).

The estimated weight of the man is 70 kg, and he appears to have suffered deep second- and third-degree flame burns over 30% of his BSA.

TABLE 12-12

Description of the Types of Burns

FIRST-DEGREE BURNS
- Microscopic destruction of **superficial layer of epidermis** (erythema of skin, as seen in sunburn)
- Of little clinical significance, because water barrier of skin remains undisturbed
- Pain is usually chief symptom; it usually resolves within 48–72 hours
- Damaged epithelium peels off in small scales after 5–10 days, leaving no scar

SECOND-DEGREE BURNS
- Damage extends **through epidermis into dermis**
- Referred to as **partial-thickness burns,** because epithelial regeneration can occur
- Blisters may be present; when burns are superficial, blisters heal within 10–14 days if not infected
- May occur in more severe form, which burns more deeply into dermis; a layer of white, nonviable dermis is seen. **Deep second-degree burns** can easily develop into third-degree burns without proper burn management to prevent surface infection

THIRD-DEGREE BURNS
- Involve **full thickness of skin down to subcutaneous tissue**
- Total, irreversible destruction of all skin, dermal appendages, and epithelial elements
- Characterized by white, waxy appearance; lack of sensation; lack of capillary refill; and leathery texture
- Require skin grafting for repair
- Deep Second- and third-degree burns are equally significant physiologically, and coverage may be estimated by the "rule of nines" see Table 12-13)

TABLE 12-13

"Rule of Nines" Used to Determine Percent of Surface Area Burned in Adults

Anatomic Area	% Body Surface
Head	9
Right upper extremity	9
Left upper extremity	9
Right lower extremity	18
Left lower extremity	18
Anterior trunk	18
Posterior trunk	18
Neck	1

TABLE 12-14

Indications for Transfer to a Burn Center

Full-thickness burn >5% BSA
Partial-thickness burn >20% BSA
Age <5 or >50 years
Burns of face, hands, feet, genitalia, perineum, or over major joints
Inhalation injury
Circumferential burns of the chest or extremities
Chemical or electrical burns

BSA = body surface area.

▷ *How is the amount of fluid replacement estimated?*

▶ The overall strategy of burn resuscitation aims **to return plasma volume to normal and sustain adequate perfusion of tissues.** Evidence supports the need for both crystalloid and colloid solutions. The Parkland formula has been adopted in many burn centers to provide specific replacement guidelines; it can be used to calculate the volume of solution necessary in the first 24 hours after the burn.

Total volume of lactated Ringer's solution = % BSA burned × weight (kg) × 4 mL/kg

where BSA = body surface area.
One-half of the solution is given over the first 8 hours, and the second half is given over the next 16 hours. **In the next 24 hours,** it is also necessary to give D_5W to replace evaporative water loss and maintain serum sodium at 140 mEq/L and administer 0.5 mL plasma/% BSA burned over 8 hours to maintain colloid oncotic pressure.

Crystalloid solutions are used to expand depleted plasma and extracellular volumes as soon as possible, which helps return cardiac output to normal. **Colloid is not given in the first 24 hours,** because the capillaries are "leaky," and most of the fluid will leak into the extracellular space very quickly. **Colloid is most effective for returning intravascular/ plasma volume to normal without adding edema.**

▷ *What is the appropriate management in the following situations?*

Case Variation 12.23.1. Need for topical treatment of burns

▶ It is important to provide an aseptic environment for topical wound care in burn patients to prevent infections. While superficial burns do not require topical antibiotics, deeper wounds do. **Silver sulfadiazine,** mafenide, and povidone-iodine ointment are some of the topical antibiotics available for use. Occlusive dressings are used to minimize exposure to air, increase the rate of epithelialization, and decrease pain. It is necessary to change the dressings at least twice daily to inhibit bacterial growth. Third-degree burns may also require regular debridement of necrotic tissue until a biologic dressing, preferably a split-thickness skin graft of the patient's own skin, is in place.

Prophylactic systemic antibiotics are not used because they select for resistant organisms. They should be used only for clearly documented infections. The most common infections are *Staphylococcus aureus, Pseudomonas, Streptococcus,* and *Candida.*

Case Variation 12.23.2. Dark urine that is positive for blood

▶ Microscopic analysis of the urine is necessary. If no RBCs are seen, the patient has **myoglobinuria** and is at risk for **acute tubular necrosis** if this condition goes unrecognized and inadequately treated. **Fluids** should be administered to ensure a urine output two to three times normal. **Alkalinization** of the urine and osmotic diuretics (e.g., mannitol) may also be used in severe cases.

If RBCs are present in the urine, the workup should include investigation into traumatic causes of hematuria. In addition, electrical injuries can cause hemolysis.

Case Variation 12.23.3. Carbonaceous sputum and hoarseness

▶ It is essential that these signs of **inhalation injury** not be overlooked, because they are indications of laryngeal edema and pulmonary injury. Other signs of inhalation injury include singed facial hair, carbon particles in the oropharynx, and a history of being burned in a closed space. Some institutions perform laryngoscopy at presentation to determine the need for intubation. The threshold for intubation should be low.

Carbon monoxide poisoning should be a consideration in every patient suspected of having inhalation injury. Levels of carboxyhemoglobin of more than 5% in nonsmokers or more than 10% in smokers indicates carbon monoxide poisoning. If this has occurred, 100% oxygen should be administered until the carboxyhemoglobin level returns to normal and symptoms resolve. Hyperbaric oxygen chambers are also used to rapidly remove carbon monoxide from the blood.

Case Variation 12.23.4. Methemoglobinemia

▶ Methemoglobin is hemoglobin with the iron oxidized to the ferric (Fe^{3+}) form rather than the normal, reduced ferrous (Fe^{2+}) state. The ferric form is unable to bind or transport oxygen. Enclosed-space fires can cause a buildup of this product, which results in a shift of the oxyhemoglobin dissociation curve to the left.

Symptoms of methemoglobinemia range from a chocolate-brown appearance of the blood and central cyanosis of the trunk and proximal extremities to generalized seizures, coma, and cardiac arrhythmias. **Pulse oximetry is unreliable as a measure of oxygen saturation,** because it cannot differentiate between methemoglobin and hemoglobin. Instead, ABG readings should be taken. If the patient is asymptomatic, supplemental oxygen is sufficient as treatment; methemoglobin will reduce to normal hemoglobin in 24–72 hours. Specific therapy for methemoglobinemia is administration of IV methylene blue (1–2 mg/kg). In extreme cases, if massive hemolysis occurs, hyperbaric oxygen therapy or exchange transfusion may be necessary.

Case Variation 12.23.5. Early deterioration of ABGs with CO_2 retention

▶ With early deterioration of ABG readings and CO_2 retention, **airway obstruction is likely.** This condition warrants prompt endotracheal intubation and mechanical ventilatory support. Added positive pressure helps prevent atelectasis and closure of lung units distal to the swollen airways.

Case Variation 12.23.6. Circumferential third-degree burn of the thorax

▶ Circumferential burns rapidly become thick and contracted, limiting motion and blood flow. In the chest, this may seriously impair ventilation, whereas in the extremities, it may create ischemia and necrosis of the muscles. An **escharotomy** helps avoid this problem (Figure 12-26).

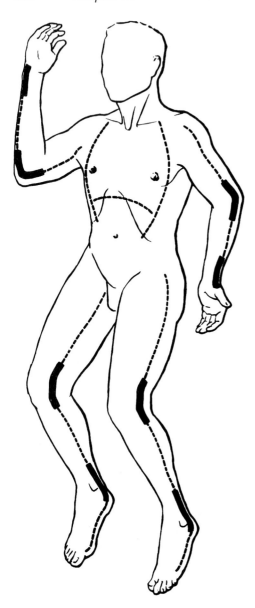

FIGURE 12-26. Preferred sites for escharotomy. Third-degree burns can cause immobility and contraction of muscular compartments and the chest. Escharotomy may be necessary if vascular or ventilatory compromise is present. (From Martin RR, Becker WK, Cioff, et al. In: Peitzman AB, Rhodes M, Schwab CW, et al. [eds]. *The trauma manual.* 2nd ed. Philadelphia: Lippincott Williams & Wilkins, 2002.)

Case Variation 12.23.7. Electrical burn

▶ Electrical burns appear benign on the surface but may be associated with large amounts of **interior damage to muscles, nerves, and vessels.** Examination for entrance and exit sites is necessary. Evaluation with an ECG and cardiac enzymes is appropriate to rule out suspected cardiac injury. Necrotic muscle results in myoglobinuria, which can cause acute renal failure. Maintaining high urine output and alkalinizing the urine can prevent such renal failure.

CASE 12.24. ▶ Total Parenteral Nutrition

A 50-year-old man who was in an automobile crash undergoes exploration for abdominal injury. He has a significant contusion to his bowel with intramural hematomas and several areas of perforation. The bowel is repaired but is very edematous. Postoperatively, you decide that enteral feeding is not safe and that total parenteral nutrition (TPN) is appropriate during the postoperative period.

▶ *What is the initial step in determining the nutritional requirements for this patient?*

▶ Nutrients may be given by TPN when the GI tract is unavailable or not functioning. TPN provides calories, amino acids, electrolytes, vitamins, trace minerals, and fatty acids through a central venous catheter. For every patient who requires TPN, it is necessary to determine the nutritional status.

QUICK CUTS   **"Nondepleted" patients** (those with a **good nutritional status**) are in a minor catabolic state. **Depleted patients were malnourished** before surgery. **Hypermetabolic patients are in a severely stressed catabolic state** (i.e., due to trauma, burn, sepsis, cancer).

Requirements for both protein and energy vary according to the patient's nutritional state. The protein requirements of patients who are considered **nondepleted** are approximately 1.0 g/kg/day, with total daily calories of 20% above **basal energy expenditure.** The protein and calorie requirements of **depleted** patients are in an intermediate zone. The protein requirements of **hypermetabolic** patients may be 2.0–2.5 g/kg/day, with total daily calories of 50%–100% above basal energy expenditure.

This patient appears to be in a nondepleted condition, in a minor catabolic state.

▶ *What is the estimated daily energy expenditure?*

▶ A patient's daily energy expenditure can be measured by a variety of methods. The most accurate is indirect calorimetry, which involves calculation of the production of O_2 (VO_2) and CO_2 (VCO_2) from the timed volumetric collection of expired O_2, CO_2, and urinary nitrogen (Table 12-15). Because indirect calorimetry requires measurements of gas volumes using sophisticated equipment (metabolic cart), it is not often performed.

  If you assume this patient was well-nourished prior to surgery and is the standard 70-kg male, his daily baseline caloric needs are about 30 kcal/kg/day × 70 kg = 2100 kcal/day.

▶ *Given this caloric estimate, how would you choose the type of TPN solution?*

▶ Protein should not serve as a calorie source when a determination of the type of TPN is made. Instead, protein is needed to replace the amino acids that are constantly being recycled in the body. Calories are derived from a mixed-energy substrate system, with approximately 70% of calories supplied as dextrose and 30% of calories supplied as fat (Table 12-16).

  In this patient, a standard TPN formula, which is a 50% dextrose solution with 4.25% amino acids, could be given (Table 12-16; Table 12-17). Fat is usually given as a 10% or 20% emulsion, separate from the TPN bag. A single infusion of 500 mL is usually given over 10–12 hours. Serum triglyceride levels must be monitored to avoid high levels. If hypertriglyceridemia occurs, the amount of lipid administered must be reduced.

  To determine the calories in 1 L of standard TPN solution, see Table 12-17. If 1000 mL of $D_{50}W$ and 500 mL of fat emulsion is given over a 24-hour period, the total nonprotein calories infused is 1700 + 550 = 2250 kcal. The TPN solution should be started at 40 mL/hr

TABLE 12-15

Estimate of Daily Baseline Metabolic Needs

WEIR FORMULA for determination of **resting energy expenditure (REE)** [kcal/min]*

$3.9(VO_2) + 1.1(VCO_2) - 2.2$(urine nitrogen [g/min])

where VO_2 is the oxygen production and VCO_2 is the carbon dioxide output.

HARRIS-BENEDICT EQUATION for determination of **basal energy expenditure (BEE)**
[kcal/24 hr]†

Males
$66 + (13.7 \times$ weight [kg]) $+ (5 \times$ height [cm]) $- (6.7 \times$ age [years])

Females
$665 + (9.6 \times$ weight [kg]) $+ (1.8 \times$ height [cm]) $- (4.7 \times$ age [years])

---

*Requires metabolic cart to measure.
†Estimate based on age, weight, height, and gender. BEE can be estimated as approximately 1400–1800 kcal/day
(30 kcal/kg/day) for baseline needs (as much as 3000 kcal/day in severely stressed patients).

the first day; this supplies 960 mL of $D_{50}W$, or just under the dextrose daily target of 1700 kcal. The fat emulsion is given as a 500-mL daily infusion.

▶ *How is the daily nitrogen requirement determined?*

▶ A patient who is critically ill and on TPN should have a positive nitrogen balance as a goal, particularly with a body weight that is 10% or more below the ideal level. Nitrogen balance is defined as nitrogen intake minus nitrogen excretion. Nitrogen intake in a patient on TPN is calculated from the contents of the solution. The protein in TPN is typically 4.25%, which means there are 4.25 grams of protein per liter. To calculate the nitrogen content of the same liter of TPN solution described in Table 12-16, use the formula grams nitrogen = grams protein ÷ 6.25. This calculation yields 4.25 g protein ÷ 6.25 = 0.68 g nitrogen per liter of TPN.

Nitrogen excretion can be partially measured and partly estimated. Up to 90% of nitrogen excretion is in the form of urea in the urine. Stool losses of nitrogen are approximately 1 g/24 hours in patients who are eating and much less in patients who are on nothing-by-mouth (NPO) feeding. A 24-hour urine collection and urea measurement allow the majority of urinary nitrogen excretion to be measured. To convert grams of urea to grams of protein, it is necessary to multiply the urea by 0.50. An additional 15% of protein is lost in the urine from nonurea compounds, including creatinine and ammonia.

Once the nitrogen balance has been determined, it is appropriate to adjust the standard TPN solution infusion rate to maintain a positive balance.

 QUICK CUTS   The more severe the injury, the more severe the catabolic state and the higher the amino acid requirement.

The response to starvation in normal individuals is to use ketones for energy, which spares protein from being metabolized. During starvation, the overall metabolic rate also

TABLE 12-16

Composition of a Standard Central Venous Solution

BASIC REQUIREMENTS FOR STANDARD TOTAL PARENTERAL NUTRITION (TPN)

Fat	9 kcal/g
Carbohydrate	3.4 kcal/g
Protein	4 kcal/g

VOLUME

10% amino acid solution	500 mL
50% dextrose solution	500 mL
Fat emulsion	—
Electrolytes	~ 50 mL
Total volume	~ 1050 mL

COMPOSITION

Amino acids	50 g
Dextrose	250 g
Total potassium	8.0 g (50 ÷ 6.25)
Dextrose kcal	840 kcal (250 g × 3.4 kcal/g)
mOsm/L	~ 2000

Electrolytes Added to TPN Solutions	Usual Concentration (mEq/L)	Range of Concentrations (mEq/L)
Sodium	60	0–150
Potassium	40	0–80
Acetate	50	50–150
Chloride	50	0–150
Phosphate	15	0–30
Calcium*	4.5	0–20
Magnesium	5	5–15

*Calcium is generally added as calcium gluconate or calcium chloride. One ampule of calcium gluconate = 1 g of calcium = 4.5 mEq.

TABLE 12-17

Calculation of Calories in Standard Total Parenteral Nutrition (TPN) Solution in Adults

$D_{50}W$ contains 500 g/L of glucose
500 g × 3.4 kcal/g = 1700 kcal/L
A 10% fat emulsion represents 1.1 kcal/mL of fat. Therefore, 500 mL contains 550 kcal
A 4.25% amino acid solution contains 4.25 g/100 mL of amino acids, or 42.5 g/L
42.5 g × 4 kcal/g = 170 kcal (not to be used for caloric calculation)

falls. In severe injury, the adaptation to ketone metabolism does not occur, and thus protein is used as a source for gluconeogenesis (Table 12-18). This creates a significant catabolic state. In addition, the resting metabolic state increases with severe injury, which also increases the need for energy and thus increases the catabolic state. The metabolic rate alters in response to various diseases (Figure 12-27).

▶ *What other molecules are also in TPN solution?*

▶ The standard composition of TPN solutions is shown in Table 12-16.

The patient has been on TPN for 2 weeks and still cannot tolerate enteral feeding.

▶ *What is the appropriate evaluation and management for the following TPN-related problems?*

Case Variation 12.24.1. Fever

▶ A temperature spike greater than 101°F may indicate an **infected catheter,** among other causes. Patients should undergo complete evaluation for all possible sources of infection. The physician should examine the catheter site for erythema, tenderness, or purulence and obtain cultures both peripherally and directly from the catheter. If **cultures are negative but fever persists,** it is necessary either to change the catheter over a wire (send tip for culture) or change the site. If you choose to change the catheter over a wire, the new catheter may remain if the fever resolves and the cultures are negative. If **cultures are positive or fever persists,** it is necessary to select a new catheter site and initiate antibiotics. Single-lumen catheters carry a 3%–5% risk of infection, whereas triple-lumen catheters have a 10% risk.

Case Variation 12.24.2. Metabolic coma

▶ **Hyperglycemic, hyperosmolar, nonketotic coma** is a common cause of coma in patients on TPN. This condition is **secondary to dehydration following excessive diuresis due to hyperglycemia.** This situation warrants discontinuation of TPN, administration of insulin, and very close monitoring of glucose and electrolytes.

Case Variation 12.24.3. Elevated bilirubin and liver enzymes

▶ Liver function tests become abnormal in as many as 30% of patients on TPN. During the first 2 weeks, transaminases rise, and a gradual increase in alkaline phosphatase occurs. Rising enzyme levels normally respond to a modest reduction in the rate of infusion. Fail-

TABLE 12-18

Daily Amino Acid Requirement for a 70-kg Man

Condition	Amino Acids Needed (g/kg/day)	Catabolic State
Uncomplicated postoperative course	1–1.5	Mild
Mild-to-moderate sepsis or injury	1.5–2.0	Moderate
Severe sepsis or burn	2.0–3.0	Severe

FIGURE 12-27. Metabolic response to surgical stress and starvation. Major burns represent the largest metabolic requirement encountered by humans. (From Wilson RF [ed]. *Handbook of trauma: pitfalls and pearls.* Philadelphia: Lippincott Williams & Wilkins, 1999: 578. After Long CL, Schaffel N. Metabolic response to injury and illness: Estimation of energy and protein needs from indirect calorimetry and nitrogen balance. *JPEN J Parenter Enteral Nutr.* 1979;3:425.)

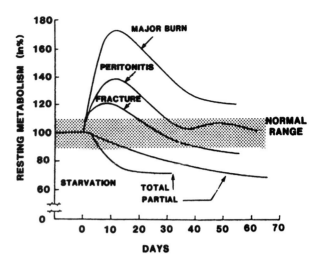

ure of the serum enzymes to plateau or return to normal within 7–14 days should suggest another etiology. Fatty liver and structural liver damage can be induced by TPN. Prolonged TPN can cause cirrhosis, but this usually occurs over years of TPN.

Case Variation 12.24.4. Dry, scaly skin

▶ This condition is indicative of free fatty acid deficiency. Administration of lipids should correct the problem.

INDEX

Page numbers in italics denote figures; those followed by a t denote tables.